Degenerative Aortic Valve Disease, its Mechanism on Progression, its Effect on the Left Ventricle and the Postoperative Results

Authored By

Wilhelm Peter Mistiaen

Artesis University College Antwerp
Department of Healthcare Sciences
University of Antwerp
Belgium

Degenerative Aortic Valve Disease, its Mechanism on Progression, its Effect on the Left Ventricle and the Postoperative Results

Author: Wilhelm Peter Mistiaen

eISBN: 978-1-60805-287-5

ISBN: 978-1-60805-605-7

CONTENTS

FOREWORD

In this book, Professor Wilhelm Peter Mistiaen; MD, ScD, PhD, has provided the current state of the art concerning the practical, clinical and technical aspects of degenerative aortic valve disease and aortic valve replacement. Dr. Mistiaen offers an exceptionally broad, important and clearly written book that is sure to be an excellent medical resource. As we are well aware, the prevalence of valvular heart disease has been steadily rising as a major health hazard in the present era, and is considered a most common form of valve disease in the western world. At present, despite decades of clinical technical and basic science progress, cardiovascular disease remains the leading cause of death worldwide.

The author, Dr. Mistiaen, is well-known in the field; he tackles confusing science of cardiovascular disorders. During his training as surgeon (1987-1994), he was involved for some years in the Department of Cardiovascular Surgery in the ZNA Hospital Middelheim (Antwerp, Belgium; head: Philip Van Cauwelaert, MD). Since he is a general surgeon, he never performed heart surgery himself, but he continued to do research in this field until today. The two research lines are postoperative complications after aortic valve replacement and mechanism leading to degenerative aortic valve disease. This resulted in a number of articles, which can be accessed through ISI Web of Knowledge. Both lines resulted in a second doctoral degree in 2009 (the first PhD was in digestive surgery, in 1999 but the subject of vagotomy has become obsolete; therefore this investigation has stopped in 2000). His current position concerns exclusively teaching and research.

Dr. Mistiaen's book offered easily understood lessons to field of aortic valve disease and aortic valve replacement that any cardiovascular researcher and/or clinician would be proud to write. The book reviewed the diverse and varied answers to challenging situations in the management of calcified aortic valve stenosis with regard to diagnostic strategies and treatments. It is not only surgical valve replacement and alternative options. Elucidation of the cellular and molecular pathogenesis of degenerative valve disease has certainly provided a basis for future therapeutic interventions to delay or prevent its progression.

Degenerative aortic valve disease is a highly prevalent disease associated with significant morbidity and mortality. We need to continuously monitor progress in cardiac diseases to measure increases, if any, for aortic valve disease control, screening, and data collection. There are now various promising techniques to diagnose and treat this problem but several issues remain, and are nicely discussed in this book. Dr. Mistiaen sufficiently addressed the current various concepts of decreasing mortality and improvement of both pre and postoperative patient conditions. If we apply all, we could improve aortic valve disease incidence rate and its mortality among the susceptible populations.

Dr. Mistiaen guides the reader through the nature of valve replacement operation, a type of surgery is usually recommended when the damage to the valve is severe enough to be potentially life-threatening. Therefore this book will be helpful to educate and inform practitioners and patients seeking knowledge about this critical area. It is generally accepted that eradicating aortic valve disease is virtually never simply a matter of using available therapies. Successful treatment needs expanded approaches and better methodologies and options. Patients and practitioners in the field must utilize all available information in this book to seek out the best possible knowledge and maximize chances for therapeutic success.

Eltyeb Abdelwahid

CBRC-Massachusetts General Hospital/Harvard Medical School
Harvard Medical School
Charlestown, MA 02129
USA

PREFACE

Half a century ago, surgical treatment of calcified aortic valve disease has been introduced. This has been only possible by the development of the necessary imaging techniques, the extracorporeal circulation, the anesthetic procedures and the proper postoperative care. This operation turns an incurable and lethal disease into a manageable condition. This evolution, however has not been straightforward. The first biological devices failed quickly and the first mechanical devices have had a high rate of thromboembolism. Nevertheless, it is fruitful to look to the past and to watch the efforts, the failures and successes of those that have explored a yet unchartered field. The Ross procedure is such an example. After its introduction, it has become out of use because of postoperative problems, but it has been rediscovered afterwards. Currently, this procedure has its place in pediatric cardiac surgery. Following such developments, it feels as if one stands on the shoulder of giants.

Understanding aortic valve degeneration requires first a knowledge of the macroscopic and microscopic features of the normal aortic valve, which is offered in the first chapters. The development of the aortic valve degeneration is displayed as a three-layered phenomenon by Yetkin in 2009. The model is further developed in this manuscript. Many events and mechanisms have some degree of cross-talk, which makes the unraveling of this process very difficult. Congenitally bicuspid aortic valve has been excuded from this discussion, since it also involves the aortic wall. There has been hope that knowledge of risk factors and mechanisms of degenerative valve disease would lead to measures in preventing the progress of the disease. The results of the first patients series, in whom statins have been tried, seemed encouraging, but this could not be confirmed in recent trials presented by Chan and by Gerdts, both in 2010.

In the last decades, imaging has developed further: echocardiography and catheterization have been supplemented by computer tomography and magnetic resonance imaging. These modalities are helpful is solving difficult problems: the low-flow low-gradient conundrum, the moderate valve disease in patients referred primarily for CABG and the ascertaining of the valvular origin of symptoms in elderly patients. The use of stress echocardiography has become very useful in that respect.

The topic of medical treatment of aortic valve disease has not been covered in the manuscript. In truly asymptomatic patients, a watchful waiting could be advocated. Angiotensin converting enzyme inhibitors could have some beneficial effects. Once patients become symptomatic, prompt valve replacement is indicated. Patients with symptoms of doubtful origin are a challenge, however.

Once the decision has been made to replace the diseased aortic valve, the choice for the most appropriate prosthesis has to be made. Few randomized trials are available, however. The series of Stassano in 2009 is the only recent one. The choice for the valve depends on many factors, which can be derived from such trials. Age of the patient is one of the most important factors, but it is not the only one. The choice between different types of valves is a joint decision between the cardiologist, the cardiac surgeon and the patient.

In the last decades, more and more octogenarians have been referred for aortic valve replacement. The decision to operate upon such patients is not always an easy one. About ten years ago, Bouma and Iung pointed out that about one third of the patients is denied surgery unjustly and that referral patterns can vary greatly between cardiologists. Several criteria, including age, left ventricular function and the EuroSCORE have been applied for this purpose. The EuroSCORE, however, should be applied with great caution, since it overestimates hospital mortality in patients with a high risk. This problem is still relevant today and the conclusion of this chapter might help in the decision making.

Once the valve has been implanted, the patient needs thorough and life-long follow-up. The adverse events all need to be defined in advance and recorded in a proper way. For every event, risk factors and predictors need to be identified. This can be helpful in quality benchmarking and in future patient selection.

Recent developments also require attention: first, the development of tissue engineered heart valves and second the development of trans-catheter aortic valve implantation. The heart valve engineering has seemed promising, especially with the introduction of stem cells. But as recently as 2005, Vesely has pointed out that there is still a long way to go. Work on this subject, published in 2010 indicates that not all steps in the development of such devices have been unraveled. It might be that the "silver bullet" will never be found.

The implantation of aortic valves through catheters also seems a promising development. Leon *et al.* published a first randomized controlled trial in 2010 in which this procedure was compared to balloon aortic valvuloplasty. The trans-catheter implantation proved to be superior to valvuloplasty, but the complication rate was high. In 2011, a second RCT has been published by Smith *et al.* The results indicate to an non-inferiority of TAVI, compared to AVR. Use of the EuroSCORE should be used cautiously in the decision making for TAVI or conventional AVR.

These recent developments show that still a lot of work has to be done. Nevertheless, the ultimate goal, curing a valve disease by a procedure which does produce as minimal side effects as possible and by a device, which has the capacity to grow along and to repair and to remodel itself and thus requires no medication might be approached or even reached.

This works aims to summarize the main findings in the field of aortic valve disease and aortic valve replacement. The area, however, is vast and rapidly expanding. Many scientific manuscripst have appeared and continue to appear. It is therefore not possible to give a complete review.

I wish to express my gratitude to my wife, Collette Emwinomwan for her patience and endurance, while this manuscript has been written. Although she never involved herself in any medical practice, she was a source of inspiration. My gratitude also goes to my parents, David and Hanna, who taught me sound principles in this life.

This book is dedicated to my children, Rebecca, Dominic and Peter.

Wilhelm P. Mistiaen

Artesis University College Antwerp
Department of Healthcare Sciences
University of Antwerp
Belgium
E-mail: wilhelm.mistiaen@ua.ac.be

List of Abbreviations

ACC : American College of Cardiology

ACE : angiotensin convering enzyme

ADL : activity of daily life

AF : atrial fibrillation

AHA : American Heart Association

AHT : arterial hypertension

AMI : acute myocardial infarction

ANOVA : analysis of variance

Apo B : apolipoprotein B

AR : aortic regurgitation

AS : aortic stenosis

ATR : angiotensin receptor

AVA : aortic valve area (native valve)

AVAI : aortic valve area index

AVB : atrio-ventricular block

AVC : aortic valve calcium

AVI : aortic valve implant

AVJ : aortoventricular junction

AVR : aortic valve replacement

BAV	: balloon aoric valvuloplasty/valvotomy
BBB	: bundle branch block (left or right RBBB, LAHB, unspecified)
BHV	: bioprosthetic heart valve
BMI	: body mass index
BMP	: bone morphogenetic factor
BNP	: B-type natriuretic peptide
BSA	: body surface area
CABG	: coronary artery bypass graft
CAD	: coronary artery disease
CAVS	: calcified aortic valve stenosis
CCT	: cross clamping time
CD	: conduction defect
CDxx	: cluster of differentiation xx
CE	: Carpentier-Edwards
CEp	: Carpentier-Edwards pericardial
CEACAM	: carcino-embryonic antigen related cell adhesion molecule
CHF	: congestive heart failure
CI	: confidence interval
CMR	: cardiac MRI
CO	: cardiac output

COPD	: chronic obstructive pulmonary disease
CRP	: C reactive protein
CVA	: cerebro-vascular accident
DM	: diabetes mellitus
DSCT	: dual source computer tomography
DVR	: double valve replacement (aortic with mitral)
EACTS	: European Society for Cardio-Thoracic surgery
EAO	: effective orifice area (valve prosthesis)
EAOI	: effective orifice area index
EMB	: electron beam tomography
EC	: endothelial cells
ECC	: extra corporeal circulation (or CBP cardiopulmonary bypass)
ECE	: endothelin converting enzyme
ECG	: electrocardiography/electrocardiogram
ECM	: extra-cellular matrix
ELI	: energy loss index (also SWL or stroke work loss)
eNOS	: endothelial nitric oxid synthase
EPC	: endothelial progenitor cells
ESC	: European Society of Cardiology
ET	: endothelin

EuroSCORE : European System for Cardiac Operative Risk Evaluation

FU : follow-up

GAG : glycosaminoglycans

HDL : high density lipoprotein

HOCM : hypertrophic obstructive cardiomyopathy

Hs-CRP : high sensitivity C reactive protein

IABP : intra-aortic balloon pump

IC : interstitial cells

ICAM : intercellular adhesion molecule

ICU : intensive care unit

IHC : immunohistochemical

IL : interleukin

INR : international normalized ratio

LDH : lactate dehydrogenase

LDL : low density lipoprotein

LF-LG : low flow-low gradient

Lp : lipoprotein

LRP 5 : lipoprotein receptor 5

LV : left ventricle

LVEDV : left ventricular end diastolic volume

LVEF : left ventricular ejection fraction

LVEFI : left ventricular ejection fraction index

LVF : left ventricular function

LVH : left ventricular hypertrophy

LVM : left ventricular mass

LVMI : left ventricular mass index

LVOT : left ventricular outflow tract

MDCT : multi-detector computer tomography

MGP : matrix gamma-carboxyglutamic acid (GLA) proteins

MHV : mechanical heart valve

MMP : matrix metalloproteinase

MR : mitral regurgitation

MRI : magnetic resonance imaging

mRNA : messenger ribonucleic acid

MSCT : multi-slice computer tomography

MVR : mitral valve replacement

NFkB : nuclear factor kappa B

NO : nitric oxide

NYHA : New York Heart Association

OPG : osteoprotergin

OPN	: osteopontin
OR	: odds ratio
PAD	: peripheral artery disease
PAHT	: pulmonary arterial hypertension
PCMW	: pulmonary capillary wedge pressure
PHV	: prosthetic heart valve
PM	: pacemaker (permanent)
PMI	: PM implant
PPAR	: peroxisome proliferative activated receptor
PTCA	: percutaneous transluminal coronary angioplasty
PVD	: prosthetic valve dysfunction
PVE	: prosthetic valve endocarditis
PPVL	: prosthetic paravalvular leak
PVT	: prosthetic valve thrombosis
QALY	: quality adjusted life of years
QoL	: quality of life
RBC	: red blood cells
RCT	: randomized controlled trial
ROC	: receiver operator characteristic
SEM	: scanning electron microscopy

SJM	: St Jude Medical Valve
SMA	: smooth muscle cell actin
SMC	: smooth muscle cells
SPV	: stentless porcine valve
SR	: sinus rhythm
STJ	: sino-tubular junction
STS	: Society of Thoracic Surgery Predicted Risk Of Mortality
SVD	: structural valve degeneration
SWL	: stroke work loss
TAVI	: transcatheter aortic valve implantation
TE	: thrombo-embolic
TEE	: trans-esophagal echocardiography
TEM	: transmission electron microscopy
TGF	: transforming growth factor
TIA	: transient ischemic attack
TIMP	: tissue inhibitor of matrix metalloproteinase
TLR	: toll like receptor
TNF	: tumour necrosis factor
TTE	: trans-thoracic echocardiography
TVG	: trans-valvular gradient
VAP	: vascular adhesion protein

VEGF	: vascular endothelial growth factor
VIC	: valve interstitial cells
VPPM	: valve – patient prosthesis mismatch
VTI	: velocity time integral
vWF	: von Willebrand factor
3VD	: three vessel disease

CLASSIFICATION OF RECOMMENDATIONS

Class I: Conditions for which there is evidence and/or general agreement that a given procedure or treatment is useful and effective.

Class II: Conditions for which there is conflicting evidence and/or a divergence of opinion about the usefulness and efficacy of a procedure or a treatment.

IIa: Weight of opinion and evidence is in favour of usefulness and efficacy.

IIb: Usefulness and efficacy is less well established by evidence and opinion.

Class III: Conditions for which there is evidence and general agreement that the procedure/treatment is not useful or effective and in some cases may be harmful.

LEVEL OF EVIDENCE

Level A: Data derived from multiple randomized clinical trials.

Level B: Data derived from a single randomized trial or from non-randomized studies.

Level C: Consensus opinion of experts.

CHAPTER 1

The Normal Aortic Valve

Abstract: The aortic valve has a deceivingly simple design. However, its macroscopic anatomy must be understood in relation to its function. This understanding also has a repercussion on the surgical treatment of aortic valve disease. A supporting structure of a valve prosthesis does not necessarily follow the line of attachment of the native leaflets.

The aortic root has to be defined properly. It is more than just a ring in a two dimensional plane. The attachment of the valvular leaflets possesses a three dimensional structure which changes in shape during the cardiac cycle.

The aortic annulus also needs full description. The diameters at the level of the STJ, the mid-sinusal level and the anatomic AVJ are part of this concept.

The microscopic and cell biological description of the aortic valve include

- The layers within the leaflets.
- The cells.
  - Endothelial cells or EC and their function.
  - Valvular interstitial cells or VIC and their function.
- The extracellular matrix.
  - The fibers: collagen and elastin.
  - The glycosaminoglycans or GAG.

A thorough description of these elements is needed for understanding of:

- The durability of the native valve during an entire human life span.
- The understanding of pathological processes.
- The construction of tissue engineered heart valves or TEHV.

Keywords: Aortoventricular junction, bone morphogenetic protein, collagen, endothelial cells, extracellular matrix, fibrosa, glycosaminoglycans, left ventricular outflow tract, nitric oxide, sinotubular junction, spongiosa, valvular interstitial cells, ventricularis.

Wilhelm Peter Mistiaen

1. MACROSCOPIC DESCRIPTION OF THE AORTIC ROOT

Although the design of the aortic valve seems simple [1], the aortic root is somehow an enigmatic structure. The AVJ can be considered as the centerpiece of the heart, and it is often referred to, but without a proper description. The aortic root represents the LVOT and surrounds and supports the leaflets. It extends from within the LV to the STJ. This structure is a cylinder where supporting ventricular structures extend into the fibro-elastic walls of the aortic sinuses. These sinuses are alternating with the intersinusal fibrous triangles. This cylinder is discordant with the leaflets of the valve itself: it is crossed by the hinge-lines of the leaflets. These lines separate the pressure curve within the LV from that within the aorta. The three sinuses can be considered as similar, except in two aspects: 1) the coronary arteries and 2) the crescent-like muscular tissue, which is incorporated at the base of these coronary sinuses. In contrast, the non-coronary sinus has only a fibrous wall. It also is continuous with the anterior leaflet of the mitral valve. Its base is located beneath the AVJ [2].

The semilunar attachment of the leaflets divide the aortic root in a supravalvular and a subvalvular part. Their bases extend proximally into the ventricle, *i.e.* these cross the anatomic AVJ. The supravalvular parts are aortic in nature, but at their base structures of ventricular origin are present. The subvalvular parts have a ventricular origin, but extend as triangles, between the semilunar lines of attachment, to the level of the STJ. The STJ can be considered as the distal end of the aortic root, being still a part of it. Hence its dilatation produces regurgitation of the aortic valve. The aortic annulus can be defined in several ways. Many define it as the remnant after the removal of the valvar leaflets. However, due to the semilunar attachment, the root should be considered as a three dimensional design. Hence the annulus can also be considered as a virtual ring, the "joining together" of the most proximal parts of each leaflet. The diameter of this ring is measured by echocardiography. Since the diameter of the root varies throughout its length, a full description of the root requires the measurement of the diameter at 1) the STJ, 2) mid-sinusal level, and 3) the anatomic AVJ. The differences between these sizes can be up to 20% and have to be taken into account [2].

One has also to take into account the difference between the native hemodynamic AVJ, which is the line of the attachment of the leaflets, and the prosthetic hemodynamic junction, which is at the site of a flat sewing ring.

2. PHYSIOLOGICAL CONSIDERATIONS

The aortic valve is most extensively studied valve and offers the best illustration of the need to understand the structure-function relationship for the development of valvular disease and for valve replacement. The structure includes the whole root, from the level of the annulus to the STJ. Therefore, the movements of all its components need proper description. The aortic valve also becomes most often diseased, and is most frequently replaced. Understanding of its structure and function can also lead to improvement of heart valve substitutions, and maybe to devices that are capable to remodel itself after implantation.

The normal adult heart valve is well adapted to its physiological environment, and is able to withstand the unique hemodynamic/mechanical stresses under normal conditions [3]. Healthy heart valves allow an unidirectional flow of blood without causing obstruction or regurgitation, hemolysis or TE. There is no concentration of excessive mechanical stress in the leaflets. This enables the aortic valve to withstand the lifelong repetition of the pressure variations of 100, 000 cycles every day. A normal valve function requires structural integrity and coordinated interactions among multiple critical components: the leaflets, the commissures, and their respective supporting structures in the aortic root [4].

The three leaflets open easily in a forward flow and close rapidly and completely when the pressure is reversed, even at a minimal degree. However, it has been shown that the opening of the valve precedes the forward movement of blood from the ventricle, rather than as a response to it. During systole, when the valve is open, the orifice is nearly circular. During closure, a high mechanical load builds on the cusps. Nevertheless, prolapse is prevented by substantial coaptation of the valve at its free edge [3, 4].

The aortic valve virtually has no metabolic activity and seems to function during an entire human life span, without the necessity of self repair. The microstructure and composition of the native aortic valve might offer an explanation for its resistance to mechanical fatigue. Although it still remains unknown exactly what makes aortic valve tissue so durable, the importance of its internal complexity is being appreciated more and more [1].

3. MICROSCOPIC ANATOMY

3.1. The Layers

The leaflets of the aortic valve are thin and opalescent. They have a specific architecture, allowing mutual support during stretching. Three different layers can be discerned: the ventricularis, the spongiosa and the fibrosa. Each of these layers has a specific ECM component. The fibers of the ECM has distinct mechanical properties depending on their orientation [5].

> The **ventricularis** is the closest to the left ventricle and has a dense collagen network with radially aligned elastic fibers. This layer allows the cusps to have a minimal surface area when the valve is open but also enables a stretching as a response to the hydrostatic pressure during diastole, when the valve is closed. This mechanism maximizes the coaptation area and prevents leaking.
>
> The central layer of the aortic valve cusp or **spongiosa** is composed of loosely arranged collagen and is abundantly present GAG [3].
>
> At the arterial side, or **fibrosa** contains mostly collagen fibers. Most likely, the organization of collagen and elastin in interconnected sheets, layers and tubules, as well as its highly nonlinear mechanics, anisotropy, and visco-elastic properties makes this valve tissue so durable [1].

The layers and their content are maintained and remodeled by VIC [6, 7]. With increase in age, the cusps become thinner and the number of adipose cells increase [5, 7, 8].

Within the valve, cells and ECM can be discerned. The ECM can be subdivided in fibers (collagen and elastin) and other elements (proteoglycans, GAG).

Healthy heart valves have no vasculature, except in their most proximal parts. When these valves thicken, it might be that, through inadequate diffusion of oxygen, neo-angiogenesis develops. These micro-vessels have also an EC lining [9].

3.2 The Cells

There are two main types of cells in the aortic valve leaflets: endothelial cells (EC) and mesenchymal cells or VIC. These cells are few in number.

3.2.1. *Endothelial Cells*

The endothelium consists of a single cell layer, which lines the entire cardiovascular system, including the heart valves. EC cover the valvular surface as a continuous mono-cellular layer, while the VIC can be found throughout the valve. EC of a normal heart valve are derived from the mesoderm and are polygonal in shape and are aligned with the collagen framework of the valve. These cells are arranged across the direction of the flow. The EC are interposed between the blood compartment and the VIC. The interaction with the latter, therefore, is regulated by these EC.

EC throughout the cardiovascular system provide several functions. This is of major importance to maintain the so-called cardiovascular homeostasis [10, 11]:

- Anticoagulation, through functionally active thrombomodulin, by providing a non-thrombogenic surface, as well as by fibrinolysis. This is of vital importance for "thromboresistance" [3, 4, 12].

- Vascular dilation/vascular tone/vascular remodeling.

- Anti-inflammation by regulating vessel permeability for macromolecules [3, 4, 13].

- Metabolism of lipids and of hormones.

- Differentiation into VIC [14].

- Balance between nitric oxide (which is protective against oxidation) and peroxonitrite (which is an oxidant).

This balance is maintained through haem oxygenase-1 and endothelial nitric oxid synthase or eNOS [15]. NO production is a surrogate for endothelial protective function. Peroxynitrite has been used as assessment of dysfunctional eNOS activity [16]. Anti-oxidant enzymes such as superoxide dismutase also protects against cardiovascular disease [17].

Functions, more specific for the valvular EC, are:

- The integrity of the EC, for the optimal valvular function [18].
- Protection of aortic VIC from early events which lead to calcification by producing nitric oxide [19].
- Communication between EC and VIC through cytokines, components of ECM, growth factors and by direct mechanical connections [20].
- Regulating its mechanical properties [21, 22].

Aortic valves have some contractile activity. Receptor systems that mediate this contractility are endothelin, thromboxane A2, alpha-2 adrenergic, histamine H1 and serotonin [21]. Serotonin causes a decrease in stiffness of the cusp, while endothelin-1 causes an increase (a contraction). Alpha-smooth muscle cell actin in adult thoracic aortic EC could be associated with atheromatosis [21].

One must keep in mind that EC from different sources (venous, arterial and valvular) behave differently, because they expose different markers/gene expressions. These differences determine the response of EC to mechanical and biochemical stimuli: isolated valvular EC derived from animals align perpendicular to a laminar flow while EC derived from the aortic wall align parallel to the flow [3].

EC from the ventricular side differ from EC at the aortic side. Over 500 genes are differently expressed *in situ* by EC if the aortic and the ventricular side are compared [3, 22].

Valvular EC and aortic EC have similar anti-oxidant and anti-inflammatory genes in response to shear stress. Valvular EC are intrinsically less inflammatory [23]. The aortic side seem to express significantly less inhibitors of calcification. Protection at this side is provided by enhanced anti-oxidative gene expression [22]. The significance of this difference is not known yet [3].

The expression of BMP of type 2, 4 and 6 as well as their antagonists is significantly higher at the ventricular EC, compared to the fibrosa side in both, calcified and non-calcified cusps. SMAD 1/5/8 (intracellular second messenger proteins which act as transcription factors) play a role in the calcified fibrosa [24].

These observations seem to indicate that both types of EC belong to a different organ system. Nevertheless, systemic endothelial dysfunction (determined by post-ischemic flow mediated dilation) is associated with aortic valve sclerosis [25].

A neuronal involvement of the EC function is made probable by the observation of nerve endings close to the EC. Neuromodulators could affect the expression of vaso-active factors, growth factors and cytokines secreted by EC. Sensory nerve ending also might detect substances released by EC. This could provide feedback control for the function of VIC [26].

EC can be altered by several stimuli. The most important are hypercholesterolemia and mechanical stress [10].

Hypercholesterolemia induces EC dysfunction, even before atherosclerosis develops: lipids infiltrate the arterial wall and leucocytes bind to the EC. The expression of VCAM-1 by EC increases soon after the initiation of high cholesterol levels. This is reversed by a diet or by medication. Hypercholesterolemia also reduces the exercise-induced vasodilatation, since in atherosclerosis, NO production by EC has been impaired. Lowering of lipids reduces influx of lipids in the arterial wall as well as inflammation, while vasodilatation regulated by EC is promoted [11].

Mechanical stress (shear, cyclic, hydrostatic pressure) has also an effect: laminar blood flow with high shear stress has a protective effect. Turbulent flow and low shear stress promote the development of atheromatosis and CAVS [27].

Other stimuli that can alter the function of EC are cytokines, complement, micro-organisms, Reactive Oxygen Species or ROS, hypothermia, hypoxia and advanced glycosylation in diabetes [10].

The responses of EC can be categorized as [10]:

- Morphologic adaptation, including altered shapes, appearance of microvilli, of discontinuous cell borders and of desquamation [28].
- Altered permeability: Alpha-smooth muscle actin in cell-to cell contact between EC could have a role in altered cell junctions [21, 22].
- Shift in antiocoagulant – procoagulant properties.
- Vasoconstriction (by action of ACE, endothelin).
- Vasodilation (by action of nitric oxide, endothelium derived relaxation factor).
- Expression of ECM (collagen and GAG).
- Inflammation with expression of IL-1, IL-6, IL-8, of adhesion molecules such as E-selectin, of VCAM-1 and ICAM-1 [22] and loss of the integrity of EC layer [29, 30].
- Expression of growth factors and of growth inhibitors.

These changes could lead to well known diseases as atheromatosis (with thromboemboli and hence infarction and stroke), hypertension and degenerative valve disease.

The changes at the aortic valve will be described in the next chapter.

3.2.2. Valve Interstitial Cells

VIC are the major cellular components of heart valve leaflets. These cells have the dual ability to secrete ECM components and to maintain valvular contractile function [31]. VIC are arranged in small bundles of 5 to 35 cells within the ventricularis. Sometimes, VIC are found as individual cells scattered throughout the valvular layers. This can be important in the understanding of the pathological processes within the valve [32].

VIC also have complex signaling mechanisms and show a remarkable plasticity: their phenotypic appearance can alter drastically. VIC are fibroblast-like cells in normal valves, but these cells can be activated, when valves are subjected to mechanical loading and other environmental stimuli. In such conditions, VIC can assume a myofibroblast-like phenotype, and mediate a connective tissue remodeling. This remodeling probably is an attempt to restore the normal stress profile in the valve tissue. When this normal stress profile is restored, the cells return to the quiescent state. However, when this profile is not achieved, activated myofibroblast-like cells persist [3].

VIC can be subdivided in:

1. Quiescent VIC: These maintain the physiological valve structure and inhibit angiogenesis in the leaflets; these VIC are mostly present in healthy valves; they look like fibroblasts.

2. Activated VIC: These contain alpha-SMA and smoothelin, for cellular repair processes including proliferation, migration, ECM synthesis and remodeling as a response to hemodynamic or pathological valve injury.

3. Progenitor VIC: These are found, in heart valve leaflets as well as in the bone marrow and in the circulation. These cells can enter the heart valve, for repair.

4. Osteoblastic VIC: If these are present in the leaflets, they cause calcification, chondrogenesis, and osteogenesis in the heart valve. They secrete alkaline phosphatase, osteocalcin, osteopontin and bone sialoprotein.

5. Furthermore, there are embryonic progenitor endothelial/mesenchymal cells which transform during fetal development into activated VIC and quiescent VIC that are present in the normal heart valve.

Some conversion from one type of VIC to another type is possible. However, this subdivision in phenotypes is useful to relate to their functions in physiological and pathological conditions. VIC become activated by inflammation in pathological conditions or hemodynamic stress and by associated cytokine signals. If these

VIC continue to promote these cellular processes, this could lead to a clinical valve disease [3, 4, 32, 33].

VIC can also become involved in contractile properties of the aortic valves [3], but the significance of this finding is uncertain *in vivo*. In a porcine model, a basal tonus of these myofibroblasts has been demonstrated. Contraction of these cells results in an increased stiffness of the leaflets, especially when these are bent in an unnatural way. In contrast, bending according to the natural curve results in a much lower increase in stiffness. This contraction of myofibroblasts could depend on the layer in which these cells are located: the mechanical properties of the ECM vary between the ventricularis and fibrosa layers. Aortic VIC contractile ability contributes considerably to aortic valve leaflet bending stiffness, which most likely serves a role in maintaining aortic valve leaflet tissue homeostasis [34].

Aortic VIC differ from pulmonary VIC in their response to certain stimuli:

1) The number of TLR, which are responsible for innate immune reaction, is more than twice as high in aortic VIC, compared to pulmonary VIC.

2) The inflammatory response to TLR stimulation in aortic VIC is also twice as high.

3) Expression of BMP-2 and runt related transcription factor 2 are essential for differentiation of VIC into osteoblasts. This differentiation is marked by increased alkaline phosphates activity, deposition of calcific nodules and osteogenesis. These events are found in aortic VIC.

Higher oxygen tension and transvalvular pressure are present at the left side of the heart. These conditions can be held responsible for the differences between aortic and pulmonic valve. The pro-osteogenic changes in VIC are complex and multi-factorial, and the TLR play a critical role herein [35].

3.3. The ECM

3.3.1. General Description

The valvular ECM is produced and maintained by VIC. The quality of the this ECM is the main factor for durability of the valve: this ECM has to maintain its pliability and integrity throughout the entire human life. Therefore, the aortic valve must undergo continuous physiologic remodeling which involves synthesis, degradation, and reorganization of its ECM. These processes depend on MMPs and a complex signaling mechanism. These mechanism allow the valves to respond to injury with a remarkable plasticity and modulation of the phenotype of VIC, even in fully matured valves [3].

The aortic valve consists of the three basic building blocks of all connective tissues: collagen fibers, elastin sheets, and GAG matrix. These elements play an essential role in the structural integrity of the native heart valve. It is the fundamental requirement for the long-term performance of a native aortic heart valve [1, 4].

> The collagen provides the biomechanical strength, stiffness and tensile strength to the valve, hence it can withstand diastolic loads.
>
> The elastin provides the resilience and enables the return of the collagen structures to their resting states between loading cycles.
>
> The GAG maintain hydration and the visco-elastic properties of the tissue and enable its withstanding to compressive forces.

It is necessary to assess the components of the ECM qualitatively and quantitatively in the TEHV. These have to be compared to the structural appearance of the native heart valve ECM which can be considered as the gold standard [4].

3.3.2. Fibres

Elliptical polarized light studies reveal that so-called meso-structures or intermediate size branched fiber bundles and membrane exist in the leaflets of the aortic valve. Size of the fibres and features of symmetry differ for each leaflet.

This additional information can be important for the understanding in the structure-function relationship in the aortic valve [36]. Collagen and elastic fibers are organized in different planes and orientations. These can be recognized for each of the layers.

1) The zona ventricularis, is the closest to the left ventricle chamber and is largely composed of elastin. This layer is able to extend in diastole and recoil in systole to minimize cusp area.

2) The zona fibrosa is the closest to the outflow surface. It rich in densely packed collagen, which is organized in radial and circumferential direction. The fibres are parallel to the free edge of the leaflet. This layer provides the strength and stiffness of the cusps and is mainly responsible for bearing diastolic stress, thereby preventing regurgitation.

3) The zona spongiosa is centrally located. It mainly consists of GAG, which are responsible for accommodation of shear forces of the cuspal layers. This layer also functions as a shock absorber during the valve cycle, but it has little structural strength.

The whole valve geometry and the microscopic fibrous network within the cusps accomplish effective transfer of the stress induced by diastolic back pressure (approximately 80 mm Hg) to the annulus and aortic wall [3].

This organization of the aortic native heart valve allows for certain unique qualities.

1) There are corrugations, or accordion-like folds present in the valve cusps. These allow the variation of the shape and dimensions of the leaflets during the cardiac cycle.

2) Microscopic collagen folding, also known as crimp, allow the lengthening of the valve at minimal stress.

3) The tissue in the leaflet displays anisotropy. This is the quality conferred by collagen architecture that permits differences in radial and circumferential extensibility.

4) The macroscopic collagen alignment enables that forces from the leaflets are transferred to the aortic wall. By employing these properties, the native heart valve avoids excess stress concentration on the leaflets and their supporting tissues. Biomechanical loads caused by repetitive deformations can be resisted.

5) Biomechanical stress may induce repair of connective tissue. In particular, when stimulated by mechanical loading, VIC become activated and mediate connective tissue remodeling. This remodeling restores a normal stress profile in the tissue. Mechanical forces acting on the valve are translated into biological responses at the tissue level, which in turn lead to a VIC response at cellular level. Intracellular signaling leads to changes such as increased VIC stiffness and increased ECM biosynthesis.

6) The higher valvular pressure gradients on the left side of the heart lead to larger local tissue stress on the VIC, which leads to higher VIC stiffness and collagen biosynthesis in the left-sided valves [4].

3.3.3. GAG

The ECM contains structural and functional proteins such as glycoproteins and proteoglycans. These components are also arranged in a tissue specific three dimensional ultra-structure. This allows attachment of cells through receptors. The ECM also acts as a reservoir for signaling factors which modulate angiogenesis, cell migration and cell proliferation [37].

Proteoglycans play an important role with respect to tissue mechanics, tissue hydration and the regulation of extra-cellular calcium homeostasis. Their large molecular weight, as well as anionic and hydrophilic nature, allow them to function as excellent lubricants and mechanical shock absorbers [38].

Hyaluronan, which is a GAG polymer, has a repeating disaccharide structure with 25, 000 elements or more. In solution, hyaluronan forms large, random coil structures that occupy large solvent volumes. When constrained within a matrix, such as a collagen network, hyaluronan traps water, and causes swelling. This induces a pressure which results in a resistance to compression, and imparts visco-elastic properties. Hyaluronan also plays a role during embryonic cardiac development as invading cells transform "cardiac jelly" into specialized cardiac structures, like the myocardium and the cardiac valves [1].

The most important factor of valve durability is the valvular ECM. Its continuous quantity and quality depend on the viability and function of VIC. These cells synthesize the several types of valvular ECM molecules. To maintain integrity and pliability, the aortic valve must undergo constant physiologic remodeling, which includes the synthesis, degradation, and reorganization of its ECM. MMP play a major role herein [3].

4. EMBRYONIC FORMATION OF THE AORTIC VALVE

Embryonal valve formation in its final stages is characterized by coordination of ECM structure in time and space. The interstitial cells are organized in compartments. The developmental programs for cusp remodeling contribute to valve growth and maintenance in postnatal life. These findings are common in all avian and mammalian species [5].

Leaflets of the valvar cusps are formed by mesenchymal outgrowths which are described as endocardial cushions. Signals from the underlying myocardium cause a subset of EC in this cushion-forming area to modify into mesenchymal cells. These acquire markers such as alpha-SMC actin, while the endothelial markers are reduced. These cells migrate into the cardiac jelly, which does not contain cells yet. There, they lose the cell-to-cell contact. This forms the endocardial cushions. This process is called endothelial-to-mesenchymal transformation and is probably regulated by TGF-beta and VEGF [3].

Even after formation of the aortic valve, cells (including alpha-SMA containing myofibroblasts) proliferate and produce the elements of the ECM. Fetal aortic valve cells contain also abundant embryonic myosin and MMP. These cells have a higher level of activity compared to a more quiet fibroblast-like VIC in adults. They are more densely present and mitotic as well as apoptotic activity is higher compared to VIC in adult valves. This might reflect a progressive adaptation to hemodynamic conditions. Furthermore, valve EC contain an embryonic form of myosin heavy chain, as well as MMP-1, MMP-13, and other markers of endothelial-activated phenotypes such as ICAM-1 and VCAM-1 [3].

When the fetal aortic valve matures, the collagen fibers align themselves. ECM remodeling occurs together with changes in the phenotype of the valvular cells and with their balancing between proliferation and apoptosis. These events continue after the formation of the valve leaflets, throughout the entire adult human life. This is called valvular homeostasis. This active process can become dysregulated in certain conditions, leading to aortic valve disease. Both ECM and cells undergo changes, which modifies the mechanical properties and the function of the valve [3].

Apoptosis or programmed cell death type I has an importance in the development of organs such as the heart by tissue sculpturing through cell proliferation on the one hand, and removal of redundant cells on the other hand [29-42].

BMP are members of a larger family of TGF-beta. BMP 2 has been shown to be tightly involved in the formation of the atrioventricular junction and valves during their development [18]. BMP 4 is involved in the development of the outflow tract of the ventricles and of the endocardial cushions. These factors seem to be associated with the differentiation and apoptosis in the endocardial cushions and with cardiac valve formation. Furthermore, apoptosis takes place in the early development of the ventricular myocardium [42].

Morphogenesis and developmental remodeling of cardiovascular tissues involves coordinated regulation of cell proliferation and apoptosis [43]. Cells can be mutually interdependent by secretion of paracrine factors. These paracrine factors allow survival and regulated growth whereas isolated cells undergo apoptosis as consequence of lack of these paracrine factors

CONCLUSIONS

The macroscopic design of the aortic valve is deceivingly simple. The aortic annulus must not be seen as a simple flat ring. Its full description is needed to understands its function.

The microscopic structure of the valve shows three layers, with their cells, fibers and other elements of the ECM.

The interstitial cells show a remarkable capacity for change in phenotype, repair and remodeling. An understanding of these processes is necessary for a description of the events occurring in CAVS.

The fibers have important biomechanical properties: collagen shows tensile strength and structural integrity, while elastin provides tissue resilience. The GAG provides resistance to compression. An understanding of these elements is necessary for the construction of TEHV.

ACKNOWLEDGEMENT

Declared none.

CONFLICT OF INTEREST

The author(s) confirm that this chapter content has no conflict of interest.

REFERENCES

[1] Vesely I. Heart valve tissue engineering. Circ Res 2005;97:743-755.
[2] Andersen RH. The surgical anatomy of the aortic root. doi:10.1510/mmcts.2006.002527.
[3] Schoen FJ. Cardiac valves and valvular pathology, Update on function, disease, repair, and replacement. Cardiovasc Pathol 2005;14:189-194.
[4] Hjortnaes J, Bouten CVC, Van Herwerden LA, *et al.* Translating Autologous Heart Valve Tissue Engineering from Bench to Bed. Tissue Eng Part B 2009;15:307-317.
5] Hinton RB Jr., Lincoln J, Deutsch GH, *et al.* Extracellular Matrix Remodeling and Organization in Developing and Diseased Aortic Valves. Circ Res 2006;98:1431-1438.
[6] Mohler ER III, Gannon F, Reynolds C, *et al.* Bone Formation and Inflammation in Cardiac Valves. Circulation 2001;103:1522-1528.
[7] Knaapen M, Somers P, Mistiaen W. Histopathology of calcified aortic valve stenosis. Acta Cardiol 2006; 61[5]:557-562.
[8] Cowell SJ, Newby DE, Boon NA, Elder AT. Review article. Calcific aortic stenosis: same old story? Age and Ageing 2004; 33: 538–544.
[9] Weind KL, Ellis CG, Boughner DR. The aortic valve blood supply. J Heart Valve Dis 2000;9:1-7.
[10] Leask RL, Jain N, Butany J. Endothelium and Valvular Diseases of the Heart. Micropscopy Research and Techniques 2003;60:129-137.
[11] Libby P, Aikawa M, Selwyn A, Ganz P. Lipid lowering improves endothelial functions Int J Cardiol 2000;74:S3-S10.

[12] Lin SJ, Hsieh FY, Chen YH, *et al.* Atorvastatin induces thrombomodulin expression in the aorta of cholesterol-fed rabbits in TNF alpha-treated human aortic endothelial cells. Histol Histopathol 2009;24:1147-1159.

[13] De Paola N, Phelps M. Shear stress gradients regulate endothelial permeability to macromolecules *in vitro*. Ann Biomed Eng 2000;28(Suppl1):S69.

[14] Arciniegas E, Ponce L, Hartt Y, *et al.* Intimal thickening involves transdifferentiation of embryonic endothelial cells. Anat Rec 2000; 258:47-57.

[15] Heeba G, Moselhy ME, Hassan M, *et al.* Anti-atherogenic effect of statins: role of nitric oxide, peroxynitrite and haem oxygenase-1. Br J Pharmacol 2009;156:1256-1266.

[16] Imanishi T, Ikejima H, Tsujioka A, *et al.* Combined effects of an 3-hydroxy-3-methylglutaryl coenzyme A reductase inhibitor and angiotensin II receptor antagonist on notric oxide bioavailability and atherosclerotic change in myocardial infarction-prone Watanabe heritable hyperlipemic rabbits. Hypertension Res 2008;31:1199-1208.

[17] Heistad DD. Oxidative stress and Vascular Disease. Arterioscl Throm Vacs Biol 2006;26:689-695.

[18] El-Hamamsy I, Balachandran K, Yacoub MH, *et al.* Endothelium-dependent Regulation of the Mechanical Properties of the Aortic Valve Cusps. J Am Coll Cardiol 2009;53:1448-1455.

[19] Kennedy JA, Hua X, Mishra K, *et al.* Inhibition of calcifying nodule formation in cultured porcine aortic valve by nitric oxide donors. Eur J Pharmacol 2009;602:28-35.

[20] Davies PF. Mechanisms involved in endothelial responses to hemodynamic forces. Atherosclerosis 1997;131(Suppl):S15-S17.

[21] Chester A, Misfeld M, Yacoub M. Receptor-mediated contraction of aortic valve leaflets. J Heart Valve Dis 2000;9:250-254.

[22] Simmons CA, Grant GR, Manduchi E, Davies PF. Spatial Heterogeneity of Endothelial Phenotypes Correlates With Side-Specific Vulnerability to Calcification in Normal Porcine Aortic Valves. Circ Res 2005;96:792-799.

[23] Butcher JT, Tressel S, Johnson T, *et al.* Transcriptional Profiles of Valvular and Vascular Endothelial Cells Reveal Phenotypic Differences. Influence of Shear Stress. Arterioscl Thromb Vac Biol 2006;26:69-77.

[24] Ankeny RF, Thourani VH, Weiss D, *et al.* Preferential Activation of SMAD1/5/8 on the Fibrosa Endothelium in Calcified Human Aortic Valves-Association with Low BMP Antagonists and SMAD6. PLoS ONE 2011;6(6): e20969. doi:10.1371/journal.pone.0020969

[25] Poggianti E, Venneri L, Chubuchny V, *et al.* Aortic valve sclerosis Is Associated with Systemic Endothelial Dysfunction. J Am Coll Cardiol 2003;41:136-141.

[26] Marron K, Yacoub MH, Polak JM, eta l. Innervation of human atrioventricular and arterial valves. Circulation 1996;94:368-375.

[27] Chiu JJ, Chien S. Effects of Disturbed Flow on Vascular Endothelium: Pathophysiological Basis and Clinical Perspectives. Phys Rev 2011;91:327-387

[28] Stein PD, Wang CH, Riddle JM, *et al.* Scanning electron microscopy of operatively excised severely regurgitant floppy mitral valves. Am J Cardiol 1989;64:392-394.

[29] Ghaisas NK, Foley JB, O'Briain DS, *et al.* Adhesion Molecules in Nonrheumatic Aortic Valve Disease: Endothelial Expression, Serum Levels and Effect of Valve Replacement. J Am Coll Cardiol 2000;36:2257-2262.

[30] Metzler SA, Pregonero CA, Butcher JT, *et al.* Cyclic Strain Regulates Pro-Infammatory Protein Expression in Porcine Valve Endothelial Cells. J Heart Valve Dis 2008;17:571-578.
[31] Yang X, Meng X, Su X, *et al.* Bone morphogenic protein 2 induces Runx2 and osteopontin expression in human aortic valve interstitial cells: Role of Smad1 and extracellular signal-regulated kinase 1/2. J Thorac Cardiovasc Surg 2009;138:1008-1015.
[32] Cimini M, Rogers KA, Boughner DR. Smoothelin-positive cells in human and porcine semilunar valves. Histochemistry and cell biology 2003;120:307-317.
[33] Liu AC, Joag VR, Gotlieb AI. Review. The Emerging Role of Valve Interstitial Cell Phenotypes in Regulating Heart Valve Pathobiology. Am J Pathol 2007, 171:1407-1418.
[34] Merryman WD, Huang HYS, Schoen FJ. Sacks MS. The effects of cellular contraction on aortic valve leaflet flexural stiffness. Journal of Biomechanics 2006;39:88-96.
[35] Yang X, Fullerton DA, Su X, Ao L, *et al.* Pro-Osteogenic Phenotype of Human Aortic Valve Interstitial Cells Is Associated With Higher Levels of Toll-Like Receptors 2 and 4 and Enhanced Expression of Bone Morphogenetic Protein 2. J Am Coll Cardiol 2009;53:491-500.
[36] Doehring TC, Kahelin M, Vesely I. Mesostructures of the aortic valve. J Heart Valve Dis 2005;14:679-686.
[37] Neuenschwander S, Hoerstrup SP. Review Heart valve tissue engineering. Transplant Immunology 2004;12:359-365.
[38] Lehmann S, Walther T, Kempfert J, *et al.* Mechanical Strain and the Aortic Valve: Influence on Fibroblasts, Extracellular Matrix, and Potential Stenosis. Ann Thorac Surg 2009;88:1476-1483.
[39] Abdelwahid E, Pelliniemi LJ, Jokinen E. Cell death and differentiation in the development of the endocardial cushion of the embryonic heart. Microscopic Res and Techn 2002;58:395-403.
[40] Abdelwahid E, Rice D, Pelliniemi LJ, Jokinen E. Overlapping and differential localization of BMP-2, BMP-4, MSX-2 and apoptosis in the endocardial cushion and adjacent tissues of the developing Mouse heart. Cell and Tissue Res 2001;305:67-78.
[41] Abdelwahid E, Eriksson M, Pelliniemi LJ, Jokinen E. Heat shock proteins, HSP 25 and HSP 70, and apoptosis in the developing endocardial cushion of the mouse heart. Histochemistry and Cell Biology 2001;115:95-104.
[42] Abdelwahid E, Pelliniemi LJ, Niinikoski H, *et al.* Apoptosis in the pattern formation of the ventricular wall during heart organogenesis. Anat Rec 1999;256:208-217.
[43] Fisher SA, Langille BL, Srivastava D. Apoptosis during cardiovascular development. Circ Res 2000;87[10]:856-864.

Send Orders of Reprints at bspsaif@emirates.net.ae
"Degenerative" Aortic Valve Stenosis, its Pathogenesis and Treatment, **2013, 21-62**

CHAPTER 2

Pathology of CAVS

Abstract: The pathological changes in CAVS are much more than a simple age related "wear and tear". There is some resemblance of CAVS with atherosclerosis, but important differences have also been authenticated. Both conditions share a number of risk factors, however

The mechanisms leading to the microscopically observable changes in CAVS include many molecules and pathways. There is a considerable "cross talk" between these mechanisms which makes their description difficult.

The unravelling of these pathways requires a description in layers.

The outer layer consists of the risk factors of which the most common are lipid disorders and hypertension.

The middle layer consists of the molecules and mediators involved. Some of these molecules are inflammatory, others are the result of mechanical or oxidative stress, still others play a role in the remodelling of the ECM.

The inner layer consists of the mechanisms, which are inflammation, calcification or ossification, angiogenesis, remodelling of the ECM and programmed cell death.

The unravelling of these processes in CAVS is an ongoing process and is still not completely understood. This understanding might have some consequences in terms of prevention or slowing down of the process.

Keywords: Angiotensin, apoptosis, atheromatosis, autophagy, calcification, Heyde's syndrome, inflammation, lipid infiltration, mechanical stress, neo-angiogenesis, osteoblastic differentiation, oxidative stress, vitamin K antagonists.

1. THE INCIDENCE AND THE NATURAL HISTORY OF CAVS

CAVS is the most frequent heart valve disease in industrialised countries today and its prevalence acutely increases with age: the prevalence in patients over 65 years is estimated at 2%. An additional 29% have aortic valve sclerosis, *i.e.*, thickening and calcification and cuspal thinning of a trileaflet aortic valve in the absence of ventricular outflow obstruction [1, 2]. Hence, with the lengthening of

Wilhelm Peter Mistiaen

life expectancy, the population of elderly patients with CAVS is expected to increase in the future. AVR still is the reference treatment for severe symptomatic CAVS and there are no explicit restrictions for intervention related to age itself. The number of operations also increases. However, the decision to operate is often difficult in old patients in whom it may not be obvious whether or not the benefit of surgery, compared to spontaneous outcome, outweighs the risk of intervention. The published results of AVR for CAVS in elderly could serve as a standard for comparison and decision making for alternatives such as medical treatment, BAV or TAVI [1].

The natural history of CAVS was highlighted half a century ago [1, 3]. When symptoms and certainly signs of CHF appear, compensatory mechanisms that maintain an adequate circulation get exhausted. Life expectancy decreases drastically from that moment on. Based on these observations, AVR should be recommended. However, the extrapolation of these findings to the elderly with CAVS may be debatable. In Ross and Braunwald's study, death occurred at an average age of 63. A more contemporary series of elderly patients with severe CAVS showed that there still is a wide range of survival rates in non-operated patients. The three predictive factors of poor spontaneous outcome were NYHA functional class III or IV, associated mitral regurgitation, and LV systolic dysfunction. The combination of these three factors has identified a subgroup at particularly high risk, with a 3 year survival rate of only 20%. On the other hand, the 3 year survival was over 80% in patients who did not have any of these three factors [1].

Hemodynamic progress has also been described. In CAVS, the obstruction to LVOT leads to a gradual increase in TVG. This reaches levels of 100 mm Hg in severe cases. This corresponds to an AVA of 0.5-1 cm^2. Cardiac output can be maintained by the development of LVH. Eventually, CHF may develop. This emphasizes on the deleterious effect of chronic pressure overload on the myocardial cells [2].

2. MACROSCOPIC AND MICROSCOPIC DESCRIPTION OF THE DISEASED VALVE

When valves are excised during surgery, they show a variety of pathological changes, macroscopically as well as microscopically.

The **macroscopic** appearance includes sclerosis with thickening of the leaflets, calcification as irregular masses at the aortic side, thrombi, fractures and sometimes even bacterial vegetations [4-7]. Calcification occurs at the bases of the cusps in the depth of the sinuses of Valsalva. This calcification extends throughout the leaflets as irregular nodules.

The **microscopic** description involves; 1) the endothelium, 2) the type and extent of calcification, 3) the collagen deposit, as well as the infiltration of 4) lipids and of 5) inflammatory cells.

2.1. Endothelium

The endothelial cell line and its basement membrane are disrupted, even in mild forms of CAVS. The intima/media thickness has increased compared to normal individuals. This relates aortic sclerosis somehow to atheromatosis [5, 6, 8]. The degenerative lesions of CAVS are subendothelial with displacement of the elastic lamina. These lesions extend into the fibrosa [9]. The focal changes of sclerosis are located on the aortic side of the leaflets. This suggests that endothelial injury from low shear stress and high tensile stress are possible initiating factors in the disease process [10].

2.2. Calcification

There is a wide spectrum of severity of CAVS: on the one end, there is sclerosis, which is more commonly observed in elderly, and which can be without clinical significance; on the other end there is a critical stenosis [9]. Calcification occurs at the base of the leaflets, in the sinuses of Valsalva and extends throughout the leaflets. Initially, these lesions can be seen as small foci consisting of calcium deficient hexagonal hydroxyl-apatite crystals. Osteopontin binds easily to these crystals [9]. At the end stage, masses of amorphous calcific nodule can be observed. Usually, the degree of calcification is correlated with the degree of valve stenosis [11].

2.3. Collagen

An excess of collagen is produced in the spongiosa layer, as a response to mechanical stress [9]. The collagen is disorganized [5]. The fibrotic mass of the valve is negatively correlated with severity of stenosis [11].

2.4. Lipid Infiltration

Large amounts of neutral lipids can be found inside and outside cells in CAVS. These lipids are not found in healthy valve leaflets. A strong association between serum lipids and CAVS has been documented. A proof of concept has been delivered by the observation that; 1) plant sterols accumulate in CAVS and 2) there is a relation to serum concentration. Lipids enter the leaflets and have their effects on the valvular interstitium [8].

2.5. Cellular Infiltration

T-lymphocytes and macrophages are scarce in the normal aortic valve. From the onset of the development of CAVS, these cells are starting to accumulate. These inflammatory cells are found closely to the deposits of oxidized lipids. These cells secrete a number of cytokines, such as TNF. These substances initiate the expression of a number of ECM proteins and of enzymes, such as MMP. This could influence a remodeling process [5, 9, 12]. It is not certain that these inflammatory cells activate calcification.

3. SIMILARITIES AND DIFFERENCES BETWEEN CAVS AND ATHEROMATOSIS

3.1. Similarities

Early lesions of CAVS are similar to atheromatosis, with lipid infiltration, inflammation and calcification. Both diseases are a consequence of an active process, in which lipid infiltration and the toxic effects of oxidized cholesterol are involved. In both, the basement membrane is disrupted and inflammatory cells, such as macrophages and T-cells, as well as calcification can be demonstrated. Both conditions have a number of risk factors in common: ageing, hypertension, use of tobacco, diabetes mellitus and hypercholesterolemia [8-11, 13-17]. There are some variations in the significant factors found for both conditions [10].

Several mechanisms can act in concert in both conditions. Elevated serum cholesterol facilitates lipid deposition after any injury of the endothelium from any cause. Use of tobacco increases permeability of endothelium and can promote lipid oxidation [10]. Furthermore, cholesterol and its oxidized form can play an important role in the differentiation of interstitial cells towards osteoblast like cells, and hence in calcification [9]. Oxidative stress is also found in both conditions [17].

3.2. Differences

There is also a considerable difference between atheromatosis and CAVS [17]. This can be deducted from the observation that in many patient series, only one of the two conditions is present.

The oxidative stress in CAVS and atheromatosis shows differerence. In CAVS, oxidative stress is due to the "uncoupled" NOS, which produces increased amounts of superoxide in calcified regions. In atheromatosis, NADH/NADPH oxidase is mainly responsible for the stress. Moreover, a compensatory increase in anti-oxidant mechanism can be found in atheromatosis. In contrast, this antioxidant activity decreases in CAVS, which is somewhat surprising [17].

Furthermore, proliferation of SMC and macrophages loaded with lipids, the so-called foam cells, are found in atheromatosis, but are absent in CAVS. Nevertheless, stenotic valve leaflets also contain lipids, which are absent in healthy valves. This lipid infiltration into the fibrosa and the spongiosa can be the consequence of mechanical injury to the endothelium, which is caused by shear stress. Calcification remains the most prominent feature of CAVS [5, 8, 9, 14].

In stenotic aortic valves, CRP and complement have been documented within the affected leaflets. This CRP activates complement, which on its turn appeals white blood cells. Anti-complement mediators are much less present. This indicates that their mitigating effect on inflammation in CAVS is insufficient, which allows inflammation to continue [18].

ACE and angiotensin II type 1 and type 2 receptors have been documented in stenotic aortic valves, implicating a role for this signaling pathway in the disease process [11].

The mode of programmed cell death is another difference between CAVS and atheromatosis. Apoptosis plays an important role in atheromatosis, but this might be different in CAVS [9].

4. THE LAYERED MODEL FOR THE PATHOGENESIS OF CAVS

The pathology of CAVS and its mechanisms is not yet fully understood. One of the difficulties is that several processes are involved and that there is a cross talk between them. An important diagram [11] indicates that there are several layers that can be discerned in the development of CAVS. The outer layer consists of the risk factors, the medium layer contains the molecules and mediators involved, and the inner layer contains the processes leading to CAVS. The two modes of programmed cell death and their mediators also need to be considered [9, 19].

The risk factors in the outer layer are summarized as follows:

- Smoking.
- Diabetes mellitus.
- Hypertension, involving mechanical stress.
- Aging.
- Infection, by Chlamydia pneumonia.
- Rheumatic heart disease, which is increasingly rare in Western societies.
- Hyperlipidemia.
- Hyperparathyroidism.

The mediators in the middle layer are molecular and include:

- Tenascin C.
- VEGF.
- TGF.
- BMP.

- Osteopontin/osteonectin.
- Adhesion molecules (ICAM, VCAM and CEACAM).
- Decrease in NO (nitric oxide).
- CRP.
- Calcium.
- Cathepsin enzymes.
- MMP.
- Cystatin C enzyme.

The mechanisms in the deepest layer have an effect on cells, tissues and the ECM.

- Inflammation.
- Osteoblastic differentiation/calcification.
- Angiogenesis.
- ECM remodelling.
- Programmed cell death such as apoptosis and autophagy.

These complicated mechanisms clearly indicate that CAVS is not a passive "wear & tear", but the result of an active process. These processes are mediated by a number of receptors such as:

- Osteoprotegerin (OPG).
- LRP5.
- TLR and other interleukin receptors.
- NOTCH-1.

- Apoptotic death receptors.

CAVS therefore, is not an inevitable consequence of aging [2]. This is also indicated by the absence of CAVS in many octogenarians [6, 10, 14].

5. INTEGRATION OF TWO LAYERS, MECHANISMS AND MEDIATORS, IN THE DEVELOPMENT OF CAVS

Each of these processes in the development of CAVS has a number of mediators [11, 16].

For **inflammation**, these are:

- CRP, which has been identified as an independent predictor, and which has been detected in explanted valves [20, 21].
- Increase in ICAM and VCAM in oxidative stress, indicating an endothelial dysfunction.
- Decrease in nitric oxide, coupled with oxidative stress.
- Adhesion molecules and interleukins, by activation of T lymphocytes.
- ACE, as an active enzyme, and angiotensin receptor I, which co-localize with oxidized LDL in plasma and concentrated in diseased valves [22, 23].
- T-lymphocyte infiltration secreting cytokines, thereby recruiting more inflammatory cells [14] such as monocytes.
- Deposits of activated complement in the valve [18].
- Endothelin 1 and its receptor ETA [24].
- BMP 2 and 4.
- NO, endothelial and inducible NOS, eNOS and iNOS [25].

For **osteogenesis**, these are [11, 16]:

- TGF-β 1, by activation of T lymphocytes.
- TNF-α, from monocytes/macrophages.
- BMP 2 and 4.
- Osteopontin/osteonectin (osteopontin activity increases by macrophages which form "foam cells" through oxidized lipids).
- RANKL.
- Cell-to-cell contact with an effect on NOTCH-1.

For **remodeling** of ECM, these are [11, 16]:

- Cystatin C.
- MMP.
- Cathepsin enzymes.
- Tenascin.
- TGF-β 1, which plays a role in osteopontin, TNF, interleukins; formation of calcium noduli and bone tissue.
- Calcium ion.

For **angiogenesis**, these are [11, 16]:

- VEGF.
- Tenascin C.
- CEACAM.
- Chondromodulin, osteonectin and osteocalcin as inhibitors.

These mediators are strongly interrelated and these complicated pathways are difficult to unravel. Some risk factors, which initiate these mechanisms are very common in the Western population and deserve a more elaborate discussion. Hypertension as cause for mechanical stress, and disorders in lipid metabolism are the main examples. The role of infection in the development of CAVS is vague.

6. RISK FACTORS FOR CAVS

6.1. Mechanisms of initiating of CAVS: Mechanical Stress

6.1.1. Effects of Mechanical Stress on EC

The flow pattern at both sides of the valve differs somehow. At the ventricular side, this pattern is unidirectional and acts as shear stress. This pattern inhibits oxidative and inflammatory responses by activating anti-oxidant enzymes and by inhibiting BMP 4, an inflammation promoting protein. This flow pattern also protects against osteogenic and chondrogenic differentiation. At the vascular or aortic side, a more complex pattern occurs, which could be compared to the flow pattern found in arterial bifurcations. Both regions may be susceptible to inflammatory disease [4]. Moreover, turbulences may result in a low shear stress, resulting in endothelial injury, disruption, lipid infiltration and inflammation as can be observed in atherosclerotic lesions [10].

At the aortic valve, the EC at the ventricular side differ from those at aortic side in several ways. These EC act as different organ systems:

1) The EC at the vascular side align themselves parallel to a unidirectional flow, those at the ventricular or valvular side align themselves perfendicular to the flow. This difference can be the result of signaling kinase enzymes, which are involved in various ways.

2) The vascular EC show a tendency to osteogenic differentiation, while the ventricular EC tend to express chondrogenic factors.

3) Moreover, the EC at the vascular side show more tendency to inflammatory response, with inflammatory markers such as VCAM-1, ICAM-1, BMP-4 and TGF beta-1.

These differences explicate why various pathological changes occur on the vascular side of the leaflet. Nevertheless, hemodynamical changes may play a comparable role in the pathogenesis of valvular and vascular diseases.

Hypertension could be held responsible for an increase in mechanical stress. The role of an increased mechanical stress is a key mechanism in the pathogenesis of CAVS. This has also been documented by the experience with bicuspid valves, which show more turbulent flow patterns and therefore suffer more shear stress on the cusps. Further support for the mechanical stress theory appears from the fact that even in tricuspid valves, the areas of calcification correspond to the areas of increased tensile stress [6, 10, 11, 26, 27].

With continuing haemodynamic stress, valvular EC can be lost. Under normal physiological conditions, the EC layer is kept intact after injury, either by mitosis of mature EC or by restoration with circulating EPC. Under pathological conditions, loss of valvular EC is no longer compensated.

Three events occur in CAVS concerning endothelial repair:

1) The EC at the aortic side are senescent with less mitotic capacity.

2) The EPC from the bone marrow have less migratory capacity.

3) There is tendency towards apoptosis, which is recognized by an increase in caspase 3 activity.

All three events contribute to a reduced reparative capacity of the EC lining at the aortic side of the valve [7]. Moreover, circulating EPC express an osteoblastic phenotype in patients with CAVS. These cells may play a role in the active process of CAVS [28].

In advanced CAVS, it might be that a hemodynamic stress promotes fractures on microscopic scale and fracture healing. This in its turn involves further changes in ECM, inflammation, oxidation, angiogenesis, calcification, and osteogenesis [4, 26, 29].

Some other changes of the EC have been documented in patients with CAVS. The plasma level of E-selectin and activated monocytes has been increased. Diseased aortic valves express more markedly several endothelial markers such as CD31, CD34, vWF, and CEACAM 1, compared to normal valves. This also supports the association between endothelial dysfunction and progression of CAVS [23].

Endothelins (ET-1, ET-2, and ET-3) are potent vasoconstrictor isopeptides, which are produced by vascular EC. ET-1 is the most important one in cardiovascular pathology. It interacts with two receptors ETA and ATB, which are found in human aortic valves. Activation of ETA causes vasoconstriction, whereas the endothelial ETB-receptor causes vasodilatation through the release of NO and of prostacyclin. Furthermore, ET-1 has growth-promoting and inflammatory effects, directly or through activated macrophages. In patients with CAVS, levels of ET-1 and its receptor ETA are increased while the level of ETB, endothelin converting enzyme 1 and eNOS are decreased. In patients with early stages of CAVS, ETA receptor antagonists might have a therapeutic potential [25].

NO is a gaseous lipophilic free radical cellular messenger, which modulates inflammation, cell growth, leukocyte adhesion, SMC proliferation, and platelet aggregation. Endothelial NOS and inducible NOS have been documented in aortic valves in patients with CAVS. Interestingly, endothelial NOS gene is significantly down-regulated in CAVS. Thus, the progressive and active processes of sclerosis and CAVS involve alterations in both the ET-1 and NO signaling pathways: ET-1 signaling appears to be increased by reduced bioavailability of protective NO. This is also the case in atherosclerosis. The down-regulated NOS activity may be one of the central factors common to cardiovascular disease, although it is unclear whether this is a cause or result of CAVS [24].

6.1.2. Effects of Mechanical Stress on VIC

Endothelial injury from any cause (smoking, mechanical shear and tensile stress) adversely affects its permeability and hence facilitates lipid deposits [5, 10]. During such injury, quiescent VIC are transformed into activated VIC. The latter cell type participates in repair and remodeling of the valve [30].

Mechanical strain may affect the aortic valve cusp, which leads to a change in ECM ultrastructure and on long term to CAVS. Proteins of the ECM can be localized in stenotic valves. Decorin and biglycan are mostly located at the inflow sides of the cusp, tenascin-C can be found in the central layer, and osteopontin, osteocalcin, and alkaline phosphatase are concentrated near the cell populations which surround the calcified areas. The intensity of this protein expression can be related to the pressure gradient. Comparable findings have been made in fibroblasts, experimentally subjected to mechanical strain.

Proteoglycans play an important role with respect to tissue mechanics, but also in CAVS. With mechanical stress, proteoglycan expression is increased within the ECM. All proteoglycans have an acid function at their endings. A concomitant increase of their negatively charged ends leads to an increase in binding sites for potential adsorption of calcium. Besides osteogenic differentiation of aortic VIC, this may be an alternative pathway to explain calcification of the aortic valve cusp, at least in the early stages. If mineralized ECM is related to CAVS still needs to be determined [29].

Tissue factor, which is involved in blood clotting, can be demonstrated in the fibrosa with experimentally induced aortic valve lesions, such as thickening of leaflets with altered valve performance in rabbits. This observation strengthens the link between CAVS and atheromatosis. Tissue factor; however is also found in EC and in myofibroblasts of normal aortic valves. Macrophage infiltration during development of CAVS may be involved in the synthesis of tissue factor. They can enrich the valve leaflet with tissue factor. This tissue factor may participate in the formation of micro-thrombi and hence embolization [31].

6.2. The Role of Lipids and of Oxidative Stress in CAVS

Among traditional risk factors for atherosclerosis, abnormalities of lipid metabolism have been frequently associated with CAVS. There is also a link between lipid disorders and oxidative stress [17]. Large amounts of neutral lipids have been found inside and outside cells in diseased valves, but not in healthy ones. A strong association between lipid metabolism and CAVS has been documented. Plant sterols accumulate in stenotic aortic valves. This effect is related to their respective serum concentrations. These observations serve as "proof of concept" that lipid metabolism is related to the development and progression of CAVS. Circulating lipids are capable of entering into aortic valve leaflets and thus to exert local effects in the interstitium of aortic valves [23].

There are two ways in which superoxide (ROS or Reactive Oxygen Species) can increase in cardiovascular disease [17]:

1) Inactivation by the dismutase enzyme.

2) Or more commonly, increase in superoxide. This increase in superoxide is due to many enzymes, such as oxidases and cyclo-oxygenase as well as to "uncoupled" NOS. Activated leukocytes also can contribute to this event.

This increase in ROS is called oxidative stress and stimulates antioxidant mechanisms, with a compensatory increase in levels of dismutase. Superoxide is increased in CAVS, especially in calcified regions, as can be found in hereditary lipid disorders. Treatment of lipid disorders reverses this increment in superoxide. Increase in oxidative stress has a causative role in the development of CAVS, since superoxide in the aortic valve increases before the valve becomes stenotic [17].

Superoxide in aortic VIC has several effects:

- Induction of nodule formation by TGF-β1 as an early manifestation of calcification in CAVS through multiple intracellular pathways [32-34].

- Activation of MMP. In the valve, MMPs may play a permissive role in the progression of calcification. Degraded fragments of collagen and elastin also may increase signals that promote calcification in VIC [17].

- Contribution to fibrosis [17].

The degree of ***cross talk between these different signaling pathways*** in different cell types is currently the subject of intense investigation [35], and multiple pathways are likely to be involved in calcific nodule formation under the influence of TGF-β1, of which superoxide formation may be but one.

Although, nodule formation by aortic VIC is followed by apoptosis [36], apoptosis does not appear to be necessary for nodule formation, since inhibition of apoptosis was unable to reduce nodule formation.

NO or nitric oxide has a protective effect in several ways:

- By inhibition of the TGF-β/SMAD effects [37], in EC and aortic VIC.
- Generation of NO in VIC *via* a calcium-sensitive constitutive NOS.
- Paracrine effect of NO from valvular EC on VIC.
- Autocrine effect of VIC.

In the latter two, statins might play a protective role by working through stimulation of endothelial NOS and production of NO [38, 39]. This is only effectual during the initial stages of CAVS [40].

6.3. The Role of Infection in CAVS

The presence of Chlamydia pneumoniae antigens has been documented in calcified aortic valves [41], in early as well as in advanced cases. This finding is suggestive for a role as "passengers that lodge in diseased tissue" but a contribution of such infection to the development of CAVS is not ruled out. The role of this infective agent is unclear since these reports have methodological discrepancies [11].

Lipopolysaccharides of C. pneumoniae can contribute to endothelial injury with subsequent inflammation. C. pneumoniae is often present in aortic valves and is associated with early lesions of aortic valve stenosis in cadavers from elderly persons [42, 43]. However, such findings must be understood with caution, [44].

Another infectious mechanism has been demonstrated in an animal model study. Recurrent low grade endocarditis from calcifying oral bacteria, particularly when occurring with synergistic strains, may be one cause of CAVS [11].

6.4. Other Conditions Related to the Calcification of the Aortic Valve

Alterations in calcium homeostasis are likely to play an important role in the progression of CAVS as suggested by the greater prevalence of CAVS in patients with renal failure [41, 45]. Renal dysfunction is more common in patients with more rapidly progressing CAVS. Some conditions, such as Paget's disease hypercalcemia, and hyperparathyroidism are some examples in which calcium metabolism is altered and where the prevalence of CAVS is increased. Some of the pathologic features of CAVS resemble atherosclerosis with calcification [41].

Several uremia-related mechanisms may contribute to the thickening of the aortic valve leaflets. Renal failure is associated with abnormal calcium-phosphate homeostasis. Hyperphosphatemia induces a low plasma calcium level and secondary hyperparathyroidism. Parathormone releases calcium from the bones. This may lead to metastatic calcification of tissues, including the aortic valve leaflets [45].

6.5. The Effect of Vitamin K Antagonists on Calcification

Matrix gamma-carboxyglutamic acid proteins or MGP are the inhibitors of calcification in the cardiovascular system. The synthesis of MGP is blocked by vitamin K antagonists, such as warfarin (which are used as oral anticoagulants). Vitamin K serves as cofactor for the transformation of selective glutamic acid residues into gamma-carboxyglutamic acid during the biosynthesis of the MGP and vitamin-K dependent coagulating factors. These residues are essential for the protein functions [46, 47].

There are several indicators for a causal relationship of oral anticoagulant medication and calcification of the aortic valve and other cardiovascular structures.

- The effect of vitamin K antagonists has been studied in short-term experiments in rats: the medication induces mild calcification. In mice, use of vitamin K antagonists down-regulate the expression of MGP [46, 47].

- Radiological and pathological studies have shown that the mean calcified area in explanted valves (during AVR) and the aortic valve calcium score are significantly higher in patients who received vitamin K antagonists, compared to those who have not received this medication [46, 47].

- Laboratory studies have shown altered plasma levels of MGP (especially the uncarboxylated form) in patients with vascular calcification and CAVS [46, 47, 48]. The correlation between plasma levels and the degree of CAVS are weak, but this protein might play a role in the decrease of the LVF and mortality [48]. High osteocalcin ratio (reflecting low vitamin K status) and high arterial calcium score are associated with uncarboxylated MGP [49].

- Epidemiological studies have discovered the use of warfarin as one of the independent predictors for calcification in patients who underwent AVR for CAVS [50]. In 1155 patients with AF, there was an association between the use of warfarin and the risk for valvular calcification, even if 13 confounding patient-related factors were taken into account. Whether this relationship is causal remains a matter for investigation [51].

Taken together, these findings suggest that vitamin K antagonists may decrease MGP level and subsequently increase aortic valve calcium score.

7. MECHANISMS OF PROGRESSION OF CAVS

CAVS can be considered as the result of several processes, which include:

1) Inflammation, as result of lipid infiltration.
2) Calcification with ossification or differentiation into osteoblasts.
3) Angiogenesis and remodeling of the ECM.
4) Programmed cell death.

For each of these processes, several mediators exist which can act at several levels. These processes act in concert, which make their comprehensive description a difficult task. Their mediators can "cross-talk" and can be viewed from different angles.

7.1. Inflammation

7.1.1. Mechanism

Lipid infiltration has been documented as a necessary step in the development of CAVS: hypercholesterolemia plays a role in CAVS in experimentally induced lipid abnormalities in animals as well as in homozygote patients [53]. Oxidation of lipids in CAVS is the result of uncoupling of endothelial NOS. This produces superoxides. Furthermore, the anti-oxidant activity has decreased [17]. Oxidized lipids induce adhesion of leucocytes and cause attraction of monocytes. In CAVS, T-lymphocytes, macrophages and mast cells accumulate. These cells secrete a host of cytokines which have an effect on VIC. These cells remodel the ECM within the valve by production of MMP.

Shear stress, which can be observed in hypertensive patients, damages the endothelial lining, making them more permeable to lipids. The endothelium mediates mechanical and humoral stimuli: inflammation occurs mainly at sites of disturbed oscillatory flow [4]. Lymphocytes, macrophages and mast cells enter the valve after endothelial injury [26].

Normal aortic valve tissue is devoid of inflammatory cells, whereas the stenotic valve has accumulation of inflammatory cells, such as T-lymphocytes, macrophages, and mast cells. The accumulation of T-cells within the cardiac valves is a likely source of cytokines which are important for the recruitment of more inflammatory cells. Expression of cytokines, such as TNF α, VAP-1, IL-1 and TGF-β 1 has been observed in stenotic valves. Inflammatory cells may activate growth factors which in turn stimulate valve myofibroblasts. These cells proliferate and express MMP, which remodel the valve matrix.

In vitro stimulation of these VIC results in an osteoblast-like cellular phenotype. Mast cells may influence MMP, release proangiogenic peptides, and activate cytokines as well as growth factors [11, 14, 52]. But it is not yet clear whether inflammation causes calcification of the valve and which molecular mechanisms may be involved. Macrophages, for example are capable of synthesizing osteopontin. This osteopontin influences further chemotaxis, cellular proliferation, inflammation and calcification [14].

7.1.2. Extracellular Mediators

CRP acts an independent predictor [20] and has been detected in explanted valves [21]. CRP has been documented in patients with CAVS but without atheromatosis in coronary, carotid or peripheral vessels. The association of high sensitivity CRP and CAVS is independent of other risk factors for atheromatosis such as BMI [11]. The level of CRP is not related to the degree of calcification.

CRP activates **complement** and attracts white blood cells through chemotaxis. Deposition of activated complement and anti-complement mediators is increased locally in the endothelium and in the ECM of calcified valves. These deposits are responsible for the ongoing inflammation [18].

Adhesion molecules and **interleukins** produced by activated T lymphocytes infiltrate the leaflets and recruit more inflammatory cells [14]. Other adhesion molecules which are expressed in CAVS are ICAM 1, VCAM and E-selectin. These molecules point to an inflammation [11].

ACE and **angiotensin receptor I** co-localize with LDL in plasma and are concentrated in diseased aortic valves [22, 23].

Angiotensin II has several pro-inflammatory effects which lend to several events:

1) Chemotaxis of monocytes.

2) Promoting proliferation of SMC.

3) Enhancing uptake of LDL.

4) Reducing efflux of cholesterol from macrophages.

5) Reducing the effectiveness of the intrinsic fibrinolytic system [22, 53].

6) Production of free radicals which modulate inflammatory reactions [48].

Other extracellular factors such as TNF, TGF β-1, BMP, RANKL have been identified. The description of their effects is related to the receptors to which these belong.

7.1.3. Receptors and Intracellular Mediators

Several cell receptors on VIC might play a role in inflammation in patient with CAVS. These receptors stimulate several intracellular pathways.

Angiotensin II activates through its receptor p38 Mitogen Activated Protein Kinase (MAPK), which is involved in cell differentiation of VIC [54].

A multitude of pro-inflammatory factors (interleukins, fragments of bacteria and of own cells) utilize TLR-2 and TLR-4, which are present on human aortic VIC [47]. These receptors are important mediators of the innate immune response and of inflammation. Inflammatory factors that act through TLR-2 might utilize pathways other than the Angiotensin II pathway. NFκB is a possible route.

T-lymphocytes are a source of cytokines such as TNF, which attract more inflammatory cells. TNF binding on its receptors activates NFκB, which has a pleiotropic effect, including proliferation and inflammation. There is also a moderate response of p38 MAPK by TNF, with comparable effects. The pro-apoptotic intracellular activation by TNF is weaker.

TGF β-1 stimulates the SMAD pathway, which ceases proliferation, induces differentiation or promotes apoptosis. TGF β-1 also plays a role inflammation. TGF β-1 also acts through the MAPK pathway. TGF β-1 initiates the calcification process in the end stage of CAVS and can remain active in the end stage [55].

BMP, which are inflammatory proteins, also acts through SMAD and MAPK pathways.

RANKL acts through osteoprotegerin (OPG) and LRP5 receptors. Inactivation of NFκB has an effect on inflammation and promotes activation of osteoclasts.

It is obvious that

- Several extracellular factors can stimulate more than one intracellular pathway.
- There is a cross-talk between several intracellular pathways.
- The effect of one extracellular factor/intracellular pathway is pleiotropic.

This makes the separation of the effects of these factors during the development of CAVS virtually impossible.

7.2. Calcification/Osteogenesis

7.2.1. Mechanisms

The differentiation of aortic valve myofibroblast into an osteoblastic phenotype can be induced by several risk factors, such as mechanical stress and lipid disorders. These events clearly illustrate that both risk factors have an effect on several levels and through several mechanisms, *i.e.* there is a ***so-called cross talk***. A probable model for CAVS shows a sequence involving active processes:

1) Activation of EC by lipid infiltration.
2) Activation of VIC by inflammation.
3) Cellular proliferation into "pro-osteoblasts" [14].
4) Conversion of VIC to osteoblasts.
5) Synthesis of ECM proteins: oteopontin, bone sialoprotein, alkaline phosphatase.
6) Mineralization of ECM [16].

Lipid infiltration may be the result of shear stress on the endothelium at the aortic side of the valve. By endothelial disruption, lipid can further infiltrate the valvular interstitium. The accumulation of LDL/oxLDL in the valve leaflets is more than a passive process [11, 23]. Oxidized lipids, including 25-hydroxycholesterol, can induce inflammation. This event contributes to neovascularization and ossification through mechanisms which involve BMP [14].

These extra-cellular lipid depositions are adjacent to matrix vesicles which are released from fibroblasts that are exposed to these oxidized and toxic lipid components. These vesicles can serve as pools for calcium deposits, nodule formation and hence promote progression of CAVS. These lipoproteins have also an affinity for the proteoglycans in the matrix. How this affinity results in an increased deposition of calcium is not yet known. These processes can induce intra-membranous ossification [5].

Calcification in CAVS consists of hydroxyl-apatite crystals, deposited on a bone-like matrix of collagen, osteopontin, and other bone matrix proteins [5, 11]. This starts with small dot-like hexagonal calcium deficient deposits. Osteopontin, which is released from macrophages [9] binds to the hydroxyl-apatite crystals.

Cells in the aortic valve produce osteonectin, osteocalcin and osteopontin [5, 10, 14]. Cholesterol is detected in the center of calcified granules in atheromatosis. This indicates that lipids are involved in the precipitation of minerals. The presence of 25-hydroxycholesterol accelerates calcification in vessels but also in valves. Apolipoprotein accumulations are also found in calcified valves [56].

Macrophages are capable to synthesize osteopontin. This pro-inflammatory glycoprotein influences events, such as chemotaxis of more macrophages, cellular proliferation, inflammation and mineralization [14, 26].

Osteopontin stimulates differentiation of VIC into osteoblasts and regulates deposition of calcium by these cells. Levels of osteopontin increase in patients with CAVS. Increased levels of plasma osteopontin are associated with the presence of CAVS in all stages. These findings suggest that osteopontin plays a functional role in the pathogenesis of CAVS [9, 26, 56-58].

7.2.2. Extracellular Mediators

Some extracellular mediators, identified in inflammation, have also been observed in osteoblastic differentiation of aortic VIC. These factors include BMP, TNF-α, interleukin-1b, TGF-β 1, RANKL (which is a member of the TNF family) and ACE/Angiotensin II. Another is NOTCH-1 (which inhibits osteogenesis and which is located on the surface of other cells and requires cell-to-cell contact for activation) and Wnt/catenin.

7.2.3. Intracellular Mechanisms

Receptors, identified in the inflammatory response of aortic VIC have also been identified in osteoblastic differentiation. These include TLR, LPR5 (as co-receptor for osteoprotegerin or OPG) and others.

Several intracellular pathways have been identified for osteoblastic differentiation. Runx2 is of much importance. Another is NFκB (whose suppression is involved in activation of osteoclasts).

Runx2, or runt-related-transcription factor 2, is the central regulator of the differentiation of VIC into osteoblasts. This Runx2 binds to DNA and regulates the production of osteocalcin and osteopontin; ***it is the master regulator of bone formation***. Its action is important in the development of CAVS [58].

Runx-2 and hence differentiation of VIC into osteoblasts are influenced by a number of factors [58]. These are described in conjunction with their receptors and intracellular systems.

BMP-2 and **BMP-4** are pro inflammatory proteins and are involved in transformation of myofibroblasts into osteoblasts and ossification. These BMP increase the expression of Runx2 and their expression is increased in VIC of calcified valves. These cells might exert a paracrine effect onadjacent VIC, which promotes calcification. The osteogenic transformation of VIC is characterized by an over-expression of alkaline phosphatase [23, 52, 53, 59].

Interleukin 1 and **TNF-α** from macrophages also have been found incalcified human valves. TNF-α and IL-1b also induce BMP by VIC *in vitro* [53, 58].

The pro-osteogenic phenotype of human aortic VIC has also been associated with higher levels of **TLR-2** and **TLR-4**. These receptors are modulators of innate immunity [59].

VIC in stenotic aortic valves contain increased levels of **LRP-5** or LDL-receptor-related protein-5. This is a member of the LDL receptor-related protein family of cell-surface receptors. These receptors are involved indiverse biologic processes, including lipid metabolism. LRP-5 plays a significant role in skeletal bone development and in the differentiation process of aortic VIC into osteoblasts. This has been confirmed in experimental conditions [40, 60]. This provides another link between lipid metabolism and aortic valve calcification [16, 23].

TGF-β 1, which is activated by T lymphocytes, links inflammation to calcification. It binds on a receptor of VIC and stimulates Runx2. TGF-β1 is an immunomodulator and also promotes fibrosis.

RANKL or receptor activator of NFκB ligand and osteoprotegerin are members of a cytokine system/TNF family and are involved in bone turnover and cardiovascular calcification. RANKL, which promotes calcification and induces expression of osteogenic phenotype, is expressed in CAVS but not in healthy valves [11, 52].

VEGF plays an important role in bone formation besides its angiogenic activity. VEGF is up-regulated at the sites of bone formation and is involved in bone healing. VEGF is an inflammatory mediator and plays a functional role in bone formation and calcification [11].

NOTCH-1 is able to prevent the development of CAVS by inhibiting BMP 2 and Runx2. It inhibits osteogenesis

Osteoprotegerin is also a cytokine and member of the TNF family. It is strongly expressed in normal aortic valves and inhibits RANKL. Its absence in mice results in cardiovascular calcification [11].

The result of the stimulation of the intracellular Runx2 machinery is the transformation of VIC into osteoblasts. These cells are capable of producing osteopontin, osteocalcin, bone sialoprotein and alkaline phosphatase. Osteopontin, a proinflammatory glycoprotein, is not only involved in differentiation of VIC into osteoblasts. It also regulates the deposition of calcium itself [9, 26, 51, 52].

7.3. Remodeling of the ECM is the Result of Following Mechanisms

The main mechanisms in remodeling of the ECM are mechanical strain, oxidative stress and inflammation.

Mechanical strain may affect the aortic valve cusp, which leads to a change in ECM ultra-structure and on long term to CAVS. Proteins of the ECM can be localized in different areas of the stenotic valves [29].

- Decorin and biglycan are mostly located at the inflow sides of the cusp.
- Tenascin-C can be found in the central layer, and

- Osteopontin, osteocalcin, and alkaline phosphatase are concentrated near the cell populations, which surround the calcified areas.

Stress also leads to an increased induction of expression of proteoglycans within the ECM. The up-regulation of negatively charged ends on ECM proteoglycans leads to an increase in potential binding sites for calcium, and hence calcification of the aortic valve cusp, at least in the early stages [29].

Oxidative stress may also activate MMP in the aortic valve and arteries [17]. In the valve, MMP may play a permissive role in the progression of calcification. Degraded fragments of collagen and elastin also may increase signals that promote calcification in VIC.

Inflammatory cells may activate growth factors which stimulate myofibroblasts to proliferate and express MMP. These enzymes remodel the ECM in the aortic valve [14].

A number of ECM proteins normally found in bone, such as osteocalcin, osteopontin, osteonectin, BMP, MMP-2, and MMP-9, are present in calcified valves. However, these enzymes are not found in normal cardiovascular tissue. MMP are a group of zinc-dependent endopeptidases (collagenases, gelatinases and stromelysins) which are secreted as inactive pro-enzymes by various cell types. MMP may degrade all components of the ECM and are inhibited mainly by TIMP. The local balance between the activity of MMP and of TIMP is thought to determine the extent of tissue remodeling. MMP-1, 2, 3, 9 and their inhibitors TIMP1, TIMP2 are involved in the pathogenesis of CAVS. MMP-1 is capable of cleaving the intact triple-helix of collagen while MMP-2 and MMP-9 may degrade damaged ECM and components of the basal membrane. MMP could also induce the production of connective tissue-associated growth factors that increase ECM synthesis [11, 44].

In addition, TIMP-2 may directly promote the proliferation of fibroblasts and other mesenchymal cells, thereby contributing to tissue thickening in aortic sclerosis, as well as in other fibrotic disorders. Although the underlying mechanism of the increased expression of MMP in stenotic valves is not clear,

MMP-1 expression is associated with the areas of leukocyte infiltration and expression of IL-1B. This suggests an interdependent regulation between MMP activity and inflammation.

Another potentially involved peptide in the pathogenesis of CAVS is TGF-β1. It stimulates the formation and deposition of ECM, modifies the response of the immune system and suppresses inflammatory processes. Exogenous TGF-beta1 induces fibrosis independently of tissue damage; inhibitors of TGF-β receptor binding reduce fibrosis. An acute, limited injury is accompanied by inadequate increase in TGF-β1, and fibrosis does not occur. With repeated injury, the increase in TGF-β1 production is sustained. This leads to the progressive deposition of ECM and tissue fibrosis. Such long lasting injury might be the case in CAVS, where the presence of TGF-β1 has been documented. TGF-β1 may contribute to the progression of CAVS by initiating the mineralization of VIC, which is associated to apoptosis. This event has been observed *in vitro* [11].

Connective tissue growth factor, which is in close association with TGF-β 1 stimulates osteoblast cells. Recently, it has been shown that connective tissue growth factor gene polymorphism is associated with the degree of CAVS [11].

In calcified valves, tenascin C is associated with MMP-2. In a culture of aortic VIC, tenascin C stimulates both MMP-2 mRNA expression and MMP-2 gelatinolytic activity. Tenascin C is a multifunctional hexameric ECM glycoprotein, which plays a role in cell proliferation, migration, differentiation and apoptosis. Tenascin C expression has increased during inflammation and tissue repair. Expression of tenascin C is associated to the degree of CAVS, as well as to the extent of calcification, angiogenesis and fibrosis [11].

Expression of cystatin C has increased in calcified aortic valves. Cystatin C is a cysteine protease inhibitor which is expressed in mature osteoblasts. The expression of cystatin C and TGF-β1 are comparable. This indicates that both factors are associated to CAVS. Increased expression of cathepsin enzymes S, K, and V and their inhibitor cystatin C in CAVS has also been documented [11].

7.4. Angiogenesis

Angiogenesis has been defined as the outgrowth of new capillaries from pre-existing capillaries. This process is regulated by a balance between angiogenic activators such as VEGF, and angiogenic inhibitors such as chondromodulin-1. Angiogenesis is essential for physiological processes, such as longitudinal bone growth, endochondral bone formation and fracture healing. VEGF is also present in tumors and other diseases, like CAVS. The presence of neoangiogenesis in all ossified valves is consistent with the hypothesis that angiogenesis facilitates endochondral bone formation in calcified cardiac valves. Angiogenesis may be a key step in remodeling of the aortic valve and eventual formation of calcified valves [11, 26, 58].

VEGF plays a major role in physiologic and pathologic conditions [11, 58]:

- Induction of migration and proliferation of EC.
- Enhancement of vascular permeability.
- Modulation of thrombogenicity.
- Induction of of the expression of MMP, which permits migration of EC.

In healthy heart valves, VEGF is outbalanced by chondromodulin-1. Hence, normal adult heart valves do not contain blood vessels. Chondromodulin-I is secreted by cultured VIC and is abundantly present in the three layers of the heart valves but not in EC. In contrast VEGF is absent in all cell layers. In regions of angiogenesis, chondromodulin-I is markedly down-regulated while VEGF is up-regulated. In genetic experiments with mice lacking chondromodulin-I, VEGF expression, angiogenesis, lipid deposition and calcification are increased and CAVS develops.

The critical step for angiogenesis might be a decreased oxygen tension caused by endothelial injury as a first phase in the development of CAVS. This leads to an abnormal deposition of ECM and a thickening of the valve. This decrease in oxygen tension induces secretion of VEGF and hence, angiogenesis. In the stromal tissue of calcified valves, markers for EC, such as CD31, CD34 and vWF are much more present. EC of stenotic valves exhibit CEACAM1, a cell adhesion molecule. This molecule is expressed in angiogenic EC, but not in quiescent EC [11, 30].

Infiltrating mast cells in CAVS contain a number of enzymes, such as MMP, serine proteinases, chymases, acid hydrolases, cathepsins, histamine, heparin, and proangiogenic peptides. These cells also contain inflammation producing molecules, such as TNF-α, prostaglandin D2, and leukotrienes [26]. In angiogenesis, several other factors have been implicated such as the activation of NFκB, which regulates protein synthesis [16]. In tissues in which angiogenesis has been observed, proliferation, migration, and recruitment of inflammatory cells occur. These cells can release large quantities of angiogenic factors under hypoxic conditions. Inflammatory mediators, such as prostaglandin E, IL 1 and IL 6 have the potential to elevate VEGF. This VEGF may attract monocytes by chemotaxis, thereby closing the circle [11].

7.5. The Role of Programmed Cell Death in CAVS: Apoptosis and Autophagy

7.5.1. Apoptosis

Apoptosis is a mode of programmed cell death of type I, and is universally present in eukaryotes. It requires specialized intracellular machinery [61]. Apoptosis is important in the development of organs such as the heart, by tissue sculpturing. This sculpturing occurs through cell proliferation on the one hand, and removal of redundant cells on the other hand [62-66].

Morphogenesis and developmental remodeling of cardiovascular tissues involve a coordinated regulation of cell proliferation and apoptosis [67]. Cells can be mutually interdependent by secretion of paracrine factors. These paracrine factors allow survival and regulate growth, whereas isolated cells undergo apoptosis as consequence of lack of these paracrine factors. Sometimes, apoptosis is protective, when a carcinoma outgrows its "paracrine supply". There is an apoptotic protection against carcinogenesis of damaged cells. The apoptotic pathway shares some properties with the mitotic pathway. Most mammalian cells express the proteins required for apoptosis, which acts on different cellular organelles in parallel. There are two distinctive pathways, in which p53 is active:

In the first apoptotic pathway, a "death receptor", belonging to the TNF class is activated. This receptor has an intra-cytoplasmatic death domain of about 80 amino acids and recruits adaptor molecules. These adaptor molecules activate pro-caspase 8 through cleavage. This caspase 8 activates caspase 3, 6 and 7. The latter degrades important cellular molecules.

The second apoptotic pathway is mitochondrial: activated caspase 8 or apoptotic stimuli (Bak proteins) from other sources can converge in the space between the two mitochondrial membranes. This could open the mitochondrial permeability transition pore. Calcium and other ions migrate inwards, the mitochondrion swells due to the oncotic pressure of the intra-mitochondrial proteins and the outer membrane ruptures. The cytotoxic Cytochrome C, which is located outside the inner membrane leaks into the cytoplasm. The caspases are subsequently activated. The electrochemical gradient of hydrogen within the mitochondria, which is of vital importance in ATP production, is lost. During respiration, mitochondria produce considerable amounts of hydrogen peroxide, which in conjunction with large iron storages can damage macromolecules such as mitochondrial DNA. This culminates in cell death.

Both apoptotic pathways converge in the final stage in which caspases are activated. Caspases are cysteine endopeptidases that cleave at least 280 structural or enzymatic proteins [61]. Examples of targeted structural proteins are actin and cardiac troponin T. Activated caspase 3 activates a subunit of the DNA fragmentation factor. This factor puts down DNA into nucleosomal fragments causing cell death.

The key morphological events in apoptosis are:

1) Shrinking of cells.

2) Loss of specialized parts of cell membranes such as microvilli.

3) Morphological conservation of most plasma organelles.

4) Breakdown of the cytoskeleton.

5) Perinuclear chromatin condensation.

6) Breakdown of the perinuclear membrane.

These cellular events can take place in less than two hours. Even if only 1% of the cells in a tissue is in the apoptotic process, this might represent a major reduction of cells.

Apoptotic bodies are cleared without inflammation [68]. TGF-β1 may contribute to the progression of CAVS by initiating the apoptosis associated mineralization of aortic VIC. These events have been observed *in vitro* [4, 11] and in animal experiments [15].

7.5.2. Autophagy

Alternatively, non-apoptotic forms of programmed cell death, such as autophagic cell death, have been described. This is the type II programmed cell death. Although, this process serves as a survival mechanism during stress [69], excessive protein degradation during autophagy could lead to cell death. This occurs when a critical threshold of cytoplasm, necessary for cell survival is digested or when regulatory proteins essential for viability are degraded [70]. Numerous autophagosomes and autolysosomes have been found in many dying cells, suggesting that autophagy indeed plays a role in programmed cell death.

The presence of nuclear chromatin and large parts of the cytoplasma in autolysosomes can be considered as evidence for this hypothesis. Apoptosis is triggered earlier than autophagy. Hence, autophagic cell death is considered to take place in cases where apoptosis is inhibited, as in some viral infections. To prevent spread of the virus, autophagic cell death then functions as a fail-safe mechanism. Both forms of programmed cell death could function complementary, through interconnected regulatory pathways. Hence, both forms of cell death are not mutually exclusive [64]. Autophagic cell death remains important, even in the presence of parallel apoptotic signalling. Autophagy is life-promoting in some circumstances and cell death-promoting in others [71].

Autophagy is induced by a signal, such as starvation or growth factor deprivation. This signal inhibits the protein called "target of rapamycin" or TOR. This protein triggers the formation of a phagophore, which is assembled from intracellular membranes. The endoplasmatic reticulum, the golgi-apparatus and the plasma membrane may be sources of phagophores; however, this is not yet clear [72-74].

Microtubule associated protein 1 light chain 3 or MAP1-LC3, plays a vital role in phagophore expansion. The binding of LC3 to the phagophore depends on the presence of other autophagic proteins, which have an activating and conjugating capacity [72-74]. Several steps can be discerned in autophagy:

- Unconjugated LC3 or LC3-I is conjugated to phosphatidylethanolamine and forms LC3-II.

- This conjugated complex is subsequently attached to the phagophore membrane.

- This phagophore expands as a double membrane and sequesters parts of the cytoplasma and organelles by wrapping itself around these. This organel is called an autophagosome [72-74].

- The completed autophagosome can conflate with early and late endosomes or with a multivesicular body, and forms an amphisome [73].

- This amphisome, on its turn, can fuse with a lysosome, to form an autolysosome. Thereafter, its contents are degraded. The autophagosome can also directly fuse with a lysosome [74].

- Membranes of autophagosomes and endosomes can nucleate actin and can catalyze its polymerization into filaments and networks. These actin filaments serve as tracks for organelles that have myosin in their membranes for transportation. This transport is a prerequisite for the fusion of autophagosomes with lysosomes [75].

- The lysosomial degradation is the last step [76]. The LC3 attached to the outer membrane of the sealed autophagosomes is removed and can be recycled. The LC3 within the autophagosome is trapped and degrades with the content by acidification and enzymatic lysosomial proteolysis [72, 73].

Progression of CAVS has been associated with calcification, in which apoptosis and TGF-β1 have been involved [5]. In CAVS, autophagy has also been identified as mode of cell death [9, 76, 77]. Oxidized lipoproteins induce a calcium load in dying cells and can evoke a process in which LC3 – a possible marker for autophagy – is involved [5]. The triggers in CAVS are different from those in atheromatosis since in CAVS, there are no necrotic areas and calcification is more intense.

Furthermore, the autophagic sequestration of intracellular components and their subsequent degradation in secondary lysosomes could suggest that autophagic cell death might play a role in the release of matrix vesicles in degenerative aortic valves.

These matrix vesicles can trigger inflammatory cells which regulate genes involved in mineralization. Nevertheless, the nature of these triggers for the enhancement of inflammatory cells is vague.

The presence of ubiquitin has been used as marker for autophagy [9]. Ubiquitin is a small 76 amino acid protein which labels other proteins, which are destined for degradation. It is unclear that the nature is of the molecules that are targeted by an increased ubiquitin production. Ubiquitination interacts with the apoptotic machinery, but this relation still has to be unraveled. For example, ubiquitination might inhibit the caspase-dependent apoptotic pathway.

These findings might explain the presence of larger amounts of ubiquitinated cells compared to apoptotic cells in severe CAVS. The overall conclusion is that autophagic cell death, rather than apoptosis, is the most important trigger for the release of matrix vesicles in CAVS [9].

The presence of a sparse number of autophagic cells within a calcified valve could be compared with a few burning coals within the ashes of a slow burning fire. However, the effect of autophagy on the rate of progression needs more investigation. This requires a prospective comparison of explanted valves from a range of between "slow" and "rapid" progressors of aortic valve degeneration. Whether autophagy is an early cause or a terminal event associated in the end stage of valve disease still needs to be ascertained [76].

7.6. The Final Common Pathway in CAVS

The activated VIC differentiates into osteoblasts, and calcification starts mainly in the zona fibrosa. The differentiation is expressed by the osteoblast genes. The runx2 system plays a central role herein. Runx2 is stimulated by several pathways (RANKL/OPG, Lpr5 and Wnt).

Lpr5 and Wnt signaling occurs through excess of circulatory LDL, accompanied by ACE.

RANKL/OPG signaling occurs through inflammatory cytokines.

Inflammation causes a vicious circle. It promotes inflammation and degradation of ECM. The ECM degradation products upregulate the action of TGFβ 1. This stimulates differentiation of VIC into myofibroblasts and hence further degradation of ECM.

The homeostasis of ECM is also influenced by mechanical stress, also through differentiation of VIC into myofibroblasts.

8. NON-CARDIAC CONSEQUENCES OF CAVS

8.1. Heyde's Syndrome

In 1958, the first observation of an association between CAVS and digestive bleeding has been reported, but without explanatory pathophysiological mechanisms [78]. Angiodysplasias have also been described but the link between these vascular malformations and CAVS has not always been accepted [79, 80].

Currently, the syndrome can be depicted as a triad: CAVS, an acquired vWF syndrome (type IIa) and anemia due to bleeding from gastrointestinal angiodysplasia [81]. The latter can be considered latent. The incidence of CAVS in patients with digestive bleeding is 1.5%, with a confounding effect of age [82].

The pathophysiology of this syndrome is supported by several observations.

- High shear stress due to CAVS could lead to a loss (clearance) of high molecular weight vWF [82-85] through an accelerated interaction with platelets [83]. The lower molecular weight multimers remain unaffected.

- This loss of vWF could lead to decrease in platelet adhesion [86].

- The role of the shear dependent vWF metalloproteinase ADAMTS13 (A Disintegrin and Metalloproteinase with Thrombospondin type 1 motif Member 13) has been discovered [87].

- Laboratory irregularities have correlated with the severity of CAVS [88]. However, the syndrome can also be present in moderate CAVS [89].

- Routine tests for the von Willebrand syndrome type IIa are usually normal, but bleeding time is prolonged [89].

- AVR corrects the laboratory defects [82], provided there is no postoperative VPPM [88]. This correction is paralleled by clinical improvements, *i.e.* disappearance of digestive bleeding [82, 90].

- AVR also corrects the time needed to form a platelet plug *in vitro* (improvement of adhesion and aggregation) in patients with CAVS [85].

This observations support the hypothesis that CAVS interacts with the platelet function [91]. AVR is the treatment of choice for Heyde's syndrome [89].

Some case reports have confirmed the long-term freedom of recurrent digestive bleeding and of the recovery of vWF, up to 10 years after AVR [84, 89, 92, 93].

The multifactorial origin of Heyde' syndrome has made the interpretation of these findings not easy.

- Few patients with CAVS have severe digestive bleeding but hemostatic abnormalities have a high prevalence [86].

- The bleeding is restricted to the digestive tract, which points to a local factor. CAVS might lead to hypoxia-induced vascular dilatation and hence to angiodysplasia [86].

- The need for more than one factor could explain the heterogeneous clinical presentation of the syndrome [86].

- There is a link between these findings, since AVR cures the bleeding tendency [86, 89].

Prevalence of both the conditions, angiodysplasia and CAVS, increase with age [84], but these conditions are not always clinically apparent. Wide variations between series have been observed [82]. Sometimes, a silent CAVS might be detected, provided the attending physician is aware of the problem. The syndrome is not always recognized [92]. One also needs to be aware that many patients with CAVS are also under anti-platelet medication. Anticoagulation should be used cautiously in patients with Heyde's syndrome [89].

The presence of Heyde's syndrome might influence the approach towards patients with CAVS. AVR might be indicated earlier in patients with Heyde's syndrome compared to the usual criteria for surgery. Furthermore, treatment decisions can become complicated [89]. With the advent of TAVI, a cure for both conditions may have been found for patients with severe co-morbid conditions.

9. THROMBEMBOLISM

Stroke seems to be associated with CAVS. This could be due to systemic embolization of calcium and thrombi. The frequency of such emboli seems to deviate. Many emboli are small and can be asymptomatic. Therefore, the true incidence of TE in patients with CAVS cannot be estimated. Catheter investigation in which the valve is crossed also could provoke emboli. Microthrombi can be the result of clotting activation by turbulent blood flow and of destruction of red blood cells. The management in such patients is still uncertain since few reports are available. Antiplatelet therapy might be recommendable [94].

Tissue factor, which is involved in blood clotting, can be demonstrated in the fibrosa by experimentally induced aortic valve lesions (leaflet thickening and altered valve performance in rabbits). This observation strengthens the link between CAVS and atheromatosis. Tissue factor, however, can also be found in EC and in myofibroblasts of normal aortic valves. Macrophage infiltration during development of CAVS may be involved in the synthesis of tissue factor. These inflammatory cells can enrich the valve leaflets with tissue factor. This tissue factor may participate in the formation of microthrombi and emboli [31].

These preoperative events might be clinically relevant since these are identified as a risk factor for long-term postoperative TE [19].

10. ADDENDUM

A congenital BAV is the most common congenital cardiac defect. It can be associated with other congenital cardiac defects such as dilation of the ascending aorta. This is due to abnormalities of the media, and does not depend on the presence of stenosis or regurgitation of the valve itself.

Complications of BAV are valve stenosis or regurgitation, endocarditis, aneurysm formation and aortic dissection. BAV is a disease of the valve as well as of the ascending aorta. When performing AVR, surgery of the root is often necessary. Life expectancy seems normal for patients with BAV [95].

There are several types of BAV. Bicuspid valves of the type non-coronary – right coronary differ from right coronary – left coronary type. These anatomical anomalies happen before the forming of the outflow tract septum. This event relies on the NO-dependent endothelial-to-mesenchymal transformation. The two types of BAV might be the result from a different genotype [96].

Considering the complex nature of this condition and the need to replace the ascending aorta in many patients with BAV, it doesn't't seem appropriate to include this pathology in the description of CAVS, its development and its treatment.

CONCLUSIONS

CAVS is not just the consequence of passive "wear and tear", related to aging. This condition is an active process, which shares a number of risk factors with atheromatosis. Both processes have some differences, however.

The unraveling of the mechanisms leading to CAVS is an ongoing process. It requires an approach in layers. It seems that the differentiation of VIC into cells with an osteoblastic phenotype is pivotal.

The full understanding of the development of CAVS might hold some promises in stopping the progress of the disease. The lipid lowering therapy is under scrutiny, but this approach is probably only useful in very early cases.

If alteration of the effect of VEGF, inhibition of angiogenesis, of ACE and of autophagy will be useful remains to be seen. If the "window of opportunity", *i.e.* the time in which these processes are active is small, a therapeutic alteration of these processes as attempt to stop the progress of CAVS seems not feasible.

Bicuspid aortic valve disease is beyond the scope of this manuscript, since it involves not only the valve itself, but also the wall of the ascending aorta.

ACKNOWLEDGEMENT

Declared none.

CONFLICT OF INTEREST

The author(s) confirm that this chapter content has no conflict of interest.

REFERENCES

[1] Iung B. Management of the elderly patient with aortic stenosis. Heart 2008;94:519-524
[2] Schoen FJ. Cardiac valves and valvular pathology, Update on function, disease, repair, and replacement. Cardiovasc Pathol 2005;14:189-194.
[3] Ross J Jr and Braunwald E. Aortic stenosis. Circulation 1968;38[Suppl 1]:S61-S67.
[4] Butcher JT, Tressel S, Johnson T, *et al.* Transcriptional Profiles of Valvular and Vascular Endothelial Cells Reveal Phenotypic Differences: Influence of Shear Stress. Arterioscler Thromb Vasc Biol 2006;26;69-77.

[5] Knaapen M, Somers P, Mistiaen W. Histopathology of calcific aortic valve stenosis. Acta Cardiol 2006; 61[5]:557-562.

[6] Cowell SJ, Newby DE, Boon NA, Elder AT. Calcific aortic stenosis: same old story? Age and Ageing 2004; 33: 538-544.

[7] Matsumoto Y, Adams V, Walther C, *et al.* Reduced number and function of endothelial progenitor cells in patients with aortic valve stenosis: a novel concept for valvular endothelial cell repair. Eur Heart J 2009;30:346-355.

[8] Parolari A, Loardi C, Mussoni L, *et al.* F. Review article. Nonrheumatic calcific aortic stenosis: an overview from basic science to pharmacological prevention. Eur J Cardio-thorac Surg 2009;35:493-504.

[9] Somers P, Knaapen M, Kockx M, *et al.* Histological Evaluation of Autophagic Cell Death in Calcified Aortic Valve Stenosis. J Heart Valve Dis 2006;15:43-48.

[10] Stewart BF, Siscovick D, Lind BK, *et al.*, for the Cardiovascular health study. Clinical Factors Associated With Calcific Aortic Valve Disease. J Am Coll Cardiol 1997;29:630-634.

[11] Yetkin E, Waltenberger J. Molecular and cellular mechanisms of aortic stenosis. Int J Cardiology 2009;135:4-13.

[12] O'Brien KD, Reichenbach DD, Marcinova SM, *et al.* Apolipoproteins B [a] and E accumulate in the morphologically early lesions of "degenerative" valvular aortic stenosis. Arteriosc1, Thromb Vasc Biol 1996;16[523-532.

[13] Otto CM, O'Brien KD. Why is there discordance between calcific aortic stenosis and coronary artery disease? Heart 2001;85:601-602.

[14] Veinot JP. Pathology of inflammatory native valvular heart disease. Cardiovasc Pathol 2006;15:243-251.

[15] Rajamannan NM, Sangiorgi G, Springett M, *et al.* Experimental hypercholesterolemia induces apoptosis in the aortic valve. J Heart Valve Dis 2001;10:371-374.

[16] Rajamannan NM. Calcific Aortic Stenosis: A Disease Ready for Prime Time. Circulation 2006;114:2007-2009.

[17] Heistad DD, Wakisaka Y, Miller J, *et al.* Novel Aspects of Oxidative Stress in Cardiovascular Diseases. Circ J 2009; 73: 201-207.

[18] ter Weeme M, Vonk ABA, Kupreishvili K, *et al.* Activated complement ismore extensively present in diseased aortic valves than naturally occurring complement inhibitors: a sign of ongoing inflammation. Eur J Clin Invest 2010;40:4-10.

[19] Mistiaen W, Van Cauwelaert Ph, Muylaert Ph, *et al.* Thrombo-embolism after aortic valve replacement in elderly with a Carpentier-Edwards perimount TM bioprosthesis. J Thorac Cardiovasc Surg 2004;127:1166-1170.

[20] Rabus MB, Kayalar N, Sareyyüpoglu B, *et al.* Hypercholesterolemia Association with Aortic Stenosis of Various Etiologies. J Card Surg 2009;24:146-150.

[21] Rajamannan NM. Calcific aortic stenosis: lessons learned from experimental and clinical studies. Arteriosclerosis, Thromb Vasc Biol 2009;29:162-168.

[22] O'Brien KD, Shavelle DM, Caulfield MT, *et al.* Association of Angiotensin-Converting Enzyme With Low-Density Lipoprotein in Aortic Valvular Lesions and in Human Plasma. Circulation 2002;106;2224-2230.

[23] Parolari A, Loardi C, Mussoni L, *et al.* Nonrheumatic calcific aortic stenosis: an overview from basic science to pharmacological prevention. Eur J Cardio-thorac Surg 2009;35:493-504.

[24] Peltonen T, Napankangas J, Vuolteenaho O, *et al.* Apelin and its receptor APJ in humam aortic valve stenosis. J Heart Valve Dis 2009;18:18:644-652.

[25] Peltonen T, Taskinen P, Napankangas J, *et al.* Increase in tissue endothelin-1 and ETA receptor levels in human aortic stenosis. Eur Heart J 2009;30:242-249.

[26] Mohler ER, Gannon F, Reynolds C, *et al.* Bone Formation and Inflammation in Cardiac Valves. Circulation 2001;103:1522-1528.

[27] Schoen FJ. New frontiers in the pathology and therapy of heart valve disease. Cardiovasc Pathol 2006, 15:271-279.

[28] Moedder UI, Gossl M, Lerman LO, *et al.* Circulating endothelial progenitor cells co-expressing an osteogenic phenotype are increased in patients with severe calcific aortic valve stenosis. Bone 2009;44:P181. doi:10.1016/j.bone.2009.03.607

[29] Lehmann S, Walther T, Kempfert J, *et al.* Mechanical Strain and the Aortic Valve: Influence on Fibroblasts, Extracellular Matrix, and Potential Stenosis. Ann Thorac Surg 2009;88:1476–83.

[30] Liu CL, Joag VR, Gotlieb AI. The Emerging Role of Valve Interstitial Cell Phenotypes in Regulating Heart Valve Pathobiology. Am J Pathol 2007;171:1407-1418.

[31] Marechaux S, Corseaux D, Vincentelli A, *et al.* Identification of tissue factor in experimental aortic valve sclerosis. Cardiovasc Pathol 2009;18:67-76.

[32] Derynck R, Zhang YE. Smad-dependent and Smad-independent pathways in TGF-beta family signaling. Nature 2003;425:557-584.

[33] Clements RT, Minnear FL, Singer HA, *et al.* RhoA and Rho-kinase dependent and independent signals mediate TGF-beta-induced pulmonary endothelial cytoskeletal reorganization and permeability. Am J Physiol – Lung Cellular Molecular Physiol 2005;288:L294-L306.

[34] Edlund S, Landstrom M, Heldin CH, Aspenstrom P. Transforming growth factor-beta-induced mobilization of actin cytoskeleton requires signaling by small GTPases Cdc42 and RhoA. Molec Biol of the cell 2002;13:902-914.

[35] Javelaud D, Mauviel A. Crosstalk mechanisms between the mitogen-activated protein kinase pathways and Smad signaling downstream of TGF-beta: implications for carcinogenesis. Oncogene 2005;37:5742-5750.

[36] Jian B, Narula N, Li QY, *et al.* Progression of aortic valve stenosis: TGF-beta 1 is present in calcified aortic valve cusps and promotes aortic valve interstitial cell calcification *via* apoptosis. Ann Thorac Surg 2003;75:457-465.

[37] Saura M, Zaragoza C, Herranz B, *et al.* Nitric oxide regulates transforming growth factor-beta signaling in endothelial cells. Circulation Res 2005;97:1115-1123.

[38] Wu B, Elmariah S, Kaplan FS, *et al.* Paradoxical effects of statins on aortic valve myofibroblasts and osteoblasts-Implications for end-stage valvular heart disease Arterioscl, Thromb Vasc Biol 2005;25:592-597.

[39] Osman L, Yacoub MH, Latif N, *et al.* Differentiation and proliferation of endothelial progenitor cells from canine peripheral blood mononuclear cells. Circulation 2006;114;1547-1552.

[40] Rajamannan NM, Subramaniam M, Caira F, *et al.* Atorvastatin inhibits hypercholesterolemia induced calcification in the aortic valves *via* the Lrp5 receptor pathway. Circulation 2005;112[suppl 9]:1229-1234.

[41] Bahler RC, Desser DR, Finkelhor RS, *et al.* Factors leading to progression of valvular aortic stenosis. Am J Cardiol 1999;84:1044-1048.

[42] Juvonen J, Laurila A, Juvonen T, *et al.* Detection of Chlamydia pneumoniae in Human Nonrheumatic Stenotic Aortic Valves. J Am Coll Cardiol 1997;29:1054-1059.

[43] Juvonen J, Juvonen T, Laurila A, *et al.* Can Degenerative Aortic Valve Stenosis Be Related to Persistent Chlamydia pneumoniae Infection. Ann Intern Med 1998;128:741-744.

[44] Kaden JJ, Haghi D, Vocke DC, *et al.* Chlamydia Pneumoniae – a new risk factor for calcific aortic stenosis Med Klinik 2005;100:334-339.

[45] Simolin MA, Pedersen TX, Bro S, *et al.* ACE inhibition attenuates uremia-induced aortic valve thickening in a novel mouse model BMC Cardiovascular Disorders 2009, 9:10 doi:10.1186/1471-2261-9-10

[46] Schurgers LJ, Aebert H, Vermeer C, *et al.* Oral anticoagulant treatment: friend or foe in cardiovascular disease. Blood 2004;104:104:3231-3232.

[47] Koos R, Krueger T, Westenfeld R, *et al.* Relation of circulating matrix-GLA protein and anticoagulation status in patients with aortic valve calcification. Thromb Haemost 2009;101:706-713.

[48] Ueland T, Gullesta L, Dahl CP, *et al.* Undercarboxylated matrix Gla protein is associated with indices of heart failure and mortality in symptomatic aortic stenosis. J Int Med 2010;268:483-492.

[49] Renneneberg RJMW, de Leeuw PJ, Kessels AGH, *et al.* Calcium scores and matrix GLA protein levels: association with vitamin K status. Eur J Clin Invest 2010;40:344-349.

[50] Ing SW, Mohler ER, Putt ME, *et al.* Correlates of valvular ossification with aortic valve stenosis. CTS – Clinical and Translational Science 2009;2:431-435.

[51] Lerner RG, Aronow WS, Sekhri A, *et al.* Warfarin use and the risk of valvular calcification. J Thromb Haemost 2009;7:2023-2027.

[52] Yang X, Meng X, Su X, *et al.* Bone morphogenic protein 2 induces Runx2 and osteopontin expression in human aortic valve interstitial cells: Role of Smad1and extracellular signal-regulated kinase 1/2. J Thorac Cardiovasc Surg 2009;138:1008-1015.

[53] Rallidis L, Naoumova RP, Thompson GR, Nihoyannopoulos P. Extent and severity of atherosclerotic involvement of the aortic valve and root in familial hypercholesterolaemia. Heart 1998;80;583-590.

[54] Rabkin SW, Lodhia P, Luong MW. P28 MAP kinase in vale interstitial cells is activated by angiotensin or nitric oxide/peroxynitrite, but reduced by Toll-like receptor-2 stimulation. J Heart Valve Dis 2009;18:653-661.

[55] Anger T, Carson W, Weygand M, *et al.* Atherosclerotic inflammation triggers osteogenic bone transformation in calcified and stenotic human aortic valves. Experimental and molecular pathology 2009;86:10-17.

[56] O'Brien KD, Kuusisto J, Reichenbach DD, *et al.* Osteopontin is expressed in human aortic valvular lesions. Circulation 1995;92:2163-2168.

[57] Yu PJ, Skolnick A, Ferrari G, *et al.* Correlation between plasma osteopontin levels and aortic valve calcification: Potential insights into the pathogenesis of aortic valve calcification and stenosis. J Thorac Cardiovasc Surg 2009;138:196-9.

[58] Hermans H, Herijgers P, Holvoet P, *et al.* Statins for Calcific Aortic Valve Stenosis: Into Oblivion After SALTIRE and SEAS? An Extensive Review from Bench to Bedside. Curr Probl Cardiol 2010;35:284-306.

[59] Yang X, Fullerton DA, Su X, *et al.* Pro-Osteogenic Phenotype of Human Aortic Valve Interstitial Cells Is Associated With Higher Levels of Toll-Like Receptors 2 and 4 and Enhanced Expression of Bone Morphogenetic Protein 2. J Am Coll Cardiol 2009;53:491-500.

[60] Caira FC, Stock SR, Gleason TG, *et al.* Human degenerative aortic valve disease is associated with up-regulation of low-density lipoprotein receptor-related protein 5 receptor-mediated bone formation. J Am Coll Cardiol 2006;47:1707-1712.

[61] Thornberry NA, Lazebnik Y. Caspases: enemies within. Science. 1998;281:1312-1316.

[62] Abdelwahid E, Pelliniemi LJ, Jokinen E. Cell death and differentiation in the development of the endocardial cushion of the embryonic heart. Microscopic Res and Techn. 2002;58:395-403.

[63] Abdelwahid E, Rice D, Pelliniemi LJ, Jokinen E. Overlapping and differential localization of BMP-2, BMP-4, MSX-2 and apoptosis in the endocardial cushion and adjacent tissues of the developing Mouse heart. Cell and Tissue Res 2001;305:67-78.

[64] Abdelwahid E, Eriksson M, Pelliniemi LJ, Jokinen E. Heat shock proteins, HSP 25 and HSP 70, and apoptosis in the developing endocardial cushion of the mouse heart. Histochem Cell Biol. 2001;115:95-104.

[65] Abdelwahid E, Pelliniemi LJ, Niinikoski H, *et al.* Apoptosis in the pattern formation of the ventricular wall during heart organogenesis. Anat Rec 1999;256:208-217.

[66] Lockshin RA, Zakerin Z. In: Programmed cell death and apoptosis: origins of the theory. Nat Rev Mol Cell Biol 2001;2:545-550.

[67] Fisher SA, Langille BL, Srivastava D. Apoptosis during cardiovascular development. Circ Res. 2000;87:856-64.

[68] Petrovski G, Zahuczky G, Majai G, Fésüs L. Phagocytosis of cells dying through autophagy evokes a pro-inflammatory response in macrophages. Autophagy 2007;3:509-511.

[69] Edinger AL, Thompson CB. Death by design: apoptosis, necrosis and autophagy. Curr Opinion in Cell Biol 2004;16:663-669.

[70] Debnath J, Baehrecke HE, Kroemer G. Does autophagy contibute to cell death? Autophagy 2005;1:66-74.

[71] Guillon-Munos A, Van Bemmelen MXP, Clarke PGH. Autophagy can be a killer even in apoptosis competent cells. Autophagy 2002;2:140-142.

[72] Eskilinen EL. Maturation of autophagic valcuoles in mammalian cells. Autophagy 2005:1:1-10.

[73] Cuervo AM, Bergamini E, Brunk TU, *et al.* Autophagy and aging: The importance of maintaining "clean" cells. Autophagy 2005;1:131-140.

[74] Klionsky DJ, Cuervo AM, Seglen PO. Methods for monitoring autophagy from yeast to human. Autophagy 2007;3:181-206.

[75] Kjeken R, Egeberg M, Habermann A, *et al.* Fusion between phagosomes, early and late endosomes: a role for actin infusion between late but not early endocytic organelles. Molec Biol of the Cell 2004;15:345-358.

[76] Mistiaen WP, Somers P, Knaapen MWM, Kockx MM. Autophagy as Mechanism for Cell Death in Degenerative Aortic Valve Disease: An Underestimated Phenomenon in Cardiovascular Diseases. Autophagy 2006;2:221-223.

[77] Mistiaen W, Knaapen M. Evaluation of Cell Death Markers in Severe Calcified Aortic Valves. Meth Enzymol 2009;453:365-379.

[78] Heyde EC. Gastrointestinal bleeding in aortic stenosis. N Engl J Med 1958; 259: 196.

[79] Greenstein RJ, McElhinney AJ, Reuben D, Greenstein AJ. Colonic vascular ectasias and aortic stenosis: coincidence or causal relationship? Am J Surg 1986; 151:347-351.

[80] Warkentin TE, Moore JC, Anand SS, *et al.* Gastrointestinal bleeding, angiodysplasia, cardiovascular disease, and acquired von Willebrand syndrome. Transfus Med Rev 2003;17:272-286.

[81] Massyn MW, Khan SA. Heyde syndrome: a common diagnosis in older patients with severe aortic stenosis. Age and Aging 2009;38:267-270.
[82] Pate GE, Chandavimoi M, Naiman SC, Webb JG. Heyde's syndrome: a review. J Heart Valve Dis 2004;13:701-712.
[83] Chow TW, Hellums JD, Moake JL, Kroll MH. Shear stress-induced von Willebrand factor binding to platelet glycoprotein Ib initiates calcium influx associated with aggregation. Blood 1992;80:113-120.
[84] Gola W, Lelonek M. Clinical implication of gastrointestinal bleeding in degenerative aortic stenosis: an update/Cardiology J 2010;17:330-334.
[85] Panzer S, Eslam RB, Schneller A, *et al.* Loss of high molecular weight von Willebrand factor multimers mainly affects platelet aggregation in patients with aortic stenosis. Thromb Haemost 2010; 103:408-414.
[86] Sucker C. Letter to the Editor. The Heyde syndrome: proposal for a unifying concept explaining the association of aortic valve stenosis, gastrointestinal angiodysplasia and bleeding. Int J Cardiol 2007;115:77-78.
[87] Tsai HM. Physiologic cleavage of von Willebrand factor by a plasma protease is dependent on its conformation and requires calcium ion. Blood 1996;87:4235-4244.
[88] Vincentelli A, Susen S, Le Tourneau T, *et al.* Acquired von Willebrand syndrome in aortic stenosis. N Engl J Med 2003;349:343-349.
[89] Floudas CS, Moyssakis I, Pappas P, *et al.* Obscure gastrointestinal bleeding and calcific aortic stenosis (Heyde's syndrome) Int J Cardiol 2008;127:292-294.
[90] King RM, Pluth JR, Guiliani ER. The association of unexplained gastrointestinal bleeding with calcific aortic stenosis. Ann Thorac Surg 1987;44:514-516.
[91] Olsson M, Hultcrantz R, Schulman S, Wallgren E. Acquired platelet dysfunction may be an etiologic factor in Heyde's syndrome – normalization of bleeding time after aortic valve replacement. J Int Med 2002;252:516-523.
[92] Warkentin TE, Moore JC, Morgan DG. Gastrointestinal angiodysplasia and aortic stenosis. N Engl J Med 2002;347:858-859.
[93] Morishima A, Marui A, Shimamoto T, *et al.* Successful aortic valve replacement for Heyde syndrome with confirmed hematologic recovery. Ann Thorac Surg 2007:83:287-288.
[94] Khetarpal V, Mahajan N, Madhavan R, *et al.* Calcific aortic valve and spontaneous embolic stroke: A review of literature. Journal of the Neurological Sciences 2009;287:32-35.
[95] Siu SC, Silversides CK. Bicuspid aortic valve disease. J Am Coll Cardiol 2010;55:2789-2880.
[96] Fernandez B, Duran AC, Fernandez-Callego T, *et al.* Bicuspid Aortic Valves With Different Spatial Orientations of the Leaflets Are Distinct Etiological Entities. J Am Coll Cardiol 2009:54:2312-2318.

CHAPTER 3

Prevention of the Progress of CAVS

Abstract: Since several risk factors for the development of CAVS have been identified, it seemed reasonable to explore the effects of their medical targeting on the rate of progress of this disease.

Especially for lipid disorders and statins, hopes have been high. Statins have a proven value for the treatment of lipid disorders in atheromatosis, which shares some risk factors with CAVS. A proof of concept could also be derived from animal models.

Early non randomized and retrospective studies have seemed to confirm these hopes. With appearance of the more recent trials (SEAS, SALTIRE and ASTRONOMER) it has become clear that these hopes are unjustified. No difference in effect have been found between statins and placebo on the rate of progression of CAVS.

Reasons for these findings are probably:

- The composition of the population: it is unethical to deny patients with lipid disorders a treatment with statins. This limitation makes it difficult to compare certain populations.
- The stage of CAVS: statins might work only very early in the course of the disease, which is asymptomatic.
- The mechanisms of action: fibrosis of the aortic valve could be induced by statins. A fibrotic cap in atheromatosis has a protective effect; in contrast, fibrosis in CAVS could impair the mobility of the leaflets and worsens the disease.

Statins have probably also no role in the prevention of SVD of bioprostheses.

Other approaches such as ACE inhibitors, ATR blocking agents and endothelin receptor antagonists need still investigations. The "window" of "opportunity" for their action might be too short.

Keywords: Angiotensin converting enzyme, aortic valve area, calcium score, end points, endothelin receptor antagonists, jet velocity, left ventricular ejection fraction low density lipoproteins, randomized controlled trials, statins, transvalvular gradient.

1. GENERAL REMARKS

CAVS is a progressive disease, which has a long asymptomatic phase. Once the disease has become symptomatic, mortality increases considerably, which makes

Wilhelm Peter Mistiaen

this symptomatic phase short [1, 2]. Slowing the progression of the disease might postpone the need for AVR. Since several risk factors for CAVS have been identified, it seemed worthwhile to explore the medical treatments in this respect

Several ways have been tried:

- Lipid lowering therapy by statins.
- ACE inhibitors and angiotensin receptor blocking agents.
- Endothelin receptor antagonists.
- Nitric oxide donors.
- Other pharmacological approach.

2. STATINS

2.1. The Effect of Statins (3-Hydroxy-3-Methylglutaryl-Coenzyme A Reductase Inhibitors)

Hypercholesterolemia has several effects on the cardiovascular system [3]:

- Dysfunction of EC, which occurs even before atherosclerosis develops.
- Increased expression of VCAM-1 by EC.
- Reduction of exercise induced vasodilatation.
- Impairment of NO production by EC.

The effect of statins are pleiotropic:

- Decreasing LDL cholesterol.
- Blocking of interaction of apolipoprotein-B containing lipoproteins with specific sub-endothelial matrix molecules (which mediate the retention of these lipoproteins) [4].

- Inhibition of the lectin-like Oxidized LDL receptor-1 (LOX-1), which could be a mechanism of reducing the lipids in the human aortic SMC and in macrophages [5].

- Inhibition of oxidation of LDL, reduction of vascular superoxide generation and formation of plaques (cholesterol fed rabbits) [6].

- Promoting NO production by stimulation of eNOS, [3] in EC, and in a lesser degree in VIC. These effects protect against calcification, but only in early stages [8-11].

- Improving endothelial function [12] and keeping the EC layer intact [13].

- Inhibiting ostegenic markers in human VIC [14].

- Reducing inflammation through CRP [15], through MHC class 2 expression, ICAM-1 interaction and other inflammatory signaling pathways [10-12, 16].

- Reducing the oxidative process [12].

- Partially neutralizing gene expressions, which occur early during the development of inflammation in CAVS. This is not through VCAM-1, TGF-beta, tenascin C, bone sialoprotein and osteocalcin [16].

- Reduction of ACE influx into valvular lesions. By reducing LDL, less lipoprotein is available to carry ACE and progression of CAVS might be decreased [17].

- Decreasing the secretion of MMP by macrophages [11].

- Inducing bone formation, BMP-2 expression and osteoblasts [18].

2.2. The Early Hopes and Doubts

Initially, there have been several reasons for optimism, based on the above mentioned pleiotropic effects of statins [19]. These pharmacological agents have been considered as first line candidates for slowing down progression of CAVS. Statins have a proven effect in primary and secondary cardiovascular prevention. It is reasonable to suppose that the use of statins might be beneficial in patients with CAVS for at least three reasons [2, 15, 20, 21].

1) CAVS shares some risk factors with atheromatosis, for which lipid lowering therapy has been successful.
2) There are pathological similarities between both conditions.
3) CAVS can be induced by a cholesterol rich diet in rodents.

One has to keep in mind, that differences exist between CAVS and atheromatosis which could influence the effect of statins.

Moreover, the beneficial effect of statins has been the reduction of plaque rupture by promoting a fibrous cap [15]. This protective fibrosis probably restricts the motion of valvular cusps. This reduces the EOA and worsens CAVS [22].

Several experiments have been performed, which mainly have focused on atheromatosis. The most experiments have involved rodents, fed with a cholesterol diet and in which statins have been tested. Arteries usually have been the focus of attention. Following observations have been made:

- Decrease of the area of atherosclerosis [23].
- Decrease of cholesterol ester content in macrophages [23].
- Improvement of the stability of plaques in aortas and coronary arteries [24].
- Reduction of the expression/secretion of MMP 1, 2, 3, and 9 by macrophages and SMC in atherosclerotic lesions [25, 26].
- Alteration of SMC and collagen content in plaques [25, 26].
- Reduction of vascular leakage and of the thrombin-induced endothelial barrier dysfunction in human umbilical veins and human aortic EC mono-layers [27].

- Increase of the expression of thrombomodulin of aortic EC by inhibiting intracellular second messengers (ERK and NFkB) [28].

- Restoration of the imbalance between nitric oxide (protective against oxidation) and peroxonitrite (which is an oxidant). The anti-atherosclerotic effects of statins are mediated by haem oxygenase-1 and eNOS. This imbalance is an indicator for EC dysfunction [29].

- Up-regulating eNOS in arteries (the NO production is a surrogate for endothelial protective function, peroxynitrite has been used as assessment of dysfunctional eNOS activity). A combination of statins and of angiotensin II receptor blocking agents have additive effect on the protection of EC [30].

- Reduction of the NO metabolites and S-nitrosothiols [31].

Lipophilic statins have also displayed some other effects:

- No inhibition the proliferation of SMC.

- Decrease the number of macrophages.

- No decrease of the ratio of fibromuscular/SMC components [32].

These results have been obtained by studies of the arteries. Few experiments have focused on the aortic valve itself. In a recently performed experimental approach, New Zealand white rabbits, have received a cholesterol diet during 30 months and statin treatment in the last 15 months. The valve function has been documented by MRI and by pathological study. Without statins, collagen deposition, lymphocyte invasion and calcification of the valves has been observed. With treatment of statins, a regression of the sclerotic process has not been noticed, however [33].

2.3. The Early Series

The effect of statins on the progression of CAVS has been studied for some years. Some studies have shown a slowing effect of statins, with a lesser increase in mean and peak TVG or a lesser decrease in AVA [11, 34, 35]. However, the benefits of statins have remained doubtful [36].

One early example has been a study published in 2001 [34]. This has been a retrospective study with a median follow-up of 21 months. Between 1996 and 2000, 147 patients have been included.

Inclusion criteria have been:

- A mild to moderate CAVS with an AVA between 1.0 and 1.8 cm^2.
- A LVEF of at least 50%.

At least two TTE have been made with an interval of at least 12 months.

Exclusion criteria have been:

- An aortic valve regurgitation with a degree of at least 2/4.
- An echographic evidence of mitral valve disease.

Fifty-seven patients have received statins and 117 have not. Their baseline LDL-cholesterol levels have been resp. 131 and 128 mg/dL, which have not differed significantly [p=0.49]. Both groups have been comparable for total and HDL-cholesterol, serum creatinin and proportion of bicuspid aortic valves. The group receiving statins has been older and had more CAD, DM and AHT.

At baseline, the degree of CAVS has also been comparable with an AVA of 1.2 cm^2 and mean TVG of 15 mmHg. The peak TVG has been 28 mm Hg in the statin group and 29 mm Hg in the non-statin group.

The decrease of AVA in the statin group has been 0.11 +/-0.18 cm^2. In the statin treated group, this has been 0.06 +/-0.16 cm^2, which has been significantly lower [p=0.03]. Peak TVG has increased less in the statin group compared to the control group.

A first meta-analysis of 9 series, has been published before December, 31, 2008. It has revealed that an overall significant effect of statins on the progression of CAVS could be observed with respect to peak aortic jet velocity, AVA, peak and mean TVG [37]. Another meta-analysis has been less clear [38]. The trials, which have been included, have been heterogeneous in several aspects. This should be taken into account when the results are interpreted [37]. Differences between these trials have been:

- The retrospective *vs.* prospective nature of the observation.
- The duration of follow-up.
- The severity of CAVS with initiation of statins.
- The presence or absence of CAD, diabetes, hypertension and triglyceride levels.
- The differences in end-points.
    - Hemodynamic progression: annual change in AVA, TVG or jet velocity.
    - Calcification on CT.
    - Appearance of symptoms or need for AVR.
    - Non-fatal AMI, angina pectoris, CHF, need for CABG, PCI, *etc.*
    - Hospitalization for severe CAVS or for any cause.
    - Mortality for cardiovascular cause or for any cause.
- The difference in statins used.
- Open label trials (*i.e.* not blinded and hence liable to bias).

No relation between LDL cholesterol and progression rate for CAVS has been observed in patients with all grades of severity of CAVS, defined by the jet velocity. There are some points of considerations, however. First, a 2 year treatment period might be too short and second, modest effects of statins could be missed. However, the recent development of reproducible technology for quantification of aortic sclerosis in patients will facilitate investigations of earlier stages of disease progression [7]. This is probably only relevant in younger patients, in whom statins might be started early in the course of CAVS and in whom a beneficial effect could be expected [2, 15].

2.4. The More Recent Trials

2.4.1. RAAVE or Rosuvastatin Affecting Aortic Valve Endothelium [35]

This has been a prospective open label and non randomized study. One hundred-twenty-one consecutive patients with asymptomatic moderate to severe CAVS have been included. They had an AVA between 1.0 and 1.5 cm^2. The mean age has been about 74 years. The mean follow-up has been 73 months.

Exclusion criteria have been:

- CAD.
- Rheumatic mitral valve disease.
- Previous use of statins.
- Congenital heart disease.
- Congenital bicuspid aortic valve.
- Subaortic obstruction.
- Mild aortic valve regurgitation.
- Previous aortic valve disease.
- Other vascular diseases and malignancies.

Sixty patients with CAVS have received rosuvastatin (20 mg/d) for elevated LDL-cholesterol (mean 160 mg/dL). They have been compared with 61 patients with CAVS who have not received a statin. The latter patients had a normal LDL-cholesterol (119 mg/dL). Baseline values for CAVS have been comparable for both groups, with a jet velocity of 3.65 and 3.62 m/s and an AVA of 1.23 and 1.20 cm^2.

The results have shown less progression of CAVS in the statin treated group: an annual change in:

- AVA of 0.05 +/-0.12 *vs.* 0.10 +/-0.09 cm^2 (p=0.041).
- Jet velocity of 0.04 +/-0.38 m/s *vs.* 0.24 +:-0.30 m/s (p=0.007).

The difference in baseline LDL between the 2 groups of patients might have an impact on the results. Since this study has not been blinded and not been randomized, it could only generate the hypothesis of beneficial effects of statins, not confirm it [12, 18, 19].

The RAAVE study has important limitations. It is not ethical to randomize patients with elevated LDL into the "no statin" arm, since the clinical benefits of lipid lowering treatment has been extensively demonstrated [20, 21, 39].

2.4.2. SALTIRE or Scottish Aortic Stenosis and Lipid Lowering Trial: Impact on Regression [2]

This has been the first prospective double blind randomized and placebo controlled RCT in 165 patients. This can be considered as a rather small population. The median follow-up has been 25 months.

Inclusion criteria have been CAVS with an aortic jet velocity of at least 2.5 m/s. Patients with advanced CAVS have also been included. Patients have received Atorvastatin 80 mg or a placebo.

Exclusion criteria have been:

- Severe mitral stenosis.
- Severe mitral or aortic valve regurgitation.
- LVEF below 35%.

- Total cholesterol higher than 150 mg/dL.

Median age (68 years for both groups), plasma LDL cholesterol (133 *vs.* 137 mg/dL), base line values for jet velocity (3.39 *vs.* 3.45 m/s), for peak TVG (47.8 *vs.* 49.5 mm Hg), for AVA (1.03 *vs.* 1.02 cm^2) and for calcium score (5424 *vs.* 6221) have been comparable for both groups.

Primary end-points have been aortic jet velocity and aortic calcium score on CT. Secondary end points have been composite death of cardiovascular disease or any cause, need for AVR, hospitalization for severe CAVS or for any cause.

Atorvastatin at 80 mg daily has reduced LDL cholesterol effectively, but it had no significant effect on progression of CAVS compared to placebo. The annual increase has been estimated for:

- TVG: this has been 0.199 *vs.* 0.203 m/s.

- Calcium score: this has been 22.3 *vs.* 21.7.

This has been true for patients with and without a lipid disorder [16].

For the secondary end-points, no significant effect of Atorvastatin has been observed, but the power of the study could have been insufficient. The follow-up duration has only been 25 months, which is short [12, 19]. One quarter of the patients in each group had severe CAVS. In those patients, the disease might be too advanced to be affected by the treatment with statins. Repetition by a large scale RCT is required, since this study had not the power to assess the benefits of statins on the secondary end-points [9, 15]. Appearance of symptoms during therapy with statins could be considered as a failure, since prompt AVR is required in these patients.

2.4.3. SEAS or Simvastatin and Ezetimibe in Aortic Stenosis [40]

This has been a placebo controlled RCT in 1763 patients with a mean age of 67 years. The median follow-up has been 52 months.

The inclusion criterion has been mild – to moderate asymptomatic CAVS with a jet velocity between 2.5 and 4.0 m/sec.

Exclusion criteria have been:

- Clinical indications for statins.
- Presence of CAD.
- DM.
- Other major valve diseases.

The placebo group has been comparable to the statin group for renal function (plasma creatinin both 1.06 mg/dL), LDL cholesterol (139 *vs.* 140 mg/dL), peak jet velocity (3.10 *vs.* 3.09 m/s), mean TVG (23.0 *vs.* 22.7 mm Hg), AVAI (0.67 v 0.68 cm^2/m^2), LVEF (66 *vs.* 67%) and % of bicuspid valves (6.3 *vs.* 5.0).

End points have been changes in parameters for CAVS, need for AVR and ischemic events. A significant reduction of ischemic cardiovascular events (especially the need for CABG) has been undeniable. This has not been true, however, for valvular events, not even in the group with the mildest CAVS.

The changes during the entire follow-up have been:

- Jet velocity: 0.62 m/s in the placebo group and 0.61 m/s in the treated group.
- Mean TVG increments: 22.5 in the placebo group and 22.2 mm Hg in the treated group [18, 40-42].

Higher values of baseline characteristics of CAVS have been predictive for both ischemic and for valvular events [42]. The earlier documented beneficial results of retrospective studies with statins for CAVS have not been confirmed [12, 21]. The current 4.3 years of study might be too short, the true benefit of statins in patients with aortic sclerosis (*i.e.* the mildest form) might need a RCT for longer time intervals. Furthermore, since patients with CAD, DM and renal failure have been excluded for SEAS, no definitive conclusion for statins in these groups have been made [42].

In any case, the negative results in the SEAS trial in low risk patients does not rule out that statins have a potential benefit in delaying CAVS in patients with multiple risk factors [37].

2.4.4. ASTRONOMER or Aortic Stenosis Progression Observation: Measuring Effects of Rosuvastatin [19, 43]

This has bene a randomized double blind, placebo controlled RCT, without other clinical indications for cholesterol lowering treatment. The trial was still ongoing in 2009 [19]. Patients have been followed for 3 to 5 years, with annual TTE. Primary end-points have been AVA, peak and mean TVG. Secondary outcomes have been AVR and death.

The inclusion criterion has been asymptomatic mild to moderate CAVS, with a jet velocity between 2.5 and 4.0 m/s.

The exclusion criteria have been:

- Any clinical indication for use of statins.
- Patients of Asian origin, for an increased risk for side effects.
- CAD and other arterial disease.
- DM.

The median age for both groups has been 58 years. Severity of CAVS in both groups has been comparable. A peak jet velocity has been 3.16 m/s in the Rosuvastatin group and 3.19 m/s in the control group. Mean TVG was resp. 22.5 mm Hg and 23.1 mm Hg. There have been more bicuspid valves compared to RAAVE and SALTIRE trials: 53.7 resp. 45.2% [19, 43].

The median FU has been 3.5 years [43], hence only statements for effects on mid-term can be made. The primary end point has been progression of CAVS, documented by changes in TVG and AVA. Secondary end points have been cardiac death or AVR.

Rosuvastatin 40 mg has reduced the LDL cholesterol concentration in the plasma by 50% or more and has reduced CRP with one sixth. However, it did not decrease:

- Annual progression of mean TVG: 6.3 mm Hg (statin) *vs.* 6.1 mm Hg (placebo).
- Annual progression of peak TVG: 3.9 mm Hg *vs.* 3.8 mm Hg.
- Annual reduction in AVA: 0.08 cm^2 *vs.* 0.07 cm^2.

Outcome (death, need for AVR, for CABG and AMI) has not differed between both groups. Inclusion of more patients with bicuspid valves might resemble the "real world" in a better way. It should be noted that patients with hypercholesterolemia have been excluded, since they need statins on other grounds!

In conclusion, statins should not be used for the sole purpose of reducing the progression of CAVS [43].

2.5. Conclusions from the Trials

The results of the RAAVE trial have been encouraging, but this could not be repeated with two major RCT, SALTIRE and SEAS [20, 21, 44]. These populations have not resembled fully the general population of patients with CAVS. The ASTRONOMER trial also has shown no effect of statins on the progression of CAVS [43].

The SEAS and the ASTRONOMER trials might provide more insight compared to RAAVE [15]. Such pioneering trials have provided valuable information for the future design of valvular heart disease trials [45], but it has become doubtful if more trials to study the effect of statins are fruitful [43].

These differences in results might be explained by several reasons [20].

1) The study populations. For ethical reasons, patients with hypercholesterolemia have been excluded from prospective RCT.

These patients have been included in retrospective non-randomized studies [20, 43].

2) CAVS shows some similarities with CAD, but only in part. Nevertheless, hypercholesterolemia is one of the main pro-inflammatory factors, with high levels of high-sensitivity CRP. Statins may inhibit lipid-mediated inflammation and reduce calcification significantly [20, 44].

Statins might delay the progression in CAVS, but probably only in patients with hypercholesterolemia [20], and probably only early in the development of CAVS [44, 45].

2.5.1. Addendum: The Role of Lipid Lowering Treatment for SVD

The role of lipid lowering therapy in the durability of implanted biological prostheses has also been a matter for investigation. In an observational study, 1193 patients have been followed with a mean duration of 4.5 years. Mean and peak TVG, as well as reoperation rate for SVD have been compared between patients receiving lipid lowering therapy and patients without such treatment. No association has been found between lipid lowering therapy, which has been started early after AVR, and a slowing of development of SVD in biological prostheses. Therefore, a RCT to study the effects of statins on the progress on SVD after AVR does not seem justified. Large cohorts and long duration for follow-up would be needed, since the current BHV have an excellent durability [46].

3. ACE INHIBITORS

ACE inhibitors and ET receptor blocking agents might have a potential role in the prevention of progression of CAVS for several reasons:

- These agents keep the endothelial layer intact [13].
- ACE could be carried into valvular lesions by LDL which contributes to inflammation and calcification [15, 17]; this event could be prevented by ACE inhibitors.

- Angiotensin II is a powerful pro-inflammatory mediator, which also promotes fibrosis. Especially in renal patients, ACE inhibitors could be useful [47].

There are other reasons to study the effect of ACE inhibitors in the management of CAVS:

1) Pressure overload on the left ventricle might induce LVH, myocardial fibrosis and apoptosis. This might accelerate left ventricular dysfunction.

2) Concomitant reduction of blood pressure might offer some relief of pressure overload on the left ventricle in patients with hypertension [15].

Because of vasodilatation, use of ACE inhibitors only seems more appropriate in patients with early CAVS. In patients with LV overload, LV dysfunction and AHT, ACE inhibitors have certainly their use.

Very recently, some experimental series dealing with the effect of ACE inhibitors on the progress of CAVS have published.

An animal model has shown some positive results: the effect of Ramipril has been evaluated in New Zealand white rabbits treated with Vitamin D. Aortic valve backscatter and outflow tract flow velocity have been documented by echocardiography. The intravalvular content of a pro-oxidant protein (thioredoxin interacting protein) and the endothelial function (asymmetric dimethyl arginine concentrations and vascular response to acetylcholine) also have been determined. With use of ACE inhibitors, the progression of aortic valve stenosis has slowed and the thioredoxin interacting protein accumulation has decreased. The endothelial dysfunction also has been limited in rabbits treated with Ramipril [48].

Clinical series have shown conflicting results, however.

Progression of CAVS (documented by a peak velocity of over 2.5 m/sec) has been investigated in patients with a normal LVF, who took ACE inhibitors, statins or both. This progress of CAVS has been documented by at least two echocardiographic examinations. Statins have seemingly decreased the rate of progression of CAVS, but ACE inhibitors have not, even when these were combined with statins [49].

Another study has revealed contrasting results. ACE inhibitors have slowed down the progression of CAVS in 194 Japanese patients with tricuspid aortic valves and mild calcification. This effect has been measured by peak aortic valve jet velocity: the annual increase has been 0.04+/-0.22 m/sec (with ACE inhibitors) *vs.* 0.20+/-0.32 m/sec (without ACE inhibitor). This retrospective study has been performed with echocardiographical documentation. Multivariate analysis has also shown an association of a decreased LVEF and a higher initial peak jet velocity as confounding factors [50].

Currently, the outcome in patients with CAVS treated with ACE inhibitors is still doubtful: some studies have shown an effect, other have not. In contrast to what was earlier assumed, ACE inhibitors are well tolerated by patients with CAVS. RCT to investigate the benefits of ACE in patients with CAVS are warranted [11].

One could wonder if the treatment with ACE inhibitors will suffer the same fate as statins have. Both approaches seemed very promising in the beginning, but for statins, it has become clear that early hopes will not be fulfilled. The study of the effect of ACE inhibitors on the progression of CAVS is still preliminary. Appropriate imaging techniques are required for the detection of subtle effects [51]. Other questions also remain. What will be the optimal timing and duration of any treatment? Are there other pathophysiological pathways to explore? No RCT for ACE inhibitors have been published [52], but can these trials be designed in an ethical way? And the risk for underreporting negative results remains!

4.OTHER APPROACHES

Endothelin receptor antagonists could counteract the effect of endothelin. Stimulation of the ETA receptor by endothelin-1 promotes inflammation and fibrosis. Experimentally, ETA-receptor blockade prevents endothelial dysfunction. In early cases of CAVS, this approach might have an effect, but the vasodilating properties in these patients could pose a problem [53].

Nitric oxide has a protective effect: NO donors are able to inhibit nodule formation by TGF-beta 1 in porcine VIC cultures. NO donors are less effective once nodules have formed. NO is an important functional antagonist of superoxide. The effects of NO donors may partially reflect superoxide scavenging [7]. Statins might also play a role herein.

Inhibition of valvular calcification may also be due to alterations in levels of vitamin D, parathyroid hormone, or other novel regulators of bone turnover. Although chronic secondary hyperparathyroidism in renal failure is associated with aortic calcification and osteopenia, intermittent treatment with exogenous parathyroid hormone is associated with increased bone mineral density and decreased vascular calcification. The key regulator of this process appears to be osteopontin, a potent inhibitor of vascular calcification, which has recently been demonstrated to have negative feedback on parathyroid hormone production when given in a pulsatile fashion. Perhaps the effects of bisphosphonates on calcification of the aortic valve are mediated by soluble osteopontin [54].

CONCLUSIONS

The discovery of risk factors for CAVS initially have indicated that treatment of these risk factors could slow down the progression of this disease. Especially for lipid lowering treatment with statins, there has been hope and animal studies as well early series have seemed to confirm this.

Animal studies, however, have mostly concerned themselves with atherosclerosis in arteries, few have focused on the aortic valve.

Early patients series have been non-randomized and partially retrospective in nature. Moreover, it has been, and still is unethical to withhold statins in patients with CAVS and lipid disorders.

More recently performed RCT have not confirmed the early beneficial effects of statins on the progress of CAVS. Moreover, fibrosis induced by statins may be beneficial through the formation of a protective cap in atheromatosis. Formation of fibrosis by statins in CAVS makes leaflets immobile and could worsen the problem.

Hence, statins should not be given solely for the purpose of slowing the progression of CAVS.

The discovery of ACE and angiotensin II deposition in calcified aortic valves has also raised hope for the use of ACE inhibitors in CAVS. No definitive conclusions could be reached yet. This investigation requires a large scale RCT.

The use of endothelin receptor antagonists for CAVS are still in an experimental phase. This type of treatment probably is only useful in very early cases. For inhibition of angiogenesis, the window of opportunity is probably too small to be of any practical use.

ACKNOWLEDGEMENT

Declared none.

CONFLICT OF INTEREST

The author(s) confirm that this chapter content has no conflict of interest.

REFERENCES

[1] Carabello BA, Paulus WJ. Aortic Stenosis. Lancet 2009;373:956-966.

[2] Cowell SJ, Newby DE, Prescott RJ, *et al.*, for the Scottish Aortic Stenosis and Lipid Lowering Trial, Impact on Regression [SALTIRE] Investigators. A Randomized Trial of Intensive Lipid-Lowering Therapy in Calcific Aortic Stenosis. N Engl J Med 2005;352:2389-2397.

[3] Libby P, Aikawa M, Selwyn A, Ganz P. Lipid lowering improves endothelial functions Int J Cardiol 2000;74:S3-S10.

[4] Tabas I, Williams KJ, Boren J. Subendothelial lipoprotein retention as the initiating process in atherosclerosis – Update and therapeutic implications. Circulation 2007;116:1832-1844.

[5] Hofnagel O, Luechtenborg B, Eschert H, *et al.* Pravastatin inhibits expression of lectin-like oxidized low-density lipoproten receptor-1 (LOX-1) in watanabe Heritable Hyperlipemic rabbits. Arterioscler Thromb Vasc Biol 2006;26:604-610.

[6] Rikitake Y, Kawashima S, Takeshita S, *et al.* Anti-oxidative properties of fluvastatin, an HMG-CoA reductase inhibitor, contribute to prevention of atherosclerosis in cholesterol-fed rabbits. Atherosclerosis 2001;154:87-96.

[7] Kennedy JA, Hua X, Mishra K, *et al.* Inhibition of calcifying nodule formation in cultured porcine aortic valve cells by nitric oxide donors. Eur J Pharmacol 2009;602:28-35.

[8] Wu B, Elmariah S, Kaplan FS, *et al.* Paradoxical Effects of Statins on Aortic Valve Myofibroblasts and Osteoblasts Implications for End-Stage Valvular Heart Disease. Arteriscl Thromb Vasc Biol 2005;25:592-597.

[9] Rajamannan NM, Subramaniam M, Stock SR, *et al.* Atorvastatin inhibits calcification and enhances nitric oxide synthase production in the hypercholesterolaemic aortic valve. Heart 2005 91:806-10.

[10] Veinot JP. Pathology of inflammatory native valvular heart disease. Cardiovasc Pathol 2006;15:243-251.

[11] Rabus MB, Kayaler N, Sareyyüpoglu B, *et al.* Hypercholesterolemia Association with Aortic Stenosis of Various Etiologies. J Card Surg 2009;24:146-150.

[12] Antonini-Canterin F, Leiballi, Enache R, *et al.* Hydroxymethylglutaryl Coenzyme-A Reductase Inhibitors Delay the Progression of Rheumatic Aortic Valve Stenosis. J Am Coll Cardiol 2009;53:1874-1879.

[13] Matsumoto Y, Adams V, Walther C, *et al.* Reduced number and function of endothelialprogenitor cells in patients with aortic valve stenosis: a novel concept for valvular endothelial cell repair. Eur Heart J 2009;30:346-355.

[14] Osman L, Yacoub MH, Latif N, *et al.* Role of Human Valve Interstitial Cells in Valve Calcification and Their Response to Atorvastatin. Circulation 2006;114:I547-I552.

[15] Newby DE, Cowell SJ, Boon NA. Emerging medical treatments for aortic stenosis: statins, angiotensin converting enzyme inhibitors, or both? Heart 2006;92:729-734.

[16] Anger T, Carson W, Weygand M, *et al.* Atherosclerotic inflammation triggers osteogenic bone transformation in calcified and stenotic human aortic valves: Still a matter of debate. Exp Molec Pathol 2009;86:10-17.

[17] O'Brien KD, Shavelle DM, Caulfield MT, *et al.* Association of Angiotensin-Converting Enzyme With Low-Density Lipoprotein in Aortic Valvular Lesions and in Human Plasma. Circulation 2002;106:2224-2230.

[18] Yetkin E, Waltenberger J. Molecular and cellular mechanisms of aortic stenosis. Int J Cardiology 2009;135:4-13.

[19] Chan KL, Teo K, Tam J, Dumesnil JG, for the Astronomer Investigators. Rationale, design, and baseline characteristics of a randomized trial to assess the effect of cholesterol lowering on the progression of aortic stenosis: The Aortic Stenosis Progression Observation: Measuring Effects of Rosuvastatin [ASTRONOMER] trial. Am Heart J 2007;153:925-231.

[20] Fang M, Wang T, Li J, Li X. Letter to the editor. Statins therapy for calcific aortic valve disease: Yes, but not all. Medical Hypotheses 2010;75:131-138.

[21] Hermans H, Herijgers P, Holvoet P, *et al.* Statins for Calcific Aortic Valve Stenosis: Into Oblivion After SALTIRE and SEAS? An Extensive Review from Bench to Bedside. Curr Probl Cardiol 2010;35:284-306.

[22] Heistad D, Wakisaka Y, Miller J, *et al.* Novel Aspects of Oxidative Stress in Cardiovascular Diseases. Circ J 2009; 73: 201-207.

[23] Kitahara M, Kanaki T, Ishii I, Saito Y. Atherosclerosis induced by chronic inhibition of the synthesis of nitric oxide in moderately hypercholesterolemic rabbits is suppressed by pivastatin. Br J Pharmacol 2010;159:1418-1428.

[24] Shiomi M, Ito T, Hirouchi Y, Enomoto M. Fibromuscular cap composition is important for the stability of established atherosclerotic plaques in mature WHHL rabbits treated with statins. Atherosclerosis 2001;157:75-84.

[25] Fukumoto Y, Libby P, Rabkin E, *et al.* Statins after smooth muscle cell accumulation and collagen content in established atheroma of Watanabe Heritable Hyperlipemic rabbits. Circulation 2001;103:993-999.

[26] Luan Z, Chase AJ, Newby AC. Statins inhibit secretion of metalloproteinases-1,-2,-3 and-9 from vascular smooth muscle cells and macrophages. Arterioscl Thromb Vasc Biol 2003;23:769-755.

[27] Van Nieuw Amerongen GP, Vermeer MA, Nègre-Aminou P, *et al.* Simvastatin improves disturbed endothelial barrier function. Circulation 2000;102:2803-2809.

[28] Lin SJ, Hsieh FY, Chen YH, *et al.* Atorvastatin induces thrombomodulin expression in the aorta of cholesterol-fed rabbits in TNF alpha-treated human aortic endothelial cells. Histol Histopathol 2009;24:1147-1159.

[29] Heeba G, Moselhy ME, Hassan M, *et al.* Anti-atherogenic effect of statins: role of nitric oxide, peroxynitrite and haem oxygenase-1. Br J Pharmacol 2009;156:1256-1266.

[30] Imanishi T, Ikejima H, Tsujioka A, *et al.* Combined effects of an 3-hydroxy-3-methylglutaryl coenzyme A reductase inhibitor and angiotensin II receptor antagonist on notric oxide bioavailability and atherosclerotic change in myocardial infarction-prone Watanabe heritable hyperlipemic rabbits. Hypertension Res 2008;31:1199-1208.

[31] Pereira EC, Bertolami MC, Faludi AA, *et al.* Effects of simvastatin and L-arginine on vasodilation, nitric oxide metabolites and endogenous NOS inhibitors in hypercholesterolemic subjects. Free Radical Research 2003;37:529-536.

[32] Shiomi M, Yamada S, Ito T. Atheroma stabilizing effects of simvastatin due to depression of macrophages or lipid accumulation in the atheromatous plaques of coronary plaque-prone WHHL rabbits. Atherosclerosis 2005;178:287-294.

[33] Hamilton AM, Boughner DR, Drangova M, Rogers KA. Statin treatement of hypercholesterolemic-induced aortic valve sclerosis. Cardiovascular Pathology 2011;20:84-92.

[34] Novaro GM, Tiong IY, Pearce GL, *et al.* Effect of hydroxymethylglutaryl coenzyme A reductase inhibitors on the progression of calcific aortic stenosis. Circulation 2001;104:2205-2209.

[35] Moura LM, Ramos SF, Zamorano JL, *et al.* Rosuvastatin affecting aortic valve endothelium to slow the progression of aortic stenosis. J Am Coll Cardiol 2007;49:554-561.

[36] Hermans H, Herijgers P, Holvoet P, *et al.* Statins for Calcific Aortic Valve Stenosis: Into Oblivion After SALTIRE and SEAS? An Extensive Review from Bench to Bedside. Curr Probl Cardiol 2010;35:284-306.

[37] Ge H, Zhang Q, Wang BY, *et al.* Bone Modifiers and the Quest to Slow Progression of Aortic Stenosis. Therapeutic effect of statin on aortic stenosis: a review with meta-analysis. Am J Cardiol 2009;104:125-127.

[38] Takagi H, Kawai N, Umemoto T. Do statins delay the progression of aortic stenosis? J Thorac Cardiovasc Surg 2009;137:e6-9.

[39] Rajamannan NM. Calcific aortic stenosis: lessons learned from experimental and clinical studies. Arterioscl Thromb Vasc Biol 2009;29:162-168.

[40] Rossebø AB, Pedersen TR, Boman K, *et al.*, for the SEAS Investigators. Intensive Lipid Lowering with Simvastatin and Ezetimibe in Aortic Stenosis. N Engl J Med 2008;359:1343-1356.

[41] Rossebø AB, Pedersen TR, Allen C, *et al.* Design and Baseline Characteristics of the Simvastatin and Ezetimibe in Aortic Stenosis [SEAS] Study. Am J Cardiol 2007;99:970-973.

[42] Gerdts E, Rossebø AB, Pedersen TR, *et al.* Impact of Baseline Severity of Aortic Valve Stenosis on Effect of Intensive Lipid Lowering Therapy [from the SEAS Study]. Am J Cardiol 2010;106:1634-1639.

[43] Chan KL, Teo K, Dumesnil JG, *et al.*, for the ASTRONOMER Investigators. Effect of Lipid Lowering With Rosuvastatin on Progression of Aortic Stenosis Results of the Aortic Stenosis Progression Observation: Measuring Effects of Rosuvastatin Trial. Circulation. 2010;121:306-314.

[44] Singh N, Patel P, Wyckoff T, Augoustides JGT. Progress in perioperative medicine: Focus on statins. J Cardiothorac Vasc Anesth 2010;24:892-896.

[45] Wierzbicky AS, Viljoen A, Chambers JB. Aortic stenosis and lipids: oed intervention work? Curr Opinion Cardiol 2010;25:379-384.

[46] Kulik A, Masters RG, Bédard P, *et al.* Postoperative lipid-lowering therapy and bioprosthesis structural valve deterioration: justification for a randomised trial? Eur J Cardio-thorac Surg 2010;37:139-144.

[47] Simolin MA, Pedersen TX, Bro S, *et al.* ACE inhibition attenuates uremia-induced aortic valve thickening in a novel mouse model. BMC Cardiovasc Disorders 2009;9:10-19.

[48] Ngo DTM, Stafford I, Sverdlov AL, *et al.* Ramipril retards development of aortic valve stenosis in a rabbit model: mechanistic considerations. Br J Pharmacol 2011;162:722-732.

[49] Rosenhek R, Rader F, Loho N, *et al.* Statins, but not angiotensin-converting enzyme inhibitors delay progression of aortic stenosis. Circulation 2004;110:1291-1295.

[50] Kana W, Takeshi T, Yoshiro N, *et al.* Administration of angiotensin-converting enzyme inhibitors is associated with slow progression of mild aortic stenosis in Japanese patients. Heart Vess 2011;26:252-257.

[51] Shavelle DM. Calcific aortic valve disease: imaging studies and therapeutic interventions. J Invest Med 2007;55:292-298.

[52] Cawley PJ, Otto CM. Prevention of aortic valve stenosis: fact or fiction? Ann Med 2009;41:100-108.

[53] Peltonen T, Taskinen P, Näpänkangas J, *et al.* Increase in tissue endothelin-1 and ETA receptor levels in human aortic valve stenosis. Eur Heart J 2009;30:242-249.

[54] Skolnick AH, Osranek M, Formica P, Kronzon I. Osteoporosis Treatment and Progression of Aortic Stenosis. Am J Cardiol 2009;104:122-124.

Send Orders of Reprints at bspsaif@emirates.net.ae

CHAPTER 4

Imaging in CAVS

Abstract: The evaluation of the aortic valve can be performed in several ways.

The main imaging techniques for heart valves are:

- Doppler-echocardiography.
- Catheter based investigation.
- Computer tomography.
- MRI-MRA.

Each of these techniques has its advantages and drawbacks.

Trans thoracic echocardiography or TTE remains the standard imaging technique. It is widely used due to its availability, low cost, non-invasive character and low radiation burden. Several modalities exists. Drawbacks of the technique are the operator dependency, difficult imaging in patients with obesity and in cases with extensive calcification. Trans-esophageal echocardiography or TEE might offer better imaging, but the technique is invasive.

The description of the valve, and calculation of hemodynamic parameters such as jet velocity, mean TVG and AVA are the important parameters to estimate the severity of CAVS. For some of thes parameters, the continuity equation can be used. These parameters allow the categorization of the severity of CAVS. Each of these parameter has its advantages and drawbacks. Flow dependency is an important issue to deal with.

In asymptomatic patients, it is useful to assess the rate of progress of CAVS. This can give an indication when AVR for a given patien might become necessary. Assessment of the LVF and LVM are also important parameters to take into account.

Catheter examination has the advantage of direct measurement of TVG. The technique is invasive and can be recommended when echocardiographic data are inconclusive or are in conflict with clinical data. Usually, there is good correlation with echocardiographic data. If the presence of CAD is suspected, coronarygraphy should be performed.

CT and CMR are valuable adjuncts in the assessment of AVA. CT also allows the scoring of the calcium load, which is an important indicator for the severity of CAVS. CMR allows the flow mapping and imaging of the LV.

Wilhelm Peter Mistiaen

Keywords: Aortic valve area, arterio-valvular impedance, calcification, cardio CT, cardio MR, catheterization, Doppler duplex, echocardiography, jet velocity, left ventricular diameter, left ventricular function, left ventricular mass, low flow low gradient, transvalvular gradient.

1. DOPPLER ECHOCARDIOGRAPHY

Auscultation is the first method to diagnose an aortic valve disease. A systolic murmur at the right second intercostal space is indicative, especially when it becomes louder while the patient is in sitting position and when the murmur propagates to the carotid arteries. Echocardiography serves as confirmation of CAVS [1]. TTE is most easily to use, but if it is necessary, TEE can serve as alternative. TEE is an invasive technique, but it provides similar results for measurements of the LVOT [2]. The classic views for TTE are the left lateral, long and short axis. Parasternal, apical and subcostal windows can be used [3, 4]. Motion or M-mode can be used to measure and calculate LV dimensions, LV wall thickness, LVM and LVMI [4].

The two most common types of Doppler Ultrasound transducers are Continuous Wave Doppler and Pulsed-Wave Doppler.

With the **Continuous Wave Doppler** technique, two crystals are necessary. One crystal sends the echoes, the other receives them, thereby detecting the shifts. An audible sound is created and recorded by either an analog recorder or spectral analyzer. Spectral analysis separates the signal into individual components and assigns a relative importance to each component. Normally, Fast Fourier Transformation is the preferred method of analysis. The technique shows the Velocity Time Integral or VTI curves and measures the height of the velocity. It provides no anatomical information. The benefits of Continuous Wave Doppler include high sensitivity for low velocities and detection of high velocities without aliasing. On the other hand, Continuous Wave Doppler cannot distinguish between the sending and receiving signals or extraneous echoes. Nor does this technique produce a precise image like Pulsed Wave Doppler.

The **Pulse Wave Doppler** can be combined with Duplex to produce images of cardiac structures. The Pulse Wave Doppler uses a pulsed echo system that is discriminating in its range. The Pulse Wave transducer both sends and receives the signal. It sends echo's in short bursts and receives signals during the time when it is not sending. The returned signal is gated in such a way that only information about the desired depth within the body is transmitted.

Duplex is a term used to describe the scanning device in most Pulse Wave Doppler systems. There are various types of scanners including mechanical sector, electronically steered scanner, electronically steered linear array, and linear array with offset. Duplex can be used with both Pulse Wave and Continuous Wave if the former is used first to find the shift location and the latter used subsequently. This is a check to guarantee that the shift detected with Pulse Wave is the highest over the entire anatomy.

With **Color Flow Duplex**, the evaluation of blood flow patterns has become much easier. This devices shows velocity and direction of blood flows by combining conventional imaging with Doppler and color. The color relates to direction of flow while the color intensity shows the velocity strength. Linear or phased array transducers analyze the signal by amplitude, phase, and frequency. Phase changes describe direction and presence of motion, hence only structures that move produce a phase shift. Frequency shift describes the velocity of motion and is depicted with varying color intensities. Objects that do not move are gray with the shade, depending on the strength of the signal.

The advantages of TTE are clear: the technique is non-invasive and there is no radiation burden. It is a first choice for diagnosing and follow-up of valvular heart disease. It has a low cost and is the gold standard in imaging of valves, great vessels, atria and ventricles [3, 5-7].

There are, however, some disadvantages: the results are not always reproducible and the technique is operator dependent. Images are more difficult to obtain in poor acoustic windows, especially in obese patients [3] or in patients with tachycardia and irregular heart rhythm [8]. TEE is an improvement but this is an invasive approach. The interpretation of the echocardiographic results requires always integration with clinical data [8], especially in difficult situations such as LFLG and doubtful symptoms in elderly patients.

There are several parameters that should be determined by TTE or TEE:

1.1. The Aortic Valve Itself

The standard diagnostic parameters for patients with CAVS include [5, 8, 9]:

- Degree of calcification.
- Mobility of the leaflets.
- Jet velocity.
- Mean TVG.
- AVA (measured by continuity equation).
- LV dimensions.
- LVF and LVEF.
- Aortic diameter.
- Mitral valve morphology and function.
- Right ventricular size.
- Pulmonary artery pressure.

1.1.1. Description of the Valve

This includes the morphology and function of the cusps: the number (two cusps in patients with a bicuspid aortic valve), the degree of calcification and the mobility. The results can be combined for scoring. Parasternal, subcostal an apical images are useful [5, 8, 9].

The **degree of calcification** can also be quantified to some degree [5]:

1) No calcification or increased reflectivity.
2) Localized area of increased reflectivity but no areas of dense calcification.

3) Markedly increased reflectivity or calcification in 1 leaflet but equal to or less than grade 2 changes in other leaflets.

4) Markedly increased reflectivity in 2 leaflets but equal to or less than grade 2 changes in the third leaflet.

5) Moderately increased reflectivity in all leaflets.

6) Severely increased reflectivity in all leaflets.

Leaflet mobility can be graded as follows [5]:

1) Normal leaflet mobility.

2) Restriction of only 1 leaflet with normal mobility of the other leaflets or mild restriction of all leaflets.

3) Marked restriction of 2 leaflets or moderate restriction of all leaflets.

4) Almost no mobility of any leaflet.

1.1.2. Jet Velocity

This parameter can be determined by continuous wave Doppler ultrasound with multiple windows [4, 5, 8]. The concept is simple: with a stenosis, the flow velocity increases, as water through a channel, when it flows through a narrowing.

The advantages are obvious:

1) The increment in velocity is directly measurable.

2) It has a strong predictive value for the outcome of CAVS.

There are also some limitations:

1) The measurement is flow dependent.

2) The values are position dependent: the direction of flow and ultrasound beam must be as parallel as possible; mal-alignment of 15°

results in an underestimation of 5% of the velocity, but this can be considered as acceptable.

The outer edge of the signal is used for the measurement of the VTI and mean TVG.

The shape of the curve is also useful: with more severe CAVS, the curve is more round and the maximum velocity occurs later during the systole. If there is a concavity, this indicates a dynamic subaortic stenosis. This could be due to excessive septal hypertrophy and hypertrophic obstructive cardiomyopathy.

1.1.3. Mean TVG [4, 5, 8]

This concept is more difficult: mean TVG can be calculated from velocity by the modified Bernoulli equation. It is the average difference between the pressure in the LV and the aorta during systole. Its calculation requires averaging of instantaneous gradients, not the calculation of the mean velocity.

This parameter has the advantage to be reliable and close to catheter based results. It needs to be determined at the level of the aortic valve.

There are some limitations, however:

1) The measurement is flow dependent: the lower the flow, the lower TVG. Stroke volume and systolic ejection time, myocardial contractility and the aortic systolic pressure have an effect. Hence, TVG can change from beat to beat [7].

2) The results are sensitive to mal-alignment and to the presence of mitral valve regurgitation.

3) Since the relationship between velocity and TVG is a square one, there is a risk for greater underestimation than with the determination of the velocity.

4) The peak LV and peak aortic pressure do not occur simultaneously. Hence the difference between those two values is less than the maximal instantaneous pressure difference.

5) There is another source for underestimation: the pressure recovery distal to the stenosis. This is caused by the conversion of kinetic energy into potential energy by the decrease in velocity. The result is an increase in pressure and thus an underestimation of TVG. Turbulence limits this phenomenon but this pressure recovery is clinically relevant in small aortas [8]. Pressure recovery also alters measurements by catheters [10].

The peak TVG is calculated from peak velocity [8]. It occurs early in the systole, when the valve is not fully open. This is in contrast with the peak-to-peak measurement during cardiac catheterization, later in the systolic phase and with a fully open valve. These events makes the mean TVG more reliable than peak TVG [7].

1.1.4. AVA [4, 5, 8]

This concept is also complicated: the calculation of AVA is based on a) the continuity equation or b) the Gorlin equation. The principle of the continuity equation is based on the fact that, at both sides of the stenotic valve the rate of mass displacement of blood is the same, provided there are no shunts in between the two areas. In practical terms, the flow from the LVOT is compared to the flow at the level of the aortic valve.

The use of AVA as parameter has some advantages:

1) It depends less on the flow, but it is not completely independent.
2) AVA is measurable in nearly all patients.
3) It is useful in conditions with high as well as low flow.

Its use is limited by measurement errors of velocity and of the diameters of LVOT.

1.1.4.1. The Continuity Equation

The continuity equation states that the flow in one area must be the same is in the following area, provide there are no shunts in between these two areas.

Practically, the flow in the LVOT is compared to the flow at the level of the aortic valve [10].

Following measurements have to be made:

1) The cross sectional area of the LVOT, which has to be performed with great care.

2) The VTI in the LVOT by pulse wave Doppler.

Multiplication of both values gives the LV stroke volume. The AVA can be calculated by dividing the LV stroke volume by VTI.

VTI can be determined by continuous wave Doppler, at the aortic valve level. This method is well validated and reliable as predictor for the clinical outcome of CAVS.

There are some concerns, however. The AVA equals the product of LV outflow cross-sectional area and the ratio between the subaortic VTI and the aortic VTI [9, 11].

1) Due to "contraction of the flow", the effective orifice becomes smaller than the anatomical orifice. It is the former value that predicts the clinical outcome.

2) The AVA can change with changes in blood flow. This effect remains limited in patients with CAVS and normal LVF. In cases with poor LVF, the opening of the aortic cusps can be diminished, even if CAVS is not severe (See the Low-Flow-Low-Gradient conundrum). In such cases, it is not the LVOT component of the continuity equation that alters.

3) As alternative for the use of LVOT cross-sectional area, which is less reliable, the velocity ratio of LVOT and aortic valve can be used. For example, if this is 0.25, AVA has reduced to 25% of its value.

4) Another alternative is AVA planimetry during systole, when the valve is open. But this is unreliable due to shadows caused by extensive

calcification [8]. It has not become the mainstream in measurement of the orifice area [10].

The LVOT can be measured during mid-systole, 4 or 5 mm distally from the aortic annulus, with a parasternal long-axis view [5]. If LVOT measurement is difficult, its diameter can be derived from a regression analysis, which involves BSA [12].

The LVOT can also be measured using 3D techniques, which improves the accuracy of the continuity equation. The intra and inter-observer variability is low in parasternal view. An apical approach is not recommended.

A dynamic change in hypertrophic obstructive cardiomyopathy has to be accounted for [13], which makes the diameter not uniform in such patients. The obstruction worsens in the second half of the systole [8]. Additional subvalvular LVOT obstruction needs to be recognized if it is present. Hence, the appropriate measures must be taken during AVR [14].

1.1.4.2. The Gorlin Formula

The Gorlin formula requires also several measurements:

1) The cardiac output (l/min).
2) The heart rate (beats/min).
3) The systolic ejection period (seconds/beat).

From these, the flow across the valve during every beat can be calculated as:

Cardiac output (l/min)/heart rate/systolic ejection period

The AVA equals the systolic flow across the aortic valve divided by the systolic pressure gradient and multiplied with a constant.

This technique has also disadvantages [13]:

1) The flow dependency: with a low flow, AVA calculation may erroneously be labeled as "stenotic".

2) The AVA determined with the Gorlin formula can be overestimated due to the pressure recovery.

The flow dependency of both methods have been confirmed by simultaneous catheter based measurements of pressure and flow [15].

1.1.5. Categorizing the Severity of CAVS

The decision to refer patients depends on the symptomatic status, but the severity of condition also plays a role, especially if co-morbid conditions are present, which makes the symptomatic status difficult to assess.

This requires measurements of maximum velocity, mean TVG and AVA, in conjunction with the symptomatic status and LVF [16, 17]. In some cases, additional measurement, such as velocity ratio values can be necessary. No single value should be relied upon for a therapeutic decision

A **severe CAVS** has:

- a jet velocity > 4.0 m/s.
- a median gradient > 40 (or 50) mm Hg.
- an AVA index of < 0.6 cm^2.
- and a velocity ratio < 0.25.

A **moderate CAVS** has:

- a jet velocity of 3.0 – 4.0 m/s.
- a median gradient 20 – 40 (or 30 – 50) mm Hg.
- an AVA index of 0.6 – 0.85 cm^2.
- and a velocity ratio 0.25 – 0.50.

A **mild CAVS** has:

- a jet velocity 2.6 – 2.9 m/s.

- a median gradient < 20 (or 30) mm Hg.

- an AVA index of > 0.85 cm².

- and a velocity ratio > 0.50.

An **aortic sclerosis** has a jet velocity of < 2.5 m/s.

A **normal aortic valve** has an AVA of 3.0 – 4.0 cm².

Indexing AVA and other values is controversial, since in obese patients, it does not necessarily reflect the reality. In small adults, indexing is important, however.

If an AVA is smaller or larger than expected for a given velocity or mean TVG, echographical values must be verified. In a next step, a high output state, LVF and severity of a co-existing aortic regurgitation must be evaluated [8, 9].

It is of vital importance to remind that AVA at rest does not always reflect the overload on the LV during daily activity [5].

Inconsistent grading of CAVS means that one parameter indicates a severe CAVS, while another parameter points to a mild-to-moderate valve disease in a patient with a normal LVEF. This is the case, for example in a patient with a small value for AVA, but a low TVG.

A plotting of AVA against mean TVG in patients with CAVS and a normal LVEF shows such inconsistencies in 30% of the patients: on the basis of AVA, CAVS has been diagnosed as severe while mean TVG indicated a mild-to-moderate condition [18].

This demonstrated that inconsistent grading of CAVS is frequent and could be due to:

- Discrepancy in cut-off values, meaning that an AVA of 1.0 cm² does not necessarily relate to a mean TVG of 40 mm Hg.

- A low flow, in spite of a normal LVEF, results in a lower TVG than could be expected on the basis of AVA.

A paradoxical low stroke volume, *i.e.* lower than 35 ml could be held responsible for such inconsistency. Such a low stroke volume occurrs more in specific patient groups with decreased LVEF, but still with a value still above 50%, and higher systemic vascular resistance [19].

The clinical relevance of a paradoxical low stroke volume in patients has been demonstrated by the reduced age and gender survival with either surgical or medical treatment. This has been documented in a retrospective way and in a rather small population. An cut-off value of LVEF of 50% in patients with CAVS and concentric LV remodeling could already reflect a decreased myocardial shortening, and hence be abnormal [19]. This abnormal LVEF, could on its turn be held responsible for a lower survival, since this has been determined as the most important predictor for long-term postoperative survival [20]. Therefore, a low flow should not be considered as unexpected or paradoxical in such patients.

Another pitfall in the diagnosis of a low flow is the use of the continuity equation for the calculation of AVA. For this parameter, the cross sectional area of the LVOT, as well as the stroke volume are needed. If the LVOT is assessed too low, stroke volume and AVA will be misleadingly small. A low-flow severe CAVS may be misdiagnosed [21].

Inconsistency in the grading of CAVS has also been observed with catheter investigations. AVA criteria, calculated by the Gorlin formula, would show a severe CAVS, while TVG criteria would not show this, even in presence of a normal flow [10, 18] or stroke volume [19]. However, inconsistency in grading occurs more frequently with echocardiography than with catheter investigation. The reason might be that the anatomical AVA, measured by catheter investigation or by planimetry is larger than the so-called effective AVA by Doppler. The reason is convergence of the flow, at a short distance and distal to the stenotic valve. Adjustment of the cut-off value of AVA determined by echocardiography might be necessary [18].

When there is any doubt concerning the severity of CAVS, LVOT size should be re-checked, since its measurement is critical for the determination of AVA and stroke volume. A TEE can be performed for this purpose. An exercise test might also be useful. The prognosis of patients with inconsistent values for CAVS is probably poor [19]. The indications for AVR are less well clear in such cases.

1.1.6. Identifying Rapid Progression of CAVS

An adequate estimation of the progression of CAVS in asymptomatic patients is vital for the planning and timing of AVR. Echocardiography is very useful to monitor this progression of CAVS. The measurement is non invasive and can be repeated often [22]. The increase of TVG or decrease of AVA can be measured. Furthermore, the degree of calcification, which is an important parameter for severity of CAVS can be estimated [5]. Rapid progression of CAVS – defined as an annual decrease in AVA of 0.1 cm^2 or more – can be detected by timely measurements.

Rapid progression of CAVS is more common in:

- Elderly.
- Male gender.
- Higher serum creatinin.
- Higher LVMI, documented on ECG as an increased QRS duration.

The only independent predictor for rapid progression of CAVS, however, is the degree of calcification. This predictor can be of assistance in the decision making for AVR in difficult cases. The degree of calcification and the mobility of the leaflets can both be used to calculate a score for the severity of CAVS. Although somehow arbitrary, extensive experience has been achieved in echocardiographic assessment of aortic leaflet pathology [5].

An additional measurement is the rate of change within one cardiac cycle. This gives information of the stiffness of the cusps and hence the degree of calcification. It is an additional measurement for severity of CAVS and has also been considered as a predictor for disease progression [23].

1.1.7. Imaging in Patients with Doubtful Symptoms

In presence of symptoms, severe CAVS is a clear indication for operation and is a Class I recommendation. Symptoms can sometimes be detected by exercise testing [10, 24]. This is the case in patients who deny their symptoms or fail to recognize them. Exercise induced hypotension and ventricular tachycardia are signs for poor outcome. These events might be indications for AVR [10].

A so-called prophylactic AVR (*i.e.* in patients without symptoms) can be performed if LVEF is below 50%, if the aortic root is dilated, or if moderate CAVS is present in patients referred for CABG. This is also a recommendation of Class I. In asymptomatic patients with maximal velocity jet over 5m/sec or with an expected rapid progression of CAVS or with an LV wall thicker than 15 mm, the indication for AVR is less clear, *i.e.* this is a recommendation of Class IIb [9].

There can be discrepancies between the measured values of aortic valve stenosis in patients with CAVS, which makes the decision making for AVR more difficult.

1) If the velocity is over 4 m/s and AVA is more than 1 cm^2, additional measurements are needed:

    a. LVOT diameters and LVOT velocity signal must be checked and be compared with previous studies, if possible.

    b. Furthermore, the AVAI should be calculated in small adults.

    c. Increased transvalvular flow as in co-existing aortic valve regurgitation and in high output states must also be excluded.

2) If the velocity is less than 4 m/s and AVA is less than 1 cm^2, following measurements also have to be made:

    d. The same procedures for LVOT measurements and for AVAI must be performed.

    e. Possible low trans-aortic flow volume must be ruled out.

    f. Mitral valve disease must also be excluded.

g. If the LVEF is less than 55%, the degree of valvular calcification must be measured and performance of a dobutamine stress echocardiography should be considered [8].

1.1.8. Additional Parameters to Estimate the Effects of CAVS

An additional parameter is the **valvulo-arterial impedance**, as measurement of the LV afterload [4]. This parameter is calculated by:

1) Adding systolic arterial pressure to the mean TVG, which results in the estimated LV systolic pressure.

2) Dividing this sum by stroke volume, indexed for the BSA.

The valvulo-arterial impedance represents the cost expressed in mm Hg for each systemic volume unit of blood, pumped by the LV during systole. This parameter is not difficult to calculate but must be indexed for the body size.

This parameter includes the reduced arterial compliance which occurs frequently in patients with CAVS and which adds to the load imposed on the LV. It is a marker for excessive LV load and a good predictor for the outcome of CVAS. It can be used for risk stratification and clinical decision making.

In this philosophy, CAVS is a part of a more complex disorder, which also includes a reduced vascular compliance and CAD, hypertension and alterations in LVF or cardiac output. Use of only "classical" parameters could lead to an underestimation of the severity of the load on the LV, whereby a "wait for symptoms attitude" could lead to an already irreversible decrease in LVF.

Calculation of the valvulo-arterial impedance, performance of a stress test and measurement of BNP can yield valuable additional parameters in patients with severe CAVS who claim to be asymptomatic. In patients with low gradient – low flow CAVS, calculation of this impedance can also be helpful to determine the load on the LV [25].

1.2. The Aortic Valve: Regurgitation

Aortic valve regurgitation can accompany CAVS, but usually this regurgitaion is mild to moderate. In patients with severe CAVS, flow rate, maximum velocity and TVG will be higher for any given AVA. For accurate clinical decision making, both stenosis and regurgitation need adequate quantification [8]. Aortic regurgitation can be graded by the jet area just proximal to the valve, on a scale from 0 to 4 [5]. A colour Doppler echocardiography is helpful [4].

A pure aortic valve regurgitation is beyond the scope of this manuscript.

1.3. The Mitral Valve

When the LV dilates, papillary muscles are displaced and the mitral valve can regurgitate by tenting. This is not a valvular but a ventricular problem, due to remodeling of the myocradium. The presence of this functional regurgitation requires an adequate description of LVF (systolic as well as diastolic), of LV size and of LV wall thickness. The severity of mitral regurgitation can affect the measurements of CAVS in two ways.

1) With low transaortic flow, TVG is reduced, even in severe CAVS.

2) A high velocity mitral regurgitation jet can be mistaken for an aortic jet.

An adequate timing of the signals is crucial [8]. The severity of mitral regurgitation can be measured by a semi-quantitative approach, using the ratio of the mitral jet area to the left atrial area [5]. Such a dynamic mitral regurgitation is a marker for a poor prognosis [26].

Mitral annular calcification can be determined from the parasternal short axis and be graded by the amount of increased echo density [5]:

1) Small localized areas of calcification on the mitral ring.

2) Involvement less than ¼ of the circumference.

3) Between ¼ and ½ of the circumference.

4) Over ½ of the circumference.

1.4. The Ventricle

The ventricular wall consists of three layers: subepicardial longitudinal, midwall circumferential and subendocardial longitudinal.

Two aspects of the LV need to be studied with echocardiography: LVF and LVM.

The pulse Doppler technique is in practical use from 1980 and can be used to estimate LVF. It analyzes the flow of blood. Diastolic LVF can be estimated by [4, 27]:

- Early and late ventricular filling waves and their ratio.
- Isovolumetric relaxation time.
- Early filling wave peak velocity.
- Deceleration time.
- Flow analysis of pulmonary veins.

LVF can also be assessed by endocardial fractional shortening. This can be calculated as

(Diastolic LV internal diameter – endsystolic internal LV diameter)/

diastolic LV internal diameter

LVEF can be assessed in a comparable manner using the volumes, derived from the subendocardial layer.

The use of the internal diameters of the LV relies on the proximity of the midwall layer to the subendocardial layer. This assumption of proximity might not be true in patiens with concentric LV remodeling and concentric LVH. These conditions often occur in patients with CAVS. In such patients, the relative wall thickness (posterior wall thickness divided by LV diastolic diameter) often exceeds 0.43 and use of the subendocardial or internal parameters can lead to overestimation of LVEF.

Taking into account the midwall parameters assumes that the ratio of inner/outer myocardial shell remains constant throughout the cardiac cycle [28].

Calculation of midwall shortening needs the measurement of the LV internal diameter, interventricular septal and posterior wall thickness during systole as well as during diastole. These values can be used to estimate end-systolic stress as primary measure of myocardial afterload. Moreover, midwall shortening seemed to be a better predictor for major cardiovascular events than endocardial fractional shortening, at least in patients with hypertension and a high LVMI [29]. A severe CAVS is also associated more closely with a midwall shortening than endocardial fractional shortening [30].

Estimation of the LVF, systolic as well as diastolic, is an important factor in the evaluation of the severity of CAVS. In a normal functioning LV, a pressure can be built up and TVG is a reliable parameter for the severity of CAVS. With a poor LVF, TVG can remain low, even in presence of severe CAVS.

The tissue Doppler technique allows the estimation of myocardial displacement velocity during a cardiac cycle and is useful in stiff and less compliant ventricles with disturbed relaxation [27] as in LVH.

The LVF and LVEF can be calculated. The segmental contractility can be described. The thickness of the wall can be measured.

> For the female pattern, the ventricular cavity is usually small, with a thicker wall. There is a diastolic dysfunction, *i.e.* there is a decrease in relaxation. Peak LV pressure and LVEF are usually higher [31]. After AVR, there is a risk for intracavitary pressure gradient as a consequence of a mid-ventricular dynamic obstruction. However, compared to males, postoperative LVEF improvement is better.
>
> In males, the LV is usually dilated with thin walls. A reduced LVEF does not always indicate a poor LVF. The stroke volume is small and for a given AVA, jet velocity and TVG are smaller than expected. The continuity equation remains adequate [5, 8, 9].

The LV dimensions include LV diameters and end-diastolic thickness of the interventricular septum and posterior wall. LVMI can be calculated. According to previous criteria, LVH has been defined when LVMI is 104-110 g/m2 for women and 116-134 g/m2 for men. The LVEDV and LVESV have been measured from the apical two-and four-chamber views, and LVEF can be calculated [4, 5].

Four different LV geometric patterns can be distinguished [32]:

- Normal geometry, with normal LVMI and normal relative wall thickness.

- Concentric remodeling with normal LVMI and increased relative wall thickness.

- Eccentric LVH with increased LVMI and normal relative wall thickness.

- Concentric LVH with both increased LVMI and relative wall thickness.

Concentric LVH is the most common LV geometric pattern in patients with CAVS. This is also the case when arterial hypertension is present in these patients [33]. The degree of CAVS, the presence of hypertension and a decreased midwall shortening of the LV are independent predictors for LVH. Such a LVH is common in even mild CAVS [9, 34]. Age, BMI and LVEF are other independent variables for LVH [35].

LVH is usually considered as a compensatory response to a pressure overload and is expected to maintain a normal wall stress and LVF. According to the law of Laplace, the LV wall stress increases with LV pressure and decreases with LV wall thickness. In concentric LVH, the LVEF can be supra-normal. If, however LVH fails to reduce the LV wall stress, LVEF will drop. LVEF is strongly and inversely correlated with LV midwall stress [36].

LVEF also correlates with relative LV wall thickness and inversely with LVMI. The indexed AVA is also independently associated with LVEF. In patients with critical CAVS, LVH is associated with lower LVEF and a higher incidence of CHF. Hence LVMI is predictive for systolic LV dysfunction and for CHF. This is independent from the severity of CAVS [37]. LVH could be considered as a maladaptive response in such patients with CAVS.

The relationship between abnormal LV geometry and clinical outcome in asymptomatic patients with mild-to-moderate CAVS is still not clear. One needs to be aware that LVH is a consequence, not only of CAVS but also of AHT. This has to be taken into account for the postoperative evaluation of the regression of LVH and for its effect on postoperative survival.

In patients with asymptomatic severe CAVS, decision making for AVR can be difficult. Parameters such as low LVEF, low mid wall shortening and high LV wall stress are at risk for adverse events and could benefit from AVR, even before symptoms develop.

2. CATHETER EXAMINATION

Catheter examination has the advantage to measure directly TVG [7]. The technique is sometimes considered as the gold standard for the assessment of the severity of CAVS and can be used as a reference procedure for non-invasive methods [38]. Catheter examination can be indicated when echocardiographic results are inconclusive or are in conflict with clinical data [7, 39]. However, a full haemodynamic study with retrograde catheterisation of the aortic valve is no longer recommended if non-invasive assessment of the valve is completely adequate to assess valve hemodynamics [10].

Nevertheless, when a patient's history, the results of a physical examination, and echocardiographic measurements are inconsistent and leave doubt about the severity of CAVS, an invasive haemodynamic study remains important for the diagnosis [10].

Sometimes, a Doppler derived TVG overestimates the degree of CAVS, up to 29 mm Hg. This can be due to the pressure recovery phenomenon in small aortic roots, where the diameter of the STJ is less than 3.0 cm, and in patients with mild to moderate degree CAVS. This phenomenon occurs less in severe CAVS, but can still be present. The TVG observed on echocardiography does not include the pressure recovery. In contrast, the TVG measured by catheter examination does.

The latter is also clinically relevant and determines the overload on the LV. Although simultaneous measurement of TVG by echocardiography and by catheter examination shows good correlation, over or underestimation of the severity of CAVS is possible in both directions [40].

Other reasons for discrepancy between catheter based and echocardiographic results are:

- Mal-alignment of the ultrasound beam.
- Eccentric aortic jets.
- Interference by mitral regurgitation.
- Other technical factors [40].

Parameters that should be determined by catheter investigation are [7, 10].

1) TVG, or the average of the area between LV and aortic pressure curve: The gradient should be measured with one catheter within the cavity of the LV, the other in the proximal aorta.
2) Flow: The mean flow rate is calculated as stroke volume/systolic ejection period.
3) Cardiac output: The Fick method is preferable over thermodilution.
4) AVA: As calculated from TVG and flow.

There are some requirements for the measurements, for timing as well as for placement of the catheter tip. TVG in catheter examination should be determined 2-3 cm above the valve, distal from the location where pressure recovery occurs. With the Doppler technique, this at the level of the valve. As in Doppler-echocardiography, the TVG is dependent on the stroke volume [7].

All parameters must be determined throughout the systole. The aortic incisura seems a better marker for the end of the systole than the cross-over of aortic and ventricular pressure curves. The pressure gradient often reverses and the gradient will be overestimated and the systolic ejection period may be underestimated, with concurrent overestimation of the flow rate. Both errors may compensate for each other in some cases, but the final error in the quantification of CAVS might be clinically relevant [38].

When TVG is used as as parameter, a cut-off level as criterion for the severity of CAVS has to be determined. A level of 50 mm Hg has been proposed and has a positive predictive value of 90%. A lower limit for TVG with 90% negative predictive value has not been observed. Hence, a mean TVG of 50 mm Hg has been documented for a wide range of severity of CAVS. Therefore, calculation of AVA is necessary to estimate the degree of CAVS [41].

Indeed, TVG as sole parameter should be considered inadequate as determinant for hemodynamic severity of CAVS. In presence of a low cardiac output, TVG can also be low, even in patients with a severe CAVS. In contrast, in high output states, TVG rises, even if CAVS is mild-to-moderate.

In low output patients, it is necessary to measure cardiac output and to calculate AVA at rest and during exercise or during a dobutamine infusion. In cases were CAVS is not severe, AVA increases with the cardiac output. In patients with severe CAVS, AVA will increase only in a minor degree [39]. The use of the aortic incisura can be a valuable alternative in the determination of the systolic period during this test [38].

Catheter examination can be used to measure left atrial pressure. Contrast injection through the catheter can be used to determine LVF and LV sizes. Cardiac output can also be calculated [7].

The catheter technique allows visualization of the coronary arteries, the number, the place and the severity of stenosis [7]. CAD is highly prevalent in patients with CAVS [10, 22], especially in elderly. A prevalence of over 60% has been documented [42, 43]. The need for a concomitant CABG can be assessed.

Catheter examination is an invasive procedure with possible complications, such as a pseudo-aneurysm at the site of access (usually the femoral artery) and embolization of atheromatous plaques in the aortic arch. The latter could lead to ischemic cerebral events. Pulmonary oedema, cardiogenic shock, arrhythmias, ventricular perforation and sudden death have also been documented [7, 22]. Caution should be exercised with the use of contrast in patients with a decreased renal function.

3. CARDIAC COMPUTER TOMOGRAPHY

MDCT is useful in heart disease since it has a high spatial and temporal resolution, compared to TTE [3, 44, 45]. The ventricle, the valves and the coronary arteries can be investigated. CT scanning has the advantage of being non-invasive [3], but it carries a radiation burden.

3.1. Direct View of the Aortic Valve

The normal aortic valve, with its 3 thin cusps is easily visible on CT. Coronal planes as well as oblique planes through the cusps yields good images [3]. CT allows visualization of the valves in three dimensions. This makes a selection possible of the plane with the smallest AVA. Due to pressure recovery, the CT method might slightly overestimate the AVA compared to the results of the continuity equation but CT has high diagnostic performance for CAVS [46].

CT can visualize the anatomic orifice but produces no information comparable to the gradient on echocardiography. CT results are comparable with those of TTE for quantifying the calcification of the valve and of the aorta. TTE could serve as basis and remains most commonly used in practice. ECG gating allows evaluation of the valve motion and coaptation of the cusps at the end of the diastole and excursion at the end of the systole [3].

In CAVS, the leaflets are thickened and calcified. During the end systolic phase, excursion and orifice area, including its size and appearance, can be estimated. Planimetric assessment of the AVA by CT is comparable to that of echocardiography [3, 45]. The Agatston calcium score correlates with the transvalvular gradient [3]. Calcification can also be quantified with electron beam CT. This parameter correlates well with the severity of CAVS. This allows monitoring of the progression of the disease [6].

Two reconstruction techniques can be used in the determination of AVA. The slice thickness is 0.625 mm. and contrast is injected in two phases.

> In the double-oblique method, aortic valve reconstructions are derived from coronal images. Sagittal and coronal oblique views are defined in the AV's orthogonal plane.
>
> In the second method, AVA is measured from 2D curved multiplanar reconstructions. Three points are positioned in the ascending aorta and LVOT, representing the section start/end and an intermediate point. The software automatically detects the centreline and provides a "luminal" view of the pre-defined region. The luminal view plane with the smallest valve aperture is chosen to delineate AVA.

For both techniques, AVA measurement can be performed orthogonally to the axis of the aortic valve aperture at the site of smallest diameter. Orifice contour delineation can be performed manually with a digital calliper. There is an agreement with the measurements with TTE with a mean difference of 0.01 cm^2. TTE correlates well with both measurements and inter and intra-observer variability are acceptable [47].

3.2. Comparison in Determination of AVA

3.2.1. With TTE/TEE

Multi Slice CT is reliable in the assessment of AVA [45]. There has been an excellent inter-observer agreement for aortic stenosis and good agreement for aortic regurgitation. A high image quality with good differentiation between contrast and the calcified valve has also been the reason for low inter-observer variability [48].

CT examination permits visualization of the heart valves in 3 dimensions, allowing selection of a plane that demonstrates the smallest valve area. Compared to TTE, CT may slightly overestimate the effective AVA, determined by the continuity equation. This is probably due to pressure recovery. Cardiac CT exhibits a high diagnostic performance for detection of CAVS, with high sensitivity and specificity [44, 46].

The correlation between AVA determined by Dual Source CT, and the AVA calculated using Doppler TTE has been strong [48]. In a meta-analysis, the values for AVA obtained by MDCT have proved accurate, compared to the TTE method. The correlation between AVA measurements by CT and by TTE has been r = 1.45. The mean difference has been 0.03 +/-0.05 [49].

3.2.2. With Catheter Investigation

Most of the series with CT imaging have compared its results either to TTE or TEE. Few studies have used MRI or cardiac catheterization as the standard of reference. These series have included probably more patients with CAD. A close correlation between the results of Dual Source CT and of invasive catheterization has been documented. A small overestimation of the AVA using Dual Source CT has been observed. One explanation for the tendency toward greater AVA values using CT compared to cardiac catheterization might be that cardiac catheterization systematically underestimates the AVA. The reason might be the area occupied by the transvalvular-guided catheter, which is not included in the calculation of the AVA [48].

3.3. Temporal Resolution Capacity of CT

The temporal resolution of CT allows also imaging of valve motion and measurement of the valve area. Strong correlations between CT based results on the one hand and results obtained by TTE, TEE, CMR, as well as cardiac catheterization on the other hand have been observed in small cohorts. Current DSCT devices provide significantly greater temporal resolution compared to previous scanner generations. DSCT has demonstrated a high diagnostic accuracy with a lower influence of the heart rate on image quality. Modern CT devices enhance the accuracy of the evaluation of the valve function. The CT technique is time consuming, however. With the current generation of devices, temporal resolution allows the omission of beta blockers. This is an advantage since the use of this medication can be undesirable in patients with CAVS [48].

The changes of AVA within one cardiac cycle can also be estimated. On the basis of a left coronal oblique view of the LVOT, anatomically appropriate cross-sectional transversal data sets are exactly aligned with the plane of the valve. A slice thickness of 1 mm can be reconstructed without overlap, at every 5% of the R-R interval during the entire systole, from 0% to 45%. According to the dimension of the valve, the field of view can be individually fitted in every patient The AVA can manually be traced and be measured in the transverse planes which have been reconstructed during the entire systole. The smallest measurable AVA at every 5% of the R-R interval can be regarded as an effective AVA at that instant. Of all cardiac phases, the largest orifices has been defined as the effective AVA and taken as the true measure of the stenotic orifice [48].

3.4. Other CT Investigations than for the Aortic Valve

3.4.1. Left Ventricle

Size, wall thickness and wall motion can be observed using CT. Long axis, two chamber short and long axis are derived from planes from TTE. The LVEF can be calculated from the motion of the LV walls. The atrial size can also be evaluated [3].

3.4.2. Coronary Arteries

DSCT provides a significantly greater temporal resolution compared to previous scanner generations, which makes administration of beta-blockers unnecessary. Consequently, the modality provides high diagnostic accuracy for the detection of significant CAD even without the additional administration of beta blockers [48]. Coronary arteries can be visualized simultaneously with the aortic valve [45]. Conventional CT has not been used for this purpose, but an ECG gated CT for coronary arteries has been proven to be useful [3].

Both CT and CMR provide better anatomical information than echocardiography about the aorta. Both CT and CMR produce better estimations of the LVM than using 2D echocardiography [9].

4. CARDIAC MRI (CMR)

Cardiac MRI is a high quality imaging with great detail. The technique is non-invasive and does not depend on ionizing radiation. It allows segmental analysis of the contractility of the LV and thickness in several planes. MRI devices are not widespread however, and imaging techniques are time consuming. This limits its use. Valves, ventricles and blood flow (valvular velocity mapping) can be imaged and quantified [3, 5].

4.1. Quantification of AVA

Several previous studies have validated AVA planimetric assessment by CMR against TEE planimetry, TTE continuity equation, and catheterization based AVA calculations by the Gorlin formula. AVA measured by CMR and by TEE are strongly correlated, but CMR has a superior image quality [44]. Both CMR and TEE can perform the measurement of AVA with planimetry and with the use of the continuity equation. However, similar to TEE, AVA determined by CMR is larger by planimetry than by continuity equation. This is consistent with the observation that the anatomical maximum opening of a stenotic aortic valve is larger than the size of the functional vena contracta [51].

CMR can potentially quantify AVA in CAVS using a single-slice phase contrast acquisition at valve level. It resolves some problems of poor image quality, underestimation of jet velocity due to mal-alignment, dependency on the operator experience and difficulties in estimating the LVOT volume by TTE when the continuity equation is used. CMR can also measure flow volumes and flow velocity. Hence it is possible to use the VTI or the continuity equation to calculate AVA, but this requires accurate data.

However, CMR has been shown to underestimate aortic flow in turbulent high velocity jets. This underestimation worsens with increasing severity of CAVS. Agreement between AVA determined by CMR at the aortic valve level and AVA measured by echocardiography improves with a reduced echo time of 1.5 ms. However, flow measurements in the aortic valve are underestimated and 95% limits of agreement remain large [52].

Transvalvular peak velocities and VTI are underestimated compared to Doppler measurements. The need for identical beat to beat flow patterns, which is necessary for phase contrast may not always be true. AVA is also overestimated with CMR, probably more in cases of severe CAVS, which could be due to the underestimation of the VTI. The location of the slice may also have an influence. Locating the vena contracta with moving valve leaflets can be difficult. Long axis cine imaging can be used to plan for short axis planimetry and optimizing slice positioning. Breath hold, or breath free positioning may also have its importance [52].

4.2. Flow Measurements

For measurement of stroke volume by CMR, the LV has been imaged from apex to base with six equally spaced short axis slices and three orthogonal long axis slices orientated at 60° increments around the LV long axis. LV cines have been obtained by ECG triggering. Breath hold takes 1.5 seconds. For quantitative flow measurements, breath hold is 20 seconds. By improving hardware, echo time could be reduced from 2.79 to 1.5 ms. The flow could be calculated through the planes across the tip of the valve leaflets, 1 cm and 2.5 cm distally and also in the LVOT [52].

Short axis cine can be used for planimetry and for optimal position to measure the flow. The long axis image goes through the valve. The initial cine slice of 6 mm thickness can be positioned at the aortic valve at end-diastole using the paired long axis cines. When the moderately-to-severely calcified valve opens during systole, and moves down towards the apex, it descends through this slice. This slice is a useful initial position for obtaining cine images for planimetry of the limiting valve orifice [52].

The aortic valve flow can be measured at the vena contracta. The optimal short axis slice position for measurement of peak trans-valvular velocities is at the vena contracta just at or beyond the anatomic valve orifice during systole. Appropriate positioning can be confirmed by checking at the paired long axis cines, where the slice transects the proximal AS jet during mid systole. This transecting is located immediately above the aortic valve leaflets. Nevertheless, there is an underestimation of the flow volume and peak velocities at and beyond the aortic valve. Stroke volume determined by phase contrast does not correspond well with stroke volume with determined by CMR. Shortening of echo time has somehow been helpful [52].

Stroke volume measured beyond the stenotic valve has been underestimated by 20% to 30%. Prior to the narrowest point of the jet, at the vena contracta, the flow accelerates and converges. After the vena contracta, the flow decelerates and diverges. Since accelerations have a stabilizing effect on turbulence, this turbulence increases after the location of the vena contracta. Shortening of the echo time, will improve the results. Assessment of the stroke volume by phase contrast will also improve [52].

All these factors have their importance in distinguishing moderate from severe CAVS and hence, in clinical decision making. Despite erroneous flow data, it is possible to obtain values for peak velocities, VTI and/or AVA which correlate moderately well with Doppler echo. However, the Phase Contrast method does seem to systematically underestimate peak velocity and VTI by approximately 10% compared with Doppler echo. Direct planimetry of AVA might be the best current method in CMR. Tracing the orifice of the stenotic valve is critical, but the boundary can be difficult to estimate due to calcification and turbulence [52].

CMR provides the anatomic orifice area and can produce haemodynamic information from flow mapping. Both CT and CMR provide better anatomical information than echocardiography about the aorta. Both CT and CMR produce better estimations of LVM than using 2D echocardiography [9].

4.3. Ventricular Imaging

LVH remodeling due to CAVS can be studied using MRI. LV volume, LVM and their ratio can also be assessed. Cardiac MRI is accurate and reproducible as mean to validate ECG criteria. No geometrical assumptions have to be made and cardiac tissue is visible with a good contrast between the ventricle and the blood within. This makes calculation of LVM and LVMI possible [53]. Cardiac MRI can also be used to document the regression of LVH after AVR [50, 54].

Unlike echocardiography, CMR has no body habitus-related limitations and can thus be used to complement echocardiography. It is an especially good alternative for clinical follow-up in patients with valvular heart disease, as it allows accurate measurement of the valvular dysfunction and the related ventricular burden. It can also be used to study the physiological course of valvular dysfunction and the response to therapeutic interventions [55].

Cardiac MRI can evaluate LVF and LV dysfunction in several conditions that can accompany CAVS such as AMI. It can assess the presence of viable myocardium in areas of LV dysfunction, such as hibernation. Radionuclide tests, dobutamine echocardiography and PET scanning are alternatives [7]. Focal fibrosis can be documented by Gadolinium contrast-enhanced CMR in LVH in patients with CAVS. In a twelve segment model, location, extent and enhancement pattern in the myocardium can be imaged. Wall thickness can also be viewed. Such focal scarring can be observed in LVH in CAVS patients [56].

5. ADDENDUM I

5.1. Imaging During the TAVI Procedure

An adequate imaging is necessary for the assessment of the anatomical requirements and for the guidance of the transcatheter implantation procedure. Medical imaging includes [57]:

- Echocardiography: TTE, TEE:
    - Detection of thrombi in the heart.
    - Assessment of the mitral valve function, calcification of the anterior leaflet.
    - Estimation of LVH and of septal hypertrophy.
    - Estimation of LVEF.
    - Assessment of aortic diameters.
- Cardiac CT [57, 58]:
    - Estimation of LVEF.
    - Measurement of AVA (selection of prosthesis size) and assessment of calcification for exact placement of the device.
    - Diameter of the aortic root and of the ascending aorta.
    - Anatomy of the coronary orifices for the prevention of occlusion.

    - Angulation between aorta and annulus.
    - Disease in the aortic arch.

- Cardiac MRI:
    - Estimation of LVEF.
    - Diameter of the aortic root and of the ascending aorta, sinused of Valsalva and STJ.
    - Angulation between aorta and annulus.
    - Disease in the aortic arch.

- Catheter investigation, including fluoroscopy:
    - Estimation of LVEF.
    - Detection of CAD.

The choice of modalities is determined by the operator preference, imaging expertise and the co-morbidity of the patient. The involvement of TEE requires general anesthesia. The TEE probe should not interfere with fluoroscopic view [57].

Imaging techniques should be helpful in diagnosing hemodynamic instability during the procedure and in treating the cause. In decreasing order of occurrence, these complications are loss of cardiac output, ventricular fibrillation (induced by rapid pacing), myocardial infarction, aortic dissection, acute vascular injury and brady-arrhythmias requiring pacing.

With TEE, following conditions can be detected when acute and severe hypotension develops:

- AMI due to coronary occlusion, documented by regional wall motion abnormalities.

- Mitral valve dysfunction, seen on color Doppler.

- Prosthetic dysfunction.

- Hemorrhage, documented by collapse of the atrial wall due to hypovolemia.

- Trauma at several levels: aorta dissection, rupture with pericardial effusion, RV tamponade.

- Arrhythmias, in combination with ECG alterations.

- Stroke.

5.2. ADDENDUM II: Imaging in Prosthetic Valve Dysfunction

Prosthetic valve obstruction can be due to pannus and to PVT. Making the distinction is of paramount importance to determine the therapeutic strategy. Echocardiography with fluoroscopy shows a restricted opening of the valve leaflets and a reduced EOA. Doppler derived prosthetic TVG is an important parameter but there is a considerable variation in values among valves of the same size and an overlap between valves of different sizes. Information concerning the motion of valve leaflet (angulation on fluoroscopy) is necessary [59], especially since PVT can be "Doppler silent" [60]. There are several reasons for this:

- Flow in MHV is hardly impaired when only one of the leaflets is blocked; hence patients sometimes have few or no symptoms.

- Doppler investigation does not show the leaflets clearly.

- Prosthetic TVG is flow dependent.

- There is a pressure recovery phenomenon with a wide variation.

CT, with its high temporal and spatial resolution, has been recommended for the detection of pannus and its distinction with thrombi. Cineradiography remains, however, the standard for the detection of abnormal prosthetic valve movement. It is, however not able to detect the cause. TTE has artefacts resulting from the movements of the leaflets and has also a lower resolution. In difficult places such as the pivot guard in SJM prosthetic valves, CT is able to detect the pannus. Pannus, however, can be accompanied by PVT. For such difficult problems, refinement of diagnostic techniques is warranted [61].

MRI also allows visualization of cardiac structures and prosthetic valves, but avoids X-ray exposure. Its potential in detecting dysfunction of MHV still needs exploration. Phase contrast MRI does not show the valve leaflets but demonstrates clearly fluid velocities of normal, stenotic and prosthetic valves. The amount of motion produces changes can be mapped. As a results, pixel brightness correlates with spatial velocity. Since these parameters are comparable to those obtained with Doppler-echocardiography, the same limitations are applicable. A standard velocity profile can be produced by cardiac MRI. A velocity ratio between lateral and central values of more than 1 is indicative of malfunction of a MHV. This parameter is flow independent and no information concerning the flow in the LVOT is needed, in contrast to the continuity equation [60].

5.4. ADDENDUM III: Stroke Work Loss and Energy Loss Index as Parameters for Severity of CAVS

TVG and velocities may not always reflect the severity of CAVS adequately. With the so-called pressure recovery distal from the stenotic valve, kinetic energy is partially conversed into potential energy. The net TVG is lower than TVG measured just distally to the stenotic valve. This difference is usually not relevant. In patients with small aortas and mild to moderate CAVS, it may become clinically important however. Accuracy can be improved by corrections of TVG based on AVA, root area's and stroke work loss.

LV stroke work can be defined as:

Mean systolic TVG/mean systolic LV pressure

SWL has been defined as the ratio of the mean TVG/mean LV pressure and is a strong predictor of clinical outcome.

The ELI is calculated from AVA and the area of the aorta at the level of the STJ (in the equation labelled as A2) as:

$$ELI = (AVA \times A2)/(A2 - AVA)/BSA$$

This reflects the portion of the LV pressure-volume work at every heart beat that is lost due to the LVOT obstruction [62].

Use of both, SWL and ELI, avoid errors due to pressure recovery. However, they these only reflect the steady component of potential energy loss and do not account for kinetic energy, pulsatile flow, or vascular compliance.

Although AVA seems like the most straightforward way to evaluate disease severity, the actual extent of leaflet opening is difficult to measure in patients with CAVS due to increased leaflet stiffness without commissural fusion.

Early in the disease process, the valve leaflets are flexible: AVA increases with the ventricular contraction. This results in an increase in stroke volume with only a modest increase in velocity. When CAVS progresses, the stiff leaflets become fixed and AVA does not increase any more, despite an increase in volume flow across the valve. However, measurement of the dynamic change in AVA is challenging because it requires precise measurements at two flow rates, and the observed changes are close to the limits of measurement variability.

Valve flexibility also can be estimated from the variability in valve opening during a single systolic ejection period. Although conceptually sound, its clinical use is problematic due to measurement variability. More sophisticated approaches to evaluation of instantaneous AVA, flow rate, and TVG have provided insight into the dynamics of CAVS but are not clinically applicable. Compared with AVA, there is no clear advantage to the concept of valve resistance, and there are some concerns with the assumptions underlying this calculation.

Direct imaging of AVA is helpful only in an occasional individual because repeated reflections and shadowing due to valve calcification limit accuracy. Even with optimal images, EOA is not identical to anatomic orifice area, due to contraction of the flow stream as it passes through the orifice, particularly when the three-dimensional valve shape is more or less flat, as seen with CAVS [39, 63]

SWL expressed as a percentage is a better indicator of severity of CAVS than peak jet velocity, mean TVG, aortic valve resistance in elderly patients [64].

SWL also could serve as an indicator for the composite outcome of cardiac death and AVR. The SWL has yet to be studied as a potential indicator of outcome from AVR for CAVS [39]. A cut-off value for SWL at 25% or more, could identify patients with CAVS at risk for adverse outcome, especially if LVEF is lower than 45%. This is true for patients with and without symptoms [64]. SWL of 25% or more as parameter can be helpful for the decision making in asymptomatic patients with CAVS.

5.4. ADDENDUM IV: Coronary Flow Changes Due to CAVS

CAD and CAVS can exist together, especially in elderly patients, since these diseases share some common risk factors [10]. Up to 60% of the patients needing AVR also need CABG [42, 43]. The deleterious effects of CAVS and CAD on the LV are additive.

Predictors for CAD in echocardiography are wall motion abnormality at rest, hibernation and stunning [65]. The degree of valvular calcification in CAVS seems to be correlated with calcified and mixed coronary plaques in CAD, but not with non-calcified plaques. This correlation can be attributed to common risk factors for both diseases. [66].

Coronary reserve is reduced in patients with severe CAVS [67]. This reduction is related to the severity of CAVS [68]. It leads to symptoms of cardiac ischemia and leads to adverse outcome, even in the absence of CAD. Endothelial dysfunction is a possible mechanism [69]. Patients with aortic valve sclerosis have impaired endothelium-dependent, post-ischemic, flow-mediated dilation [70].

Reduced coronary perfusion pressure and increased myocardial metabolic demands can be held responsible for LV dysfunction. At an EOA of 1.0 cm^2, the coronary reserve is already markedly reduced. At an EOA of 0.5 to 0.6 cm^2, the coronary reserve is exhausted [71]. Coronary perfusion pressure is reduced, especially in the subendocardial region [71, 72]. The reduction of the systolic coronary perfusion is due to perivascular compression. The reduction of the diastolic coronary perfusion is due to changes in diastolic perfusion time, which is the primary contributor to the impairment of coronary microcirculation.

With the development of LVH, symptoms can be attributed to the reduction of the number of resistance vessels per unit weight of myocardium. Perimyocyte fibrosis in LVH may add to this reduction [67].

Coronary perfusion pressure improves soon after AVR and this improvement is sustained during long-term follow-up. Decreased wall stress, lower LV mean pressure and decrease of LVEDP allow better coronary perfusion during diastole [72]. Changes in diastolic perfusion time and AVA have a more profound effect on the improvement of coronary vasodilator reserve than regression of LVH after AVR. This could explain why anginal symptoms after AVR regress before LVH does. This improvement of coronary microcirculation could be involved in the re-remodelling of the LV after AVR [67, 72].

CONCLUSIONS

Estimating correctly the severity of CAVS has important therapeutic consequences. The standard method is TTE, which visualizes the valve and determines parameters such as flow velocity, TVG and AVA.

It is important, however, to avoid pitfalls such as the flow dependency when AVA is calculated.

Several other methods can be used, but the data can be inconclusive or conflicting.

TTE offers a better imaging quality but is invasive. Determination of the rate of change within one cardiac cycle is clinically sound but not routinely applied.

Cardiac catheter investigation might be useful and is certainly indicated when CAD is suspected, since it allows visualization of the coronary arteries by coronarography.

AVA can also be determined by CT or CMR. CT allows also scoring of the calcium load and CMR allow flow mapping and imaging of the LV.

ACKNOWLEDGEMENT

Declared none.

CONFLICT OF INTEREST

The author(s) confirm that this chapter content has no conflict of interest.

REFERENCES

[1] Iung B. Management of the elderly patient with aortic valve stenosis. Heart 2008;94;519-524.

[2] Shiran A, Adawi S, Ganaeem M, Asmer E. Accuracy and reproducibility of left ventricular outflow tract diameter measurement using transthoracic when compared with transesophageal echocardiography in systole and diastole. Eur J Echocardiogr 2009;10:319-324.

[3] Manghat E, Rachapalli V, Van Lingen R, *et al.* Imaging the heart valves using ECG-gated 64-detector row cardiac CT. Br J Radiol 2008;81:275-290.

[4] Delgado V, Tops LF, van Bommel RJ, *et al.* Strain analysis in patients with severe aortic stenosis and preserved left ventricular ejection fraction undergoing surgical valve replacement. Eur Heart J 2009. doi:10.1093/eurheartj/ehp351.

[5] Bahler RC, Desser DR, Finkelhor RS, *et al.* Factors Leading to Progression of Valvular Aortic Stenosis. Am J Cardiol 1999;84:1044–1048.

[6] Shavelle D, Budoff MJ, Buljubasic N, *et al.* Usefulness of Aortic Valve Calcium Scores by Electron Beam Computed Tomography as a Marker for Aortic Stenosis. Am J Cardiol 2003;92:349-353.

[7] Rajamannan NM, Bonow RM, Rahimtoola SH. Calcific aortic stenosis: an update. Nature Clinical Practice 2007;4:254-262.

[8] Baumgartner H, Hung J, Bermejo J, *et al.* Echocardiographic assessment of valve stenosis: EAE/ASE recommendations for clinical practice. Eur J Echocardiogr 2009;10:1-25.

[9] Chambers JB. Aortic stenosis. Eur J Echocardiogr 2009;10:i11-i19.

[10] Carabello BA, Paulus WJ. Aortic stenosis. Lancet 2009; 373: 956-966

[11] Burwash LG. Thomas DD, Sadahiro M, *et al.* Dependence of Gorlin formula and continuity equation valve area on transvalvular volume flow rate in valvular aortic stenosis. Circulation 2004;89:827-835.

[12] Leye M, Brochet E, Lepage L, *et al.* Size-adjusted left ventricular outflow tract diameter reference values: a safeguard for the evaluation of the severity of aortic stenosis. J Am Soc Echocardiogr 2009;22:445-451.

[13] Khaw AV, von Bardeleben RS, Strasser C, *et al.* Direct measurement of left ventricular outflow tract by transthoracic real-time 3D-echocardiography increases accuracy in assessment of aortic valve stenosis. Int J Cardiol 2009;136:64-71.

[14] Bach DS. Subvalvular left ventricular outflow obstruction for patients undergoing aortic valve replacement for aortic stenosis: echocardiographic recognition and identification of patients at risk. J Am Soc Echocardiogr 2005;18:1155-1162.

[15] Burwash LG, Pearlman AS, Kraft CD, *et al.* flow dependence of measures of aortic stenosis severity during exercise. J Am Coll Cardiol 1994;24:1342-1350.

[16] Bonow RO, Carabello BA, Kanu C, *et al.* ACC/AHA 2006 guidelines for the management of patients with valvular heart disease. Circulation 2006;114:e84-e231.

[17] Vahanian A, Baumgartner H, Bax J, *et al.* Guidelines on the management of valvular heart disease. The task force on the management of valvular heart disease of the European Society of Cardiology. Eur Heart J 2007;28:230-268.

[18] Minners J, Allgeier M, Gohlke-Bärwolf C, *et al.* Inconsistencies of echocardiographic criteria for the grading of aortic valve stenosis. Eur Heart J 2008;29:1043-1048.

[19] Hachicha Z, Dumesnil JG, Bogaty P, Pibarot P. Paradoxical low-flow low-gradient severe aortic stenosis despite preserved ejection fraction is associated with higher afterload and reduced survival. Circulation 2007;115:2856-2864.

[20] Mistiaen W, Van Cauwelaert Ph, Muylaert Ph, *et al.* Determinants of survival after aortic valve replacement as treatment for symptomatic aortic valve disease in elderly. J Heart valve Dis 2001;10:354-360

[21] Doddamani S, Bello R, Friedman MA, *et al.* Demostration of left ventricular outflow tract eccentricity by real time 3D echocardiography: implications for the determination of the aortic valve area. Echocardiography 2007;24:860-866.

[22] Fazal IA, Alfakih K, Wilcox RG, Walsh JT. Retrograde catheterisation *vs.* Doppler echocardiographic evaluation of aortic stenosis-A survey of contemporary UK practice. doi:10.1016/j.ijcard.2007.12.049.

[23] Lester SJ, McElhinney DB, Miller JP, *et al.* Rate of change in aortic valve area during a cardiac cycle can predict the rate of hemodynamic progression of aortic stenosis. Circulation 2000;101:1947-1952

[24] Leurent G, Donal E, de Place C, *et al.* Argument for a Doppler echocardiography during exercise is assessing asymptomatic patients with severe aortic stenosis. Eur J Echocardiogr 2009;10:69-73.

[25] Hachicha Z, Dumesnil JG, Pibarot P. Usefulness of the Valvuloarterial Impedance to Predict Adverse Outcome in Asymptomatic Aortic Stenosis. J Am Coll Cardiol 2009;54:1003-1011.

[26] Monin JL. Stress echo and valvular heart disease. Arch Malad Coeur Vaiss 2005;3:15-20.

[27] Danzmann LC, Bodanese LC, Köhler I, Torres MR. Left atrioventricular remodeling in the assessment of the left ventricle diastolic function in patients with heart failure: a review of the currently studied echocardiographic variables. Cardiovascular Ultrasound 2008;6:56 doi:10.1186/1476-7120-6-56.

[28] Shimizu G, Hirota Y, Kita Y, *et al.* Left ventricular midwall mechanics in systemic arterial hypertension. Myocardial function is depressed in pressure-overload hypertrophy. Circulation 1991;83:1676-1684.

[29] De Simone G, Devereux RB, Koren MJ, *et al.* Mid wall left ventricular mecahnics: an independent predictor of cardiovascular risk in arterial hypertension. Circulation 1996;93:259-265.

[30] Wachtell K, Gerdts E, Cramariuc D, *et al.* Systolic left ventricular dysfunction in patients with asymptomatic and mild aortic stenosis: the SEAS study. World Congress of Cardiology, 2-6 September 2006, Barcelona, Spain. Abstract P5544.

[31] Aurigemma GP, Silver KH, McLaughlin M, *et al.* Impact of chamber geometry and gender on left ventricular systolic function in patients > 60 years of age with aortic stenosis. Am J Cardiol 1994:74:794-798.

[32] Ganau A, Devereux RB, Roman MJ, *et al.* Patterns of left ventricular hypertrophy and geometric remodeling in essential hypertension. J Am Coll Cardiol 1992;19:1550-1558.

[33] Antonini-Canterin F, Hunag G, Cervesato E, *et al.* Symptomatic aortic stenosis. Does systemic hypertension play an additional role? Hypertension 2003;41:1268-1272.

[34] Cramariuc D, Rieck AE, Staal EM, *et al.* Factors influencing left ventricular structure and stress-corrected systolic function in men and women with asymptomatic aortic valve stenosis [a SEAS substudy]. Am J Cardiol 2008;101:510-515.

[35] Gerdts E, Cramariuc C, Rieck AE, *et al.* Left ventricular structure in different types of chronic pressure-overload [Abstract 3150]. Circulation 2006;144[suppl II]:666.

[36] Gunther S, Grossman W. Determinants of ventricular function in pressure-overload hypertrophy in Man. Circulation 1979;59:679-688.

[37] Kupari M, Turto H, Lommi J. Left ventricular hypertrophy in aortic valve stenosis: preventative or promotive of systolic dysfunction and heart failure? Eur Heart J 2005;26:1790-1976.

[38] Bermejo J, Rojo-Álvarez LJ, Antoranz JC, *et al.* Estimation of the End of Ejection in Aortic Stenosis: An Unreported Source of Error in the Invasive Assessment of Severity. Circulation. 2004;110:1114-1120.

[39] Weerasinghe A, Yusuf M, Athanasiou T, *et al.* Role of Transvalvular Gradient in Outcome From Valve Replacement for Aortic Stenosis. Ann Thorac Surg 2004;77:1266-1271.

[40] Parameswaran AC, Reisner D, Amanullah A. Discrepancy between Gradients Derived by Cardiac Catheterization and by Doppler Echocardiography in Aortic Stenosis: How Often Does Pressure Recovery Play a Role? Echocardiography: CV Ultrasound & Allied Tech 2009;26:1000-1005.

[41] Rajamannan NM, Gersh B, Bonow RO. Calcific Aortic stenosis: from bench to bedside – Emerging clinical and cellular concepts. Heart 2003;89:801-805.

[42] Mistiaen W, Vissers D. Risk factors for postoperative pulmonary complications after aortic valve replacement within the hospital: an observational study. Austr J Physiotherapy 2008; 54: 119-124.

[43] Mistiaen W, Van Cauwelaert P, Muylaert P, De Worm E. 1000 pericardial valves in aortic position: risk factors for postoperative acute renal function impairment in elderly. J Cardiovasc Surg 2009;50:233-237.

[44] Bruder O, Jochims M, Hunold P, *et al.* Comparison of Aortic Valve Area Measured by Magnetic Resonance Imaging and Dual-Source Computed Tomography. Acta Radiologica 2009. DOI 10.1080/02841850902902540

[45] Abdulla J, Sivertsen J, Kofoed KF, *et al.* Evaluation of aortic valve stenosis by cardiac multi-slice computed tomography compared with echography: a systematic review and meta-analysis. J Heart Valve Dis 2009;18:634-643.

[46] LaBounty TM, Glasofer S, Devereux RB, *et al.* Comparison of Cardiac Computed Tomographic Angiography to Transesophageal Echocardiography for Evaluation of Patients With Native Valvular Heart Disease. Am J Cardiol 2009;104:1421-1428.

[47] Leborgne L, Choplin Y, Renard C, *et al.* Quantification of aortic valve area with ECG-gated multi-detector spiral computed tomography in patients with aortic stenosis and comparison of two image analysis methods. doi:10.1016/j.ijcard.2008.03.095.

[48] Ropers D, Ropers U, Marwan M, *et al.* Comparison of Dual-Source Computed Tomography for the Quantification of the Aortic Valve Area in Patients With Aortic Stenosis *Versus* Transthoracic Echocardiography and Invasive Hemodynamic Assessment Am J Cardiol 2009;104:1561-1567.

[49] Shah RG, Novaro GM, Blandon RJ, *et al.* Aortic valve area: meta-analysis of diagnostic performance of multi-detector computed tomography for aortic valve area measurements as compared to transthoracic echocardiography. Int J Cardiovasc Imaging 2009;6:601-609.

[50] Gocol R, Jasinski M, Ulbrych P, *et al.* Assessment of postoperative remodelling of left ventricle in randomized trial comparing aortic stentless prosthesis and aortic stent prosthesis using cardiac magnetic resonance [CMR]. Kardiochirurgia I Torachirurgia Polska 2008;5:122-125.

[51] Pouleur AC, de Waroux JBL, Pasquet A, *et al.* Planimetric and continuity equation assessment of aortic valve area: Head to head comparison between cardiac magnetic resonance and echocardiography. J Magn Resonance Imag 2007;26:1436-1443.

[52] O'Brien KR, Gabriel RS, Greiser A, *et al.* Aortic valve stenotic area calculation from phase contrast cardiovascular magnetic resonance: the importance of short echo time. J Cardiovasc Magn Resonance 2009;11:49-61.

[53] Buchner S, Debl K, Haimerl J, *et al.* Electrocardiographic diagnosis of left ventricular hypertrophy in aortic valve disease: evaluation of ECG criteria by cardiovascular magnetic resonance. J Cardiovasc Magn Resonance 2009;11:18.

[54] Sensky PR, Loubani M, Keal RP, *et al.* Does the type of prosthesis influence early left ventricular mass regression after aortic valve replacement? Assessment with magnetic resonance imaging. Am Heart J 2003;146:e13.

[55] Koskenvuo JW, Jarvinen V, Parkka JP, *et al.* Cardiac magnetic resonance imaging in valvular heart disease. Clin Physiol Functional Imaging 2009;29:220-240.

[56] Debl K, Djavidani B, Buchner S, *et al.* Delayed hyperenhancement in magnetic resonsnace imaging of left ventricular hypertrophy caused by aortic stenosis and hypertrophic cardiomyopathy: visualization of focal fibrosis. Heart 2006;92:1447-1451.

[57] Chin D. Echocardiography for transcatheter aortic valve implantation. Eur J Echocardiography 2009;10:i21-29.

[58] Rivard AL, Bartel T, Bianco RW, *et al.* Evaluation of Aortic Root and Valve Calcifications by Multi-Detector Computed Tomography. J Heart Valve Dis 2009;18:662-670.

[59] Aoyagi S, Nishimi M, Kawano H, *et al.* Obstruction of St Jude medical valves in the aortic position: significance of a combination of cineradiography and echocardiography. J Thorac Cardiovasc Surg 2000;120:142-147.

[60] Smadi O, Fenech M, Hassan I, Kadem L. Flow through a defective mechanical heart valve: A steady flow analysis. Medical Engineering & Physics 2009;31:295-305.

[61] Teshima H, Hayashida N, Fukunaga S, *et al.* Usefulness of a Multidetector-Row Computed Tomography Scanner for Detecting Pannus Formation. Ann Thorac Surg 2004;77:523-526.

[62] Tobin JR Jr., Rahimtoola SH, Blundell PE, Swan HJC. Percentage of left ventricular stroke work loss. A simple hemodynamic concept for estimation of severity of valvular aortic stenosis. Circulation 1967;35:868-679.

[63] Otto CM. Valvular aortic stenosis – Disease severity and timing of intervention. J Am Coll Cardiol 2006;47:2141-2151.

[64] Bermejo J, Odreman R, Feijoo J, *et al.* Clinical efficacy of Doppler-echocardiographic indices of aortic valve stenosis: a comparative test-based analysis of outcome. J Am Coll Cardiol 2003;41:142-151.

[65] Chang SM, Hakeem A, Nagueh SF. Predicting clinically unrecognized coronary artery disease: use of two-dimensional echocardiography. Cardiovascular Ultrasound 2009, 7:10 doi:10.1186/1476-7120-7-10.

[66] Mahabadi AA, Bamberg F, Toepker M, *et al.* Association of aortic valve calcification to the presence, extent, and composition of coronary artery plaque burden: From the Rule Out Myocardial Infarction using Computer Assisted Tomography [ROMICAT] trial. Am Heart J 2009;158:562-568.

[67] Rajappan K, Rimoldi OE, Camici PG, *et al.* Functional Changes in Coronary Microcirculation After Valve Replacement in Patients With Aortic Stenosis Circulation 2003;107:3170-3175.

[68] Burwash IG, Lortie M, Pibarot P, *et al.* Myocardial blood flow with low-flow, low-grade aortic stenosis: differences between true and pseudo-severe aortic stenosis. Results from the multicentre TOPAS [Truly or Pseudo-Severe Aortic Stenosis] study. Heart 2008;94:1627-1633.

[69] Yetkin E, Waltenberger J. Molecular and cellular mechanisms of aortic stenosis. Int J Cardiology 2009;135:4-13.

[70] Parolari A, Loardi C, Mussoni L, *et al.* Review article. Nonrheumatic calcific aortic stenosis: an overview from basic science to pharmacological prevention. Eur J Cardio-thorac Surg 2009;35:493-504.

[71] Garcia D, Camici PG, Durand LG, *et al.* Impairment of coronary flow reserve in aortic stenosis. J Appl Physiology 2009;106:112-121.

[72] Miyagawa S, Masai T, Fukuda H, *et al.* Coronary microcirculatory dysfunction in aortic stenosis: myocardial contrast echocardiography study. Ann Thorac Surg 2009;87:715-719.

Send Orders of Reprints at bspsaif@emirates.net.ae
"Degenerative" Aortic Valve Stenosis, its Pathogenesis and Treatment, **2013, 125-141**

CHAPTER 5

Challenges for Imaging in CAVS

Abstract: In some patients with CAVS, it can be difficult to decide if referral of AVR is warranted. There are several reasons for this.

In the low flow – low gradient conundrum, a conventional parameter, such as AVA, is insufficient to distinguish a truly severe CAVS from pseudo-severe CAVS. Additional diagnostic procedures such as a stress-echocardiography can be necessary.

In patients referred for CABG, a mild to moderate CAVS might be detected coincidentally. Must this valve be replaced? To answer this question, the outcome of a concomitant AVR must be carefully balanced against the outcome of isolated CABG and the risk of a second cardiac operation on short or mid-term.

In elderly patients, especially in those with co-morbid conditions, it can be notoriously difficult to assess the symptomatic status and to ascertain the valvular origin of their symptoms. Nevertheless, this is of vital importance in the decision making for referral of AVR. A stress test can also be useful.

The rate of progression of CAVS varies widely. Nevertheless, it can be useful to identify asymptomatic patients with a rapid progressing CAVS. Once these patients become symptomatic, they will need an AVR and the symptomatic phase of the disease should be kept as short as possible. Conventional echocardiography might offer some clues.

The referral pattern is determined, not only by the severity of CAVS, but also by age, LVF and the presence of co-morbid conditions. Nevertheless, denial of AVR is not always appropriate.

Keywords: Age, aortic valve area, B-type natriuretic peptide, contractile reserve, EuroSCORE, guidelines, left ventricular function, low flow low gradient, stress echocardiography, symptomatic status, transvalvular gradient.

1. DEFINITIONS

A proper definition avoids confusion and allows the use of guidelines for the application of AVR in difficult situations. Underuse (patients to whom AVR is denied but still need it) and overuse (patients who receive AVR while not needing it) of this operation should be avoided.

However, even adherence to the ACC/AHA guidelines does not guarantee appropriate application of AVR. Some definitions need to be agreed upon

Wilhelm Peter Mistiaen

beforehand. Definitions of the severity of CAVS are repeated here for the sake of clarity. Guidelines from the ESC differ slightly from those of AHA/ACC.

A **severe CAVS** has:

- a jet velocity > 4.0 m/s.
- a median TVG > 40 or 50 mm Hg.
- an AVA index of < 0.6 cm^2.
- and a velocity ratio < 0.25.

A **moderate CAVS** has:

- a jet velocity of 3.0 – 4.0 m/s.
- a median TVG 20 – 40 or 30 – 50 mm Hg.
- an AVA index of 0.6 – 0.85 cm^2.
- and a velocity ratio 0.25 – 0.50.

A **mild CAVS** has:

- a jet velocity 2.6 – 2.9 m/s.
- a median TVG < 20 to 30 mm Hg.
- an AVA index of > 0.85 cm^2.
- and a velocity ratio > 0.50.

An **aortic valve sclerosis** has a jet velocity of < 2.5 m/s.

A **normal aortic valve** has an AVA of 3.0 – 4.0 cm^2.

Some other definitions also need to be added.

- Asymptomatic: this means being in NYHA functional class I, having no angina [1] and no syncope.

- Rapid progress of CAVS: annual decrease of AVA of 0.2 cm^2 or more [2].

2. THE LOW-FLOW LOW-GRADIENT (LFLG) CONUNDRUM

A part of CAVS patients has a LFLG problem. In case of severe CAVS, the LV cannot generate sufficient pressure to open the diseased valve, which has a relatively fixed AVA. One major reason for impaired LVEF is the co-existence of CAD. Another reason is the exhaustion of the left ventricle. Hence, the TVG and maximal velocity jet remain low, in spite of truly severe CAVS.

A small AVA, due to severe CAVS has to be differentiated from patients with a pseudo-severe CAVS. In these patients, the weakened LV is not capable of opening the aortic valve completely. This results in an overestimation of CAVS if AVA is used as sole parameter. The LFLG state results in a small AVA, seemingly qualifying for severe CAVS [3-6].

Usually, a LFLG conundrum can be suspected when the following combination is present:

- A LVEF below 35 or 40%.

- An AVA of less than 1cm^2.

- A mean TVG below 30 or 40 mmHg.

Severe and pseudo-severe CAVS cannot be distinguished by echocardiography at rest. The degree of calcification on CT might be helpful to solve this problem. This distinction between severe and pseudo-severe CAVS, however, is of major importance: patients with a true CAVS require AVR, patients with a pseudo-severe CAVS do not. On the contrary, the operative risk is much higher in patients with pseudo-severe CAVS [3-6].

Exercise echocardiography assesses the functional status of the patient, the symptoms, the LVF and the severity of CAVS. This test provides information about the exercise tolerance and hemodynamics [5], but it is not recommended in routine clinical decision making [7]. A stepwise increase in exercise can quantify the physiological response. This test can also be used to investigate the progress of CAVS [8, 9].

With a dobutamine infusion, myocardial contractility, cardiac output and blood flow increase [7, 10, 11]. Aortic velocity, mean TVG, AVA and LVEF have to be monitored at every incremental step.

1) With increase of cardiac output or stroke volume with at least 20%, a contractile reserve is present.

    a. If the mean TVG rises, or if AVA is relatively fixed (*i.e.* an increase with less than 0.3 cm^2 and a final value of less than 1.0 cm^2), CAVS is severe and AVR is indicated.

    b. If AVA reaches a value of over 1cm^2, the ventricle will push the aortic valve further open, the increase of TVG is limited and CAVS is not severe. In these patients, AVR is not beneficial [3-6].

2) If LVEF does not increase, there is no contractile reserve. In such patients, AVR carries a high risk anyway [7].

The effect of an abnormal left ventricular contractility on the test results has to be taken into account. A simple dichotomy is an oversimplification. The results of this test depend largely on how much the flow increases during dobutamine stimulation. This increment in flow varies considerably between patients. Therefore, changes in AVA and gradients need to be normalized against the flow increase. To overcome this limitation, a new echocardiographic parameter has been proposed: the projected AVA at a standardized normal flow rate. A projected AVA of less than 1.0 cm^2 is considered as an indicator of severe CAVS.

Side effects during stress echocardiography such as arrhythmias, ventricular fibrillation and asystole can occur in up to 20% in patients with pseudo-severe CAVS. Direct arrhythmic effect, ischemia and stimulation of mechanoreceptors can be responsible, especially if LVH co-exists. Low dose dobutamine and stage duration of 5 to 8 minutes, before progressing to the next stage, are required to avoid these side effects and to reach a steady state required for echocardiographic measurements [5].

The prognosis in patients with LFLG is poor. Referral for AVR of such patients is usually less frequent, compared to those with a normal gradient. Underestimating of the severity of CAVS might be one reason.

The operative mortality in these patients is high. Its predictors are:

- TVG of less than 20 mm Hg.
- Previous cardiac operations and
- Absence of a contractile reserve and
- Presence of CAD.

The long-term survival is also reduced. For long-term mortality, predictors are:

- Low mean TVG.
- High EuroSCORE.
- AF.
- Multi-vessel CAD.

Prior AMI also has an effect. Nevertheless, some benefit of AVR might be expected. A long-term survival of 49% at 5 years could be reached in some series [4]. AVR offers relief of the pressure overload on the ventricle, but postoperative VPPM must be avoided at any cost [6]!

With medical treatment, pressure overload caused by the calcified valve on a diseased ventricle persists and mortality is high [12].

3. MILD TO MODERATE CAVS IN CAD PATIENTS REFERRED FOR CABG

CAVS and CAD can co-exist since these conditions have comparable risk factors [6]. Up to 60% of patients with CAVS in whom concomitant CABG is needed, also have CAD [13, 14]. Conversely, a decision to add AVR to a CABG is challenging in patients, in whom a mild-to-moderate CAVS has coincidentally been detected, during diagnostic work-up for CAD. The outcome in terms of survival, QoL and complications of an unoperated CAVS must be balanced against the outcome, in terms of survival and short and long-term complications of AVR added to CABG [1].

Measurement of AVA and TVG can be helpful in the decision making. Performing AVR with CABG is of no advantage if AVA is over 1.50 cm^2 [6]. A mean TVG between 30 and 50mm Hg has been given a class IIa recommendation in favor of AVR by the ACC/AHA guidelines. For a TVG less than 30mm Hg, this is a class IIb recommendation, against performing AVR.

Age, however, should also play a role in the decision making. For a patient of 70 years, AVR could be recommended if peak TVG is over 25mm Hg. For a patient of 85, the cut-off level is set at 50mm Hg [15].

Reasons to perform AVR with CABG are:

- Reduction of the risk for sudden death; this risk, however, is also present in aortic valve sclerosis [9], which is, obviously no reason to perform AVR.

- Avoidance of a second operation, in case severe and symptomatic CAVS develops rapidly. This occurs in 75% of the patients within 5 years [9, 16].

- Improvement of long-term survival, especially when AVA is between 1.0 and 1.5 cm^2.

- Life expectancy exceeding the time needed to develop symptomatic CAVS, knowing that patients become older and usually become sicker when referred for a second operation.

The last reason implies identification of a rapidly progressing CAVS, which is not always easy since the rate of progression varies widely [6]. Indications for rapid progression are the degree of calcification, the low mobility of the cusps [15] and the baseline jet velocity [8, 9]. Ascertaining the valvular origin of symptoms can also be difficult in these patients.

Reasons for not associating AVR to CABG are:

- Higher 30 day mortality, but this view is not shared by all authors.
- Risk for long-term valve related complications, such as reoperation for PVT and PVE; this is in balance with the reoperation rate.
- In case of MHV, need of anticoagulant medication [15, 16].
- Life expectancy shorter than the time needed to develop symptomatic CAVS [6].

A previous CABG is not always considered as a risk for AVR, although the mortality for repeat operations in the past has been higher than that for a combined procedure [16].

Recently, the outcome in terms of mortality for both options seemed to approach both of them [15].

A repair or decalcification of the valve is not considered an option, since the results are disappointing and the procedure does not decrease the progress of CAVS [16].

4. ARE ASYMPTOMATIC ELDERLY PATIENTS WITH CAVS TRULY ASYMPTOMATIC?

4.1. Symptomatic Status and Indication for AVR

Symptoms of CAVS, such as dyspnea may develop slowly and many patients are unaware of subtle changes in exercise tolerance. These changes may be mistaken for consequences of "getting old" and of de-conditioning. Even a careful and detailed anamnesis might not be sufficient to expose these symptoms, since these patients tend to limit their physical activity slowly. Nevertheless, the symptomatic status is a cornerstone in the decision making for AVR. Exercise stress tests, which are contra-indicated in symptomatic patients, are useful here [5].

The risks of AVR and of medical treatment have to be balanced. The operative mortality after AVR is reported to be 1 to 2% in some centers, thereby approaching the risk (which is about 1% per year) for sudden death in patients with severe but asymptomatic CAVS. The postoperative morbidity, however, exceeds that of medical management for asymptomatic CAVS, since valve related complications can appear. Hence, one condition is transformed into another. This problem is particularly relevant in our aging Western populations [17].

The management of asymptomatic patients with severe CAVS needs further evaluation, since the use of AVR remains controversial [17].

There is conflicting evidence in favor of operating (a class II a recommendation) in the presence of:

- Systolic LV dysfunction.

- Abnormal response to a stress test (symptoms or signs on ECG) [1, 5, 17].

There is conflicting evidence in favor of not operating (a class IIb recommendation) in the presence of only:

- Ventricular tachycardia.

- Marked or excessive LVH.

- An AVA of 0.60 cm^2 [1, 18].

Co-morbid conditions in patients with asymptomatic CAVS could be considered as contra-indication for AVR.

4.2. Additional Testing

Additional diagnostic procedures can be performed. These include:

- A stress test.

- Catheter investigation.

- Plasma levels of BNP.

4.2.1. The Stress Test

In difficult cases, a stress test with echography can safely be performed in controlled conditions [1, 5, 17-19]. This diagnostic procedure has also been advised by ACC/AHA and ESC guidelines [5].

Predictors for future adverse events, related to CAVS are:

- Development of symptoms during the test.
- Drop in blood pressure of 20mm Hg or more.
- Electrocardiographic changes.
- Inadequate increase in cardiac output.
- Inadequate increase in AVA.
- Impaired LV contractility.

The symptomatic status in patients with CAVS might be related to the compliance of the valve. The stiffness of the cusps in rest is difficult to estimate, since the degree of calcification is poorly visualized on echocardiography. A compliant valve correlates with a negative exercise test and points to a better prognosis. This means there is a lower risk with medical treatment than for AVR. With severely calcified and stiff valves, cardiac output and LVEF during exercise will not adapt adequately, which allows attribution of unclear symptoms to CAVS. In such cases, an increase in TVG can be observed. In these patients, outcome of AVR is favorable compared to medical treatment of CAVS [5, 17, 18].

A stress test can be used for 1) risk stratification, 2) discernment between symptomatic and asymptomatic patients and 3) timing for AVR in asymptomatic patients with severe CAVS [17]. However, care has to be taken with so-called positive tests to attribute the results to an underlying CAVS, especially in patients who are not used to performing physical exercise [5]. Conversely, no patients with CAVS and a negative exercise stress test have experienced sudden death, according to the results of a large meta-analysis [17].

4.2.2. Catheter Investigation

Valvular resistance, SWL, valvulo-arterial impedance and ELI as hemodynamical indices do not seem to be able to replace transvalvular cardiac output as parameter in patients with CAVS [18].

If echocardiography is inconclusive for the severity of CAVS or for its effect on the LV, a catheter investigation can be performed. This method can also confirm the presence of CAD, if this is suspected [1].

4.2.3. B-type Natriuretic Peptide, BNP

The plasma level of BNP is another indicator for the prognosis in patients with CAVS. A high level of BNP is found in patients with:

- Symptomatic CAVS, compared to asymptomatic valve disease.
- CAD.
- Low LVEF.

A high level of BNP has been associated with a higher mortality. The predictive value of BNP can be improved if it is combined with the symptomatic status. A level of 100 picogram/ml could discriminate cardiac from non cardiac symptoms. However, elevated levels of BNP have also been found in asymptomatic patients.

An increase of BNP seems to be indicative for the development of symptoms within one year. Varying levels between 58 and 190 picogram/ml have been proposed as levels for cut-off. Lower levels are safe for follow-up, higher levels require exercise testing if symptoms are doubtful [20, 21].

5. DETECTION OF RAPIDLY PROGRESSING CAVS

The progression of a mild to moderate CAVS shows a wide range [2, 6]. In asymptomatic patients, it is important to predict the rate of progress, since this can identify patients who will need AVR soon. This predictive ability is of importance in patients referred for CABG and in whom a mild-to-moderate CAVS has been coincidentally detected.

The symptomatic phase of CAVS should be kept as short as possible for prognostic reasons. The average annual decrease of AVA is probably 0.1 cm^2, which can be compared to an annual increase of peak instantaneous TVG with 10mm Hg. There is, however no level for initial AVA that can be associated with a rapid progression of CAVS. Nevertheless, patients with rapid progressing CAVS usually have a larger initial AVA: these patients "have more to lose" [2].

In adults with asymptomatic CAVS, the rate of hemodynamic progression and of clinical outcome can be predicted by [9]:

- Jet velocity, especially if this is over 4.0 m/s.
- The rate of change in jet velocity measured by repeated echocardiography.

The change of AVA within one cardiac cycle could also be used as a parameter to predict the rate of progression of CAVS. In patients with CAVS, the aortic valve opens and closes more slowly. There is no relationship between the rate of change of AVA during ejection and the commonly used parameters for the severity of CAVS at a given moment (*e.g.* AVA determined at peak velocity).

This means that AVA measured at peak velocity in 2 different patients can mean 2 different things. If a valve opens more slowly, there is less time for the LV to eject blood at maximal opening and the burden on the LV increases. For the same AVA at peak velocity, the stenosis is worse. The rate of change of AVA in one cycle has been proposed as an estimation for the progress of CAVS [2].

In patients with asymptomatic CAVS and with an AVA of 0.9 cm^2 and maximum jet velocity of at least 2.5 m/sec, the AVA ratio can be calculated as:

AVA ratio = AVA mid deceleration/AVA mid acceleration

This parameter has a low intra and inter-observer variability. With a ratio of 1.25 or more, there is a three-fold increase for rapid progression of CAVS (*i.e.* an annual decrease of AVA at least 0.2 cm^2). This is especially the case when CAVS is mild, with an AVA at least 1.20 cm^2. The slower valve motion serves as an important parameter. It seems that more energy is required to start the opening of a valve than to further open an already moving valve. Valves with a slower rate of change during systole indicate a more serious CAVS.

With increasing thickening and calcification of the valve, the cusps may become completely immobile. The rate of change becomes zero. Therefore, the AVA ratio seems only useful if AVA is larger than 0.90 cm^2. In mild CAVS, the AVA ratio can be used as a continuous variable, in moderate CAVS (AVA between 0.90 and 1.20 cm^2) a cut-off value of 1.25 is recommended. The AVA rate can be helpful to determine how far asymptomatic patients with CAVS are from the point where AVA decreases dramatically. This point is related to a high risk of sudden death. It should, therefore, be predicted in an adequate way [2].

6. INAPPROPRIATE DENIAL OF AVR

There is a consensus to refer symptomatic patients with CAVS for AVR. Survival, as well as functional status improves with this operation [22]. In elderly, especially in those with low LVEF and presence of co-morbid conditions, this is less evident. These patients could have a higher postoperative morbidity and mortality rate. Nevertheless, one year survival after AVR in these patients is higher than that with medical treatment.

In a nationwide survey of cardiologists in a small West-European country, several referral patterns have been discerned [22]:

- Age oriented.
- Multivariate pattern: age + severity of CAVS + LVF.
- LVF oriented.
- AVA oriented.
- Type of hospital (more referral in university hospitals and in institutions with a department for cardiac surgery).

Other and partially overlapping reasons than above, mentioned for non-referral have been a:

- High operative risk.
- Underestimation of the severity of CAVS.
- High EuroSCORE.
- High age.

In some patients, the reasons for non-referral are unclear. In spite of ACC/AHA/ESC guidelines, lack of knowledge about symptoms, severity of disease and results of surgery seem to be more important reasons for non-referral. Interdisciplinary meetings between cardiologists and surgeons seem necessary to improve the referral practice [23].

Based on another study, which included 5001 patients, AVR has been denied in 33% of the elderly patients with symptomatic CAVS [1]. LVEF lower than 50%, age and neurological dysfunction have been the predictors significantly related to the decision to deny patients the option of AVR. For other co-morbid factors, such as the Charlson co-morbidity index, no relationship has been detected [1, 22].

There is a trend to offer such patients TAVI. Initial results seem encouraging: a comparison with AVR shows good results, at least for the short-term results. TAVI might be considered as an alternative for AVR in very old patients, but it remains to be seen if its indication can be expanded.

There is a change observable in surgical practice: octogenarians are operated upon with increasing success. A low LVEF is not always considered to be a major factor for early mortality [25]. With increasing age, preoperative co-morbid conditions are also on the rise. The effects of high age and co-morbid conditions on the postoperative results are not easy to untangle. It seems, however, that only non-cardiac postoperative complications have increased, while hospital mortality and cardiac events have not altered significantly [26].

Moreover, the EuroSCORE (logistic as well as additive) does not predict the risk of AVR in an adequate way, since this instrument was developed for use in CABG in the nineties of the twentieth century, and not for valve surgery. The STS score is usually half of the EuroSCORE in a given patient, and even this score overestimates the risk [22, 25].

Some additional remarks must be made:

1) Age is a predictor for poor outcome after AVR, but the survival of operated elderly is comparable to the survival of an aged and gender matched population: therefore, age is not a contra-indication for AVR in itself. Poor postoperative results can even be considered as a self fulfilling prophecy. Hence, age is a poor basis for decision making [22, 27].

2) Symptoms in elderly patients can be underestimated [22], even with focused anamnesis. Exercise testing can be needed.

3) LVF is a double-edged problem. Decreased LVF is also a predictor for decreased short and long-term survival. Nevertheless, LVEF below 30% is rare. Even then, patients with a truly severe CAVS can benefit from AVR since the dysfunctional LV is relieved from pressure overload.

4) In patients with a decreased LVEF, the severity of CAVS can be underestimated if a low gradient – low flow conundrum exists.

5) Co-morbid conditions have an impact on postoperative survival, but their impact has been smaller on decision making. Only neurological conditions had a real impact. EuroSCORE significantly overestimates the risk of AVR [22].

6) Clinically significant CAD is a reason for cardiac surgery. Hence it is a confounding factor in the decision making for AVR, since CAD and CAVS occur together in many patients.

7) Patient refusal is rarely mentioned as a factor [24], but has been estimated to be around 9% [22].

8) In 20% of the patients, the reason for non referral is unclear [22].

Decision making for AVR should be based on knowledge of these predictors for poor outcome. Clinical judgment in individual cases remains the most important instrument, however. There is no reliable method to identify patients that will have the greatest benefit from AVR [24]. Comparison of medically treated and surgically treated patients is not helpful in this matter because of a selection bias: both groups have different characteristics. Usually, patients with a real poor prognosis are left for medical treatment. Only historical series can provide some comparative data.

CONCLUSIONS

There are some difficult situations in the management of CAVS. Such cases need additional diagnostic procedures.

In the case of the LF-LG conundrum, a truly severe CAVS cannot be distinguished from a milder CAVS by AVA alone. In the latter, a weakened ventricle is not capable to open the affected aortic valve. A stress echocardiography might offer a solution for many patients with this problem.

A stress test can also be useful in patients whose symptoms are doubtful. This is true especially for elderly patients with co-morbid conditions and who avoid physical exercise for whatever reason. A stress test also helps to ascertain the valvular origin of these symptoms. Other diagnostic procedures, such as cardiac catheter investigation and determination of the plasma BNP level, add information, needed in the decision making.

In patients referred for CABG and in whom a mild to moderate CAVS has been detected, the outcome of concomitant AVR has to be balanced against the outcome of an isolated CABG and the risk of a second cardiac operation on short or mid-term. The mortality of a combined operation as well as for a second cardiac operation has decreased with the improvement of operative and postoperative care. Much depends on the balance between postoperative valve related events on the one hand, and the risk for morbidity or sudden death with an affected aortic valve left in its place on the other hand.

Closely related to this problem is the identification of patients in whom an asymptomatic CAVS will progress rapidly. Conventional parameters such as the degree of calcification, the mobility of leaflets and baseline values of jet velocity might offer a clue. The AVA ratio is also helpful in identifying patients with rapidly worsening CAVS, but this method does not seem easy to be used in daily practice.

In spite of all these diagnostic options, AVR is denied in too many patients who need this procedure. Several reasons have been identified. Age, LVF and co-morbidity are such reasons. Individual clinical judgment remains of utmost importance to identify those patients that will benefit from AVR.

ACKNOWLEDGEMENT

Declared none.

CONFLICT OF INTEREST

The author(s) confirm that this chapter content has no conflict of interest.

REFERENCES

[1] Iung B, Messika-Zeitoun D, Cachier A, *et al.* Actual management of patients with asymptomatic aortic valve disease: How practice fits with guidelines. Am Heart J 2007;153:696-703.

[2] Lester SJ, McElhinney DB, Miller JP, *et al.* Rate of Change in Aortic Valve Area During a Cardiac Cycle Can Predict the Rate of Hemodynamic Progression of Aortic Stenosis. Circulation 2000;101:1947-1952.

[3] Otto CM. Valvular aortic stenosis – Disease severity and timing of intervention. J Am Coll Cardiol 2006;47:2141-2151.

[4] Levy F, Laurent M, Monin JL, *et al.* Aortic Valve Replacement for Low-Flow/Low-Gradient Aortic Stenosis. Operative Risk Stratification and Long-Term Outcome: A European Multicenter Study. J Am Coll Cardiol 2008;51:1466–1472.

[5] Picano E, Pibarot P, Lancellotti P, *et al.* The Emerging Role of Exercise Testing and Stress Echocardiography in Valvular Heart Disease. J Am Coll Cardiol 2009;54:2251-2260.

[6] Carabello BA, Paulus WJ. Aortic stenosis. Lancet 2009; 373: 956-966.

[7] Baumgartner H, Hung J, Bermejo J, *et al.* Echocardiographic assessment of valve stenosis: EAE/ASE recommendations for clinical practice. Eur J Echocardiogr 2009;10:1-25.

[8] Otto CM, Pearlman AS, Kraft CD, *et al.* Physiological changes with maximal exercises in asymptomatic valvular aortic stenosis assessed by Doppler echocardiography. J Am Coll Cardiol 1992;20:1160-1167.

[9] Otto CM, Burwash IG, Leggett ME, *et al.* Prospective study of asymptomatic valvular aortic stenosis – Clinical, echocardiographic and exercise predictors of outcvome. Circulation 1997;95:2262-2270.

[10] Burwash LG, Pearlman AS, Kraft CD, *et al.* flow dependence of measures of aortic stenosis severity during exercise. J Am Coll Cardiol 1994;24:1342-1350.

[11] Khaw AV, von Bardeleben RS, Strasser C, *et al.* Direct measurement of left ventricular outflow tract by transthoracic real-time 3D-echocardiography increases accuracy in assessment of aortic valve stenosis. Int J Cardiol 2009;136:64-71.

[12] Kapoor R, Kapoor JR. Letter to the editor. Nature Clinical Practice 2009;373:2023.

[13] Mistiaen W, Vissers D. Risk factors for postoperative pulmonary complications after aortic valve replacement within the hospital: an observational study. Austr J Physiotherapy 2008;54: 119-124.

[14] Mistiaen W, Van Cauwelaert P, Muylaert P, De Worm E. 1000 pericardial valves in aortic position: risk factors for postoperative acute renal function impairment in elderly. J Cardiovasc Surg 2009;50:233-237.

[15] Sareyyupoglu B, Sundt TM III, Schaff HV, *et al.* Management of Mild Aortic Stenosis at the Time of Coronary Artery Bypass Surgery: Should the Valve Be Replaced? Ann Thorac Surg 2009;88:1224-1231.

[16] Ahmed AAM, Graham ANJ, Lovell D, O'Kane HO. Management of mild to moderate aortic valve disease during coronary artery bypass grafting. Eur J Cardio-thorac Surgery 2003;24:535-540.

[17] Rafique AM, Biner S, Ray I, *et al.* Meta-Analysis of Prognostic Value of Stress Testing in Patients With Asymptomatic Severe Aortic Stenosis. Am J Cardiol 2009;104:972-977.

[18] Leurent G, Donal E, de Place C, *et al.* Argument for a Doppler echocardiography during exercise in assessing asymptomatic patients with severe aortic stenosis. Eur J Echocardiogr 2009;10:69-73.

[19] Lafitte S, Perlant M, Reant P, *et al.* Impact of impaired myocardial deformations on exercise tolerance and prognosis in patients with asymptomatic aortic stenosis. Eur L Echocardiogr 2009;10:414-419.

[20] Nessmith MG, Fukuta H, Brucks S, Little WC. Usefulness of an Elevated B-Type Natriuretic Peptide in Predicting Survival in Patients With Aortic Stenosis Treated Without Surgery. Am J Cardiol 2005;96:1445-1448.

[21] Rajani R, Rimington H, Chambers J. B-Type natriuretic peptide and tissue Doppler for predicting symptoms on treadmill exercise in apparently asymptomatic aortic stenosis. J Heart Valve Dis 2009;18:565-571.

[22] Bouma BJ, van der Meulen JPH, van den Brink RBH, *et al.* Variability in treatment advice for elderly patients with aortic stenosis: a nationwide survey in the Netherlands. Heart 2001;85:196-201.

[23] van Geldorp MWA, van Gameren M, Kappetein AP, *et al.* Therapeutic decisions for patients with symptomatic severe aortic stenosis: room for improvement? Eur J Cardio-thorac Surg 2009;35: 953-959.

[24] Iung B, Cachier A, Baron G, *et al.* Decision-making in elderly patients with severe aortic stenosis: why are so many denied surgery? Eur Heart J 2005:26, 2714-2720.

[25] Antunes MJ. Therapeutic decisions for patients with symptomatic severe aortic stenosis. Much still to do! doi:10.1016/j.ejcts.2009.02.028.

[26] Mistiaen W, Van Cauwelaert P, Muylaert P, De Worm E. 1000 Carpentier-Edwards pericardial valves in aortic position: what changed in the last 20 years and what are the effects on hospital complications. J Heart Valve Dis 2007;16:417-422.

[27] Mistiaen W, Van Cauwelaert Ph, Muylaert Ph, *et al.* Risk factors and survival after aortic valve replacement in octogenarians. J Heart Valve Dis. 2004;13:538-544.

Send Orders of Reprints at bspsaif@emirates.net.ae

CHAPTER 6

Choice of A Valve Prosthesis

Abstract: Aortic valve replacement has been applied for over half a century. Two classes of devices have been developed: mechanical and biological valve prostheses. For biological devices, autografts, homografts and xenografts (porcine and pericardial) have been developed. For mechanical devices, cage ball, tilted disc and bi-leaflet valves have been designed.

For BHV, the main drawback is a limited durability, the main advantage is the low rate for TE events, which obviates the need for peroral anticoagulation. Age is a major determinant for durability. In contrast, MHV are very durable, but they require a life-long anticoagulation with all their side effects. The choice for a valve in each individual patients depends on several factors: age and life expectancy are the main factors.

In difficult situations, *i.e.* an age between 55 and 70 years, results of comparative studies might be helpful in the decision making. Comparison should include contemporary devices and techniques. Use of historical series are confounded by changes and improvements in peri and postoperative care. A RCT remains the gold standard, but these are few in numbers.

The only recent RCT did not change much: the outcome is still more dependent on patient related factors than on the type of the valve, except 1) for bleeding, which is more common with MHV and 2) for SVD, which is observed with BHV. These observations are hardly surprising.

Results for a twenty-year follow-up might be needed. The preference of physician and patients for the choice of a valve is important. The dilemma between anticoagulation related bleeding and SVD remains for the time being.

Keywords: Anticoagulation, autografts, biological heart valve prosthesis, bleeding, calcification, effective orifice area, homografts, mechanical heart valve prosthesis, mortality, stentless xenografts, structural valve degeneration, thrombembolism, transvalvular gradient, tissue engineered heart valves, valve prosthesis patient mismatch.

1. HISTORICAL PERSPECTIVES

The concept of heart valve prosthesis is the replacement of a diseased native valve, and hence to avoid the sequelae of the malfunctioning valve. The ideal valve prosthesis should have following qualities [1].

Wilhelm Peter Mistiaen

1) An excellent hemodynamics, similar to the native valve.

2) Lasts a life time.

3) Is free of SVD.

4) Requires no medical therapy such as anticoagulation.

Such a device is not yet available.

Early surgical treatment of CAVS has been decalcification of the cusps, but already in 1964, it has become clear that this technique is not adequate to relieve the aortic stenosis. Valve repair by implantation of artificial leaflets such as Teflon, also has been inadequate to resolve the problem. These leaflets have shown shrivelling, calcification and tearing at the suture lines. This has resulted in severe aortic regurgitation [2].

Surgical heart valve replacement has been performed for the first time only 50 years ago and is therefore relatively recent. Two major options whave been developed: mechanical and biological devices. A caged ball MHV has been the standard in the first decade after its introduction. Homografts and autografts (in the Ross procedure) have been introduced as BHV in the same era [1]. Both options have undergone further development and over 50 types of valves have become available in 2005 [3].

Currently, three types of MHV exist: caged ball, tilting disc and bi-leaflet. BHV also can be subdivided into several types [4, 5]:

- Autografts (the pulmonary valve is used in the Ross procedure).
- Homografts or allografts from human origin.
- Xenografts of animal origin.
  - Porcine aortic valves: stented or stentless.
  - Bovine pericardial tissue mounted on a stent.

- Tissue engineered heart valves.

All these types of valves differ with respect to hemodynamic effects and adverse events. For MHV, these adverse events are PVT and TE. For BHV, the problem is is mainly durability. Even in one class of valves, differences in rates for adverse events can be observed [5].

A major issue is to decide which valve is most fitting for an individual patient. For this reason, the different types of valves are described. Comparing the different types of BHV and MHV requires proper randomization. Use of historical series for this purpose has a disadvantage: these series are from another time frame, with older designs and different surgical techniques and postoperative procedures. These diffrences might have an confounding effect on the postoperative results [1].

2. AUTOGRAFTS

Autografts are devices derived from the patients' own tissue: the pulmonary valve is used as a substitute in aortic position. This procedure has been introduced by Ross [1] and turns a single valve disease into a double valve condition. The Ross procedure offers the advantage of possible growth and absence of immune reaction [6]. Moreover, it has hemodynamic benefits [7] and anticoagulation is not needed. In middle aged and elderly patients, the Ross procedure has provided excellent hemodynamic results. RVOT problems have not been observed in patients over 50 years, suggesting that this procedure could be used in CAVS [8]. Stenosis of the pulmonary homograft has been observed, however [7]. Results in terms of operative mortality, long-term survival and absence of valve related complications such as TE, PVE, SVD, and reoperation rate, have been acceptable [9].

Currently, the Ross procedure is usually used in pediatric populations, in which CAVS is virtually absent [6]. Hence, this procedure is beyond the scope of this manuscript. This surgical approach places biological tissues in new configurations, but it cannot be considered as tissue engineering. There is little manipulation to the internal molecular structure for the purpose of enhancing their biological performance [4].

As early as 1960, alternative, autologous tissue valves have been constructed from alternative sources within the operation room. These tissues have been derived from pericardium, fascia lata and dura mater [1]. In a more recent series, the patient's own pericardium has been tanned in glutaraldehyde and mounted on a stent without suturing. The device has been tested immediately in the operation room The device has been implanted elderly patients, mostly for CAVS. Operative mortality and hemodynamic data have been acceptable and no degeneration has been observed in the first postoperative year of follow-up. The follow-up has been short an incomplete [10]. Therefore, the long-term durability needs to be confirmed before application of the technique could be generalized.

3. HOMOGRAFTS

The homograft valves are intact human valves obtained from organ and tissue donors, usually stored cryopreserved as entire aortic or pulmonary root, and trimmed to the desired size and shape before implantation in the recipient [2, 4, 6, 11].

One of the earliest series has consisted of 44 patients, who have been followed for some months. The age of the patients and reason of homograft implantation has varied: stenosis due to CAVS and regurgitation after previous attempt to repair the diseased valve. The grafts have been harvested from cadavers. After sterilization in betapropriolactone these grafts have been brought into a culture medium with penicillin and streptomycin at 4°C for one week. Thereafter these grafts have been freeze-dried. Bacterial control cultures have been performed.

The sinuses of Valsalva have been excised and the graft has been implanted in subcoronary position, using a double suture. The most proximal suture line has been placed first, while the graft was inverted; after pull-up, the graft has been attached to the aortic wall, whereby the proximal suture line was buried. Clinical function of the grafts after 15 months has been satisfactory [2]. Since homografts copied the anatomical and physiological features of the native valves, they have been intuitively attractive.

Early enthusiasm has decreased due to failures (high rate of SVD and reoperation), for which harvesting and preservation protocols could be responsible. There are a number of past and contemporary improvements for processing and storage of homografts. Today, SVD is still a major and not fully resolved issue for this type of valve replacement.

Harvesting and preservation protocols include issues such as:

- Cadaver *vs.* brain dead donor; the latter has been considered to be a better option [11], but this has been questioned [6, 12]. Factors to take into account are:
    - Immune reaction due to MHC mismatch [11].
    - Matching of age of donor and of recipient [12].
    - Transmission of infectious disease [11], which has not been observed.
    - Duration of warm ischemia in donors.
- Homo-vital *vs.* cryopreserved (liquid nitrogen) grafts.
    - Thawing and freezing protocols which can have an effect on:
        - Viability of cells, which progressively decreased [11].
        - Integrity of the ECM [5, 11].
        - Chemical cross-linking [5].
        - Calcification, not in leaflets but mainly in the wall [5].
    - Sterilization techniques by irradiation or antibiotics [5, 11].
- Preservation techniques.

One should keep in mind that, in contrast to xenografts, homografts are not "off the shelve" available. Moreover, the quality of the homografts is debatable. This has become evident with an autopsy series from persons between 15 and 40 years, without a history of illness. These patients have died from a trauma. The microscopic study of the heart valves have shown that over half of the specimens were not suitable for implantation as homograft. This has been more common with increasing age of the potential donor [13].

Contemporary results in term of survival rate and of reoperation rate after implantation of homografts have been considered as acceptable [12] to excellent [14] and better than for porcine BHV [5]. The reoperation rate have matched those of any other non-mechanical device. Others have found a considerable variation of 10 year freedom from SVD (57-78%) and from reoperation (38-81%) [6]. Use of a free root replacement would improve the results [12].

Independent predictors for reoperation have been:

- Large implanted valves.
- Re-exploration for bleeding and
- Previous cardiac surgery [14].

Explantation after some years has shown thinner cusps, layers without distinctive features and no stainable EC or VIC. Calcifications within the cusps have seemed absent or limited, but this has been much more extensive in the wall itself [5].

Comparison with the results after implantation of MHV have shown a comparable survival. Bleeding events have been more common with MHV, while SVD – as can be expected – has been more common with homografts. Severe long-term complication have seemed to occur more in MHV than in homografts [15, 16]. Hemodynamic results at rest and in exercise have been better in homografts, compared to MHV [16, 17] or stented BHV [18].

When comparing the results of homografts with those of other BHV, one needs to keep in mind that the indication for homografts often include complex procedures or subcoronary implantation, which could increase hospital mortality. This is the case in endocarditis and PVE [5, 11, 19, 20], pathology of the aortic root and small aortic annuli. In institutions with a large experience, hospital mortality could be as low as 2.8%, with survival rates of 77% at 10 years and 45% at 20 years [11].

ACC/AHA guidelines give no specific recommendations for the use of homografts. Patients with CAVS are usually a minority in patient series [20].

4. STENTLESS XENOGRAFTS

Stentless xenografts have been the first BHV, used to substitute the diseased aortic valve. These devices seemed ideal because of the resemblance with the native valve. Moreover, mechanical substitutes were still under development. Durability, however has been a serious problem, since appropriate chemical treatment for sterilization and preservation was not fully developed. The first xenografts has been abandoned quickly, and the use of human material had no reproducible success, partly because of technical issues of implantation [5].

Advances in the methods of xenograft valve production are fixation with glutaraldehyde under low-to zero-pressure and anti-mineralisation treatment [6]. This has resulted in cross-linking in valve tissues, which has reduced their antigenic properties and protected the tissue against the proteolytic degradation following implantation. Durability has also been improved by impregnation with anti-mineralizing chemical agents [4].

Stentless valves nowadays are obtained by removing the entire aortic root in one piece, together with adjacent tissue, including the origins of the coronary arteries. The device can be trimmed as requested. Current examples are the Toronto Stentless porcine valve, Freestyle valve, CryoLife O'Brien valve and Medtronic freestyle valve. Stentless BHV have the advantage of an almost normal hemodynamic physiology after implantation [5].

SVD, calcification, and reoperation rate are still an issue for BHV.

On the one hand, calcific stenosis could be more important in stentless devices since greater portions of the aortic wall are exposed to the circulating blood. Calcification of the wall has been observed. The root can become more stiff after implantation. It might be that a synthetic fabric at the outer side of the device protects against damage by inflammatory cells, root dilation and regurgitation of the device [5].

On the other hand, improved durability can be due to a decreased mechanical shear stress: freedom from SVD in aortic freehand homografts is better compared to stented homografts. The durability depends also on the stabilization of the STJ. Toronto SPV and Biocor have a durability inferior to stented BHV, due to the dilatation of the STJ and the increase of shear stress on the leaflets. Other models such as Medtronic Freestyle, Edwards Prima Plus, have been inserted with modified subcoronary techniques. These techniques stabilize the STJ, and the stentless devices seem currently as durable as stented BHV [6].

Stentless BHV are also supposed to have a low TVG and a large EOAI, compared to their stented counterparts. These hemodynamical properties might have a beneficial effect on postoperative regression of LVH and on survival. It also would allow a more active lifestyle and hence, an improved QoL, especially in elderly patients with CAVS. A major advantage is the unlimited availability in all sizes. These devices would also be valuable in patients with CAVS and reduced LVF. A reduced LV function might recover more rapidly [6].

The operative mortality of AVR is between 1 and 8% and depends mostly on age. The more complex implantation technique does not add to it in experienced hands. The implantation is difficult, compared to stented valves. Technical problems might lead to non structural dysfunction which makes this device less popular compared to stented BHV. Newly designed xenografts, using simplified single-suture or interrupted suture implant may allow a broader use of stentless valves [6]. Long-term survival and freedom from other valve-related events such as TE, bleeding, PVE, compares favourably with estimates derived from experience with stented bioprostheses [6].

5. STENTED XENOGRAFTS

In 1964, Duran and Gunning have replaced an aortic valve in a patient using a porcine xenograft device. SVD has been a major problem. This has been the reason for the abandonment of this device. Carpentier and associates have revived interest in xenograft valves by fixating porcine valves with glutaraldehyde. In addition, they also have mounted the aortic pig valves on a stent. From then on, Carpentier-Edwards (CE) porcine valves and Hancock and Angell-Shiley bioprostheses have become more and more popular and have been implanted in large numbers of patients. In 1979, a pericardial valve has been developed in an attempt to improve upon the earlier valve designs. The aortic CE pericardial valve has been introduced to clinical use in 1981. In September 1991, the devices has been approved by the FDA for U.S. commercial distribution [1].

The current porcine xenograft valve consists of an intact pig aortic valve which is preserved in low-concentration glutaraldehyde solution. These valves are incorporated within a sewing cuff. This is a cobalt-nickel alloy covered with Dacron and allows an easy implantation. Occasionally, these valves are assembled from up to 3 separate segments of aorta and the associated cusp material in an effort to improve valve symmetry and hence, performance. Durability of these valves is 10 – 15 years and more [4, 5, 11].

The current bovine pericardial valve is biomechanically engineered from up to 3 separate pieces of glutaraldehyde-treated calf pericardium, fixed to a supporting stent and a sewing cuff. The configuration is very similar to the porcine xenograft. The design is comparable to porcine valve. A difference is the location of the small metal cylinder, which joins the ends of the wire stents together.

The hemodynamics of pericardial valves is excellent and their durability equals and probably exceeds this of porcine valves. There is virtually no regurgitation. Nevertheless, the stent narrows the lumen [1, 4, 5, 11]. Whether this leads to VPPM is still a matter for investigation [5]. VPPM could be a major problem in patients with low LVEF. Recently developed flexible low profile stents improve the hemodynamic results but the mode of SVD has remained the same. Higher compliance of tissues has led to a failure, related to abrasion in some designs [5].

The primary advantage of BHV is absence of need for anticoagulation [11]. The main problem, however, are SVD and reoperation rate. This seems worse in younger patients and for valves in mitral position. SVD is usually due to degeneration with calcification. This leads to regurgitation and in a lesser degree to stenosis [1, 11].

By 1995, the 10-year performance of the pericardial valves could be assessed. Durability at 10 year after AVR would be over 90%. With these satisfactory results, use of CE pericardial valves has become more popular, and in many centres across the country it has become the biological valve of choice in the aortic position. However, the 10-year test is relatively easy to pass. Relative freedom from SVD at 20 years will be the important milestone [1, 5].

6. MECHANICAL HEART VALVE, MHV

MHV have an excellent durability, superior to BHV. MHV is indicated in those patients whose life expectancy exceeds the durability of BHV [5, 11]. However, fractures in the housing or of other components, due to stress is possible [21].

An ideal heart valve from an engineering perspective would have:

- Large EOA and hence small TVG.
- Small regurgitation volumes.
- Minimial turbulence.
- Reduce prevalence of high stresses.
- Absence of flow separations in the vicinity of the valve.

Three types of MHV are available: cage ball, tilting disc and bi-leaflet, each with several modifications [11].

The first artificial heart valve has been the **caged-ball**. This has been the standard for almost a decade. This valve utilizes a metal cage to house a silicone elastomer ball. The first valves of this type have been implanted in 1952. When blood pressure in the LV exceeds the intra-aortic pressure, the ball is pushed against the cage and allows blood to flow. At diastole, the LV pressure drops below the intra-aortic pressure, so the ball moves back against the base of the valve, forming a seal. Its hemodynamic characteristics are:

- Limited regurgitation.

- High flow velocity and high TVG.
- Flow separation: high-velocity reverse flow, surrounded by stagnant flow.
- A high shear stress with tendency to cell damage resulting in thrombosis and hemolysis.
- High durability.

The valve allows a near normal age and gender specific survival, provided VPPM is avoided [21, 22].

Soon thereafter, **tilting-disc** valves have been developed. The first clinically available tilting disk valve has been the Bjork-Shiley valve. This valve has undergone several significant design changes since its introduction in 1969. Tilting disk valves have a single circular occluder controlled by a metal strut. They are made of a metal ring covered by a Teflon or dacron, for suturing. The metal ring holds, by means of two metal supports, a disc which opens and closes with systole and diastole. The disc is usually made of an extremely hard pyrolytic carbon, which resists fatigue and allows the valve to function for years without wearing out. The Medtronic-Hall model is the most common tilting-disc design in the US.

Its characteristics are:

- The EOAI is somewhat lower than in bi-leaflet valves.
- The regurgitation is somewhat less compared to bi-leaflet valves [23, 24].
- The flow separation behind the valve struts and disc is a result of a combination of high velocity and stagnant flows.

The **bi-leaflet valves** consist of two semicircular leaflets that rotate about struts attached to the valve housing. This design has been introduced in 1979. Currently, it is the most widely implanted MHV.

Its characteristics are:

- A larger EOAI and a lower TVG compared to caged-ball or tilting-disc implants [23, 24].
- Some degree of regurgitation with high stress.
- There is less stasis of the forward flow.
- The need for anticoagulation is less [3].
- The hinge area is the most critical part of bileaflets; the PVT is usually starts in this location.

The main advantage of MHV, which is the durability, comes at a cost. All MHV models are vulnerable to thrombus formation due to non physiological flow patterns: high shear stress, stagnation, and flow separation [21]. Several mechanisms play a role: tissue factor exposure, platelet activation, or contact activation by foreign materials.

- Rupture of cells release tissue factor which binds to clotting factor VII; this starts a chain of events in which factors Xa, Va, thrombin, factor VIII and platelets are involved.
- Platelets are damaged by stress. These damaged platelets bind to the vWF at the glycoprotein Ib; these glycoproteins are activated through a calcium influx.
- Glycoprotein IIb-IIIa facilitates the formation of a platelet plug during amplification.
- When factor XII binds to a surface which promotes coagulation, prekallikrein is also activated and binds to factor XI. This on its turn activates factor IX and more platelets.

To prevent PVT and TE, a life-long anticoagulation is needed. This is the main disadvantage of MHV. Anticoagulation requires a tight control since patients with

MHV balance between bleeding and thrombosis. Patient compliance is of major importance [5, 11]. Computational fluid dynamics are helpful in explaining flow and shear stress as causes for these events in MHV [3, 21].

Visibility of MHV on fluoroscopy allows evaluation of its function. Leaflet positioning during the operation is also facilitated [25]. Echocardiography is the standard way to evaluate a valve for EOAI and TVG [23, 24].

Hemolysis is the result of damaged red blood cells and is also the consequence of these flow patterns. This event can be documented by serum LDH, serum haptoglobin, schistocytes and reticulocytes. Hemolysis also depends on the type of MHV [26]. Hemolysis is not related to the size of the prosthesis or to EOA [27]. In BHV, hemolysis is rare [28]. Decompensated hemolysis could be a reason for re-replacement of a valve prosthesis.

7. MHV *VERSUS* BHV

7.1. The Debate

The debate on the choice between a mechanical *versus* tissue valve continues for decades. The results of valve replacement, however, does not only depend on the type of valve but also on patient-related factors [9]. The primary problem of BHV is durability [29] and hence need for reoperation, especially in younger patients. TE and PVT are the most important events for MHV. Although some guidelines are available for choosing one valve type over another, no definitive criteria yet exist [1, 25]. Age, however could be considered as an important determining factor the choice for a certain type of valve [30].

Improvements have been made for BHV as well as for MHV:

> On the one hand, hemodynamic properties have improved for MHV. Thrombogenicity and hence, the level of anticoagulation could be reduced [1], resulting in some advantage over BHV. Moreover, self control of INR improved the postoperative results markedly [31].
>
> On the other hand, attempts were made to improve the durability and hemodynamic performance of BHV. In 1995, the favourable 10 year

outcome of the CE-p valve could be documented. This device has become the valve of choice in many centres for AVR [1].

With many types of both MHV and BHV available, the decision to place a particular valve may not be easy, and often is not based on solid scientific data. Over 50 types of prosthetic heart valves have become available, which does not facilitate the debate. Moreover, comparison of large BHV and MHV populations by age groups revealed that regardless of the differences in the freedom from SVD, the freedom from treatment failure (defined as valve related mortality and permanent impairment due to TE, bleeding, and septal emboli from PVE) is essentially the same for MHV and BHV at 10 years [1, 25].

Comparative studies, preferably RCT, are needed to make an adequate choice. Several comparative studies have appeared but there is not yet a general conclusion. This could be due to different populations, especially in relation to age, different designs in study, different outcomes and comparison of older and more contemporary valves. All these differences have to be taken into account. There are several other considerations. Different complications have different time related incidence rates. Moreover, not all so-called valve related complications are really valve related. TE can also have a non-valvular source: the left atrium, the LV, the aortic arch and other arteries [22, 32].

Conclusions of several comparative studies between MHV and BHV are summarized. Two approaches could be discerned.

7.2. The Focus on the Type of Valve with a Global Description of the Results

7.2.1. Some Studies Indicated a Superiority of BHV

The use of MHV (Carbomedics) and BHV (CE-p) has been compared in patients between 55 and 65 years of age. With MHV, there have been significantly more valve related events and survival has been poorer (66 *vs.* 75%) [29].

In patients aged over 70, long-term survival between patients with BHV and MHV has not differed significantly. SVD in BHV has been rare, but bleeding events have occurred more in MHV. Long-term survival has been dominated by non-valvular factors. It seems for patients in this age group, that BHV is preferable for its durability and low rate of bleeding events [33].

7.2.2. Other Studies Pointed to Superior Results in MHV

Implantation of MHV in patients between 50 and 70 years of age (SJM bi-leaflet) has resulted in a survival advantage compared to matched patients who received BHV (CE). Freedom of reoperation has also been better for MHV. Implantation of BHV in younger patients might be questioned [34].

Using a MHV in aortic position has resulted in a better 15 year outcome (with a lower reoperation rate but a higher bleeding rate compared to a BHV). The main reason for superiority of MHV has been the absence of primary valve failure. SVD of BHV has occurred in patients younger than 65 years. In elderly, valve failure has not significantly been more present in BHV compared to MHV [35]. Lowering a cut-off age below 65 years for implantation of BHV, therefore is not warranted [36].

Sometimes MHV have been implanted in octogenarians. Even in those patients, a survival advantage has been observed, compared to BHV. QoL, however has been unaffected [37].

7.2.3. Some Studies could not find Significant Advantages of One Valve Prosthesis Over the Other

Comparing stentless BHV (freestyle) with MHV (SJM), no significant differences have been found between both groups. In patients over 75 years, major bleeding have occurred more frequently after implantation of a MHV. BHV in elderly had demonstrated one major advantage: the QoL has improved, since no anticoagulation is needed [38].

MHV in aortic position have shown initially more valve related complications (especially bleeding). After 10 years, however, the number of reoperation for BHV has increased, as a "trade-off". The risk for reoperation with implantation of a BHV has increased with time. The type of valve, however has not seemed to affect survival [39].

In patients aged 69-71 years, implantation of MHV has resulted in more bleeding while after the use of BHV, more reoperation has been necessary. Life expectancy, even in elderly needs to be taken into account for the assessment of future events. BHV should only be used in men over 74 years and in women over 78 years [40].

No differences in hospital and long-term survival have been found between patients who have received a MHV (at mean age 65) and BHV (at mean age 71). Patient related factors such as age and renal failure have been predictors for long-term mortality [30].

The last study is a typical example of a effect of age as a confounding factor on survival as outcome. Only a few certainties can be derived from these studies.

1) In younger patients, the use of BHV should be avoided, unless their life expectancy is limited for other reasons.

2) In elderly patients, the risk for anticoagulation related bleeding must be carefully balanced against the rather low risk for reoperation after SVD if a BHV is chosen.

3) One needs to take into consideration the increased life expectancy in elderly and the need for anticoagulation for other reasons, such as AF.

For the very young and the very old, the case seems to be clear. A dilemma in choice of prosthetic valve remains in patients between 55 and 65 years or even between 55 to 70 years [41]. It also seems that the lower limit of age for use of BHV is rising. Age alone, however should not be the sole determinant of the choice between MHV and BHV [30]. Patients related factor such as age and co-morbid conditions have also an impact on survival.

One also has to be aware that current guidelines for the choice of the valve are the result of studies from valves implanted in the late 1970s and early 1980s. Since then, surgical techniques, valve design and concomitant medications have improved substantially. Updating of clinical data with current practices would be of great value [42].

Nevertheless, good results have been achieved using older valve types during the 1960s and 1970s. In patients with severe CAVS and NYHA functional classes III and IV or with CHF, AVR has resulted in a considerable improvement in terms of survival, NYHA functional class and LVEF. Moreover, the frequency of postoperative CHF has decreased.

Ten-year mortality and complication rates have been described in detail in patients in whom various prosthetic heart valves have been implanted. There have been no major differences in patient outcomes with use of the various prosthetic heart valves among MHV (such as the Starr-Edwards and SJM) and among BHV (such as the older standard Hancock, Hancock MO, CE porcine and stentless porcine valves). There is no good evidence that, in patients with similar baseline characteristics, patient outcomes are better with "newer good" than with "older good" prosthetic heart valves [9].

7.3. The Focus on the Type of Complication [9]

7.3.1. Mortality

The 10-and 15-year mortality range after AVR is wide, even with the use of the same brand of prosthetic heart valve. This indicates that factors other than the type of valve are important for the postoperative results.

Several risk factors for long-term mortality have been included in studies: age, LV dysfunction, CHF, NYHA functional classes III and IV, CAD, previous and concomitant CABG, valve regurgitation, arrhythmias, male gender, PAHT, and co-morbid conditions such as renal failure, COPD, AHT, and DM.

To complicate matters more, older patients are more likely to have clinically significant co-morbid conditions. Both, age and co-morbidity, are known to adversely affect survival after prosthetic heart valve. Patient characteristics at baseline are a major determinant of long-term mortality after valve replacement. Therefore, the preoperative patient profile needs to be properly described in any study [9].

7.3.2. TE

The risk for TE after implantation of a MHV is low in absence of patient related risk factors. These risk factors include an abnormal heart rhythm, a low LVF, presence of risk factors for atheromatosis and of atheromatosis itself, a history of previous thrombotic events and of clotting disorders [9].

7.3.3. Bleeding

The bleeding rates associated with a variety of mechanical aortic and mitral valves have been similar. Comparisons also have been made with bleeding rates in elderly patients treated with anticoagulation for AF, but the follow-up times were shorter. Age, co-morbidity and the level of INR still are major confounding factors in the study for bleeding rate [9].

7.3.4. SVD

The rate of SVD of BHV after implantation in aortic position is largely related to the age of the patient at time of the valve implantation: the 10 and 15 year freedom of SVD increases with age at implantation. The type of BHV could also play a role: results for pericardial valves seemed somewhat better than for porcine valves. The rate of SVD of newer porcine valves (Hancock MO and the stentless porcine valve) at nine years is within the range of SVD of earlier stented porcine valves, indicating that, at present, all porcine valves have similar rates of SVD [9].

7.3.5. VPPM

VPPM will be discussed in detail in later chapter. Its clinical relevancy is doubtful in some cases. VPPM can be considered to be present when the EOAI, after insertion of the valve prosthesis, is less than that of a healthy native valve. The reduced EOAI is usually mild to moderate and often of no immediate clinical significance. EOAI could be reduced during the postoperative course by formation of pannus.

However, VPPM can occasionally be a severe problem because the patient may be hemodynamic and symptomatically worse after valve replacement. VPPM may result in higher TVG at rest and on exercise. Other consequences might be a suboptimal reduction of LVM, an insufficient exercise tolerance, a higher NYHA functional class, a higher rate of CHF and a higher mortality. CAD, and hence, a need for a concomitant CABG can have a negative effect the postoperative outcome in patients who suffer the effects of VPPM. Hence, the need for concomitant CABG should be taken into account for the evaluation of VPPM.

7.3.6. Concluding Remarks

A major review (comprising a follow-up of 187, 220 patient years for MHV and 132, 519 for BHV) has confirmed that there were no major differences in outcome between the different brands of MHV and of BHV. The risk for TE has been lower in BHV, but this complication has not been absent. The risk for SVD with MHV has been negligible. However, the complication rate has varied widely for every valve prosthesis under study. These findings reconfirm that, with the use of FDA approved prosthetic heart valves, postoperative complications are largely related to factors other than the type of valve [43].

7.4. Evidence of RCT

A RCT is the preferred way to give strong evidence for a choice of a prosthesis. Thus far only three RCT have appeared, two older and one more contemporary [35, 41, 44]. The two older are ***Edinburgh heart valve trial*** and the ***Veterans affair cooperative study***.

7.4.1. Edinburgh Heart Valve Trial

The randomization has been between 1975 and 1979, for AVR. Some conclusions could be drawn after a mean follow-up of 12 year.

1) There has been a trend towards better survival with the MHV.

2) At 5 year follow-up, reoperation rate has been low, but this has increased at 12 years for porcine valves, especially in younger patients.

3) The rate of TE and PVE has not differed between MHV and BHV.

4) The bleeding rate has been higher for MHV.

7.4.2. Dept Veterans Affairs (DVA) trial

A total of 575 men have been randomized between 1997 to 1982; 394 had AVR. The average follow-up was 15 years. The principal long-term findings for AVR were:

1) With MHV, there has been a lower mortality (with only 40% valve related).

2) The difference between MHV and BHV have become apparent after 10 year follow-up.

3) With MHV, there has been no SVD and reoperation rate also has been lower.

4) SVD, after implantation of BHV, has occurred more in younger patients. This event has started at 7 to 8 years, but a follow-up of over 10 years is needed to determine the incidence and effects of SVD.

5) SVD has not occured more frequently in elderly who received a BHV.

6) The rate of TE and other valve related events has not differed between MHV and BHV.

7) The bleeding rate has been higher for MHV.

The bleeding rate with MHV is an important issue. It has been higher in the DVA trial. Therefore, some points need consideration:

- Have all bleeding events been recorded, or only the major bleeding events?

- Has the level of anticoagulation in different series been comparable, and how has this been controlled?

- Have other indications for anticoagulation such as AF been taken into account, for both MHV and BHV?

The only recent RCT [41] has shown an improved peri-operative mortality but no major changes in long-term outcome have been documented, even with the more modern valve prostheses. The use of MHV and BHV has been compared for hospital mortality, long-term survival, rate of TE, bleeding, PVE and other major events. Concomitant CABG has been comparable for both groups.

The age limits in the choice for the valve have been as follows: for patients under 55 years a MHV has been chosen (SJM bi-leaflet); for patients over 70 years, a BHV was been implanted (CE SAV or CE-p). The choice for the valve in patients between 55 and 70 years has been the matter for research. The conclusions of the RCT have been [41]:

- The postoperative results for MHV and for BHV have been comparable.

- Implantation of BHV has resulted in a significantly higher risk for SVD and reoperation after 10 years.

- Predictors of long-term mortality have been patient related: these were NYHA class, need for concomitant CABG and presence of AF.

- Over 20% of the patients who received a BHV have taken anticoagulation, for other reasons than for the MHV.

- The bleeding rate in patients who received a BHV and received no peroral anticoagulation has been lower than the bleeding rate in patients who received a MHV.

- For the BHV group as a whole, only a trend to less bleeding has been documented.

The bleeding rate also has been an issue in this RCT: the results after implantation of BHV in the two older trials could only be confirmed after comparing patients who took long-term anticoagulation for co-morbid conditions, with patients who did not take anticoagulating medication at all. Hence, the use of anticoagulants has been much more important as factor for bleeding than the type of the valve itself.

The second issue, the rate of SVD (and related to it, the reoperation rate), still has to be awaited. Even elderly patients have a long life expectancy! Moreover, the 10 year durability test for BHV is easy to pass. Twenty year follow-up is the next milestone.

Hence, little has changed in the choice for a valve. The preference of physician and patients remains important. The dilemma between anticoagulation related bleeding and SVD remains for this moment.

8. TEHV AS ALTERNATIVE?

The valve technology, operative and postoperative care have evolved, thereby improving the postoperative outcome. Durability for BHV has been the main problem to solve in the development of valves. A lifelong durability obviates the need for reoperation with its risks. There are reasons to choose for a modern BHV. The CE-p and the currently available homografts have an excellent durability of 10 to 15 and even to 20 years in elderly but this is less in younger patients. The mortality after reoperation can be considered lower than the cumulative risk for TE, which is associated with the implantation of a MHV. The current BHV also provide an excellent QoL.

Therefore, manufacturers of prosthetic heart valves and surgeons could have become reluctant to implant a potentially better but still unproven device. It is possible that the clinical outcome is worse, as has been observed in several series.

- Cusp abrasion with perforation (Carbomedics Photofix-alpha valve).
- Increased risk for TE (Medtronic Parallel mechanical valve).
- Tissue necrosis with subsequent PPVL (St Jude Silzone coating).

A new device, such as a TEHV has to compete with "proven values" such as a CE-pericardial valve. Long duration means also that deliverance for proof of superior quality takes a time span of a human generation.

Therefore, there might not be an immediate need for a TEHV in elderly patients. Comparison between TEHV and currently available BHV for adults could be ethically questionable. In the pediatric population, this is different (because of the potential for somatic growth and for remodelling of TEHV), but this discussion is beyond the scope of this manuscript. RCT in which TEHV is included in patient series are not to be expected for the near future [4, 45].

CONCLUSIONS

From the data cited, the following general conclusions can be drafted.

1) Advances in prosthetic heart valves have mostly occurred in small steps: old "good" valves might be comparable to new "good" valves. Glutaraldehyde fixation is one of the few major leaps.

2) Patient related factors play a considerable role in the postoperative outcome, hence these should be described in full detail in every manuscript.

3) 10 to 15 year outcomes are needed to reach firm conclusions for any complication.

4) There is no evidence that MHV are superior to BHV or *vice versa*, if patients have comparable baseline characteristics. The dilemma between anticoagulation related bleeding and SVD remains in certain age groups.

5) There is no evidence that any porcine valve is superior to another porcine valv. This remark applies also to different brands of MHV. A follow-up of at least 15 years is needed to establish any difference.

6) Mortality: 10 to 15 year mortality after AVR is valve related, but age and co-morbid conditions have also a high impact.

7) SVD.

    a. SVD occurs almost solely with BHV.

    b. SVD occurs sooner in younger patients.

    c. SVD with MHV is virtually absent.

    d. SVD in homografts and stentless porcine valves seems to be similar compared to SVD in stented porcine valves.

    e. Pericardial valves seem to be superior to porcine valves.

8) TE/Bleeding.

a. The risk for TE after implantation of MHV is similar to BHV if a proper anticoagulation protocol is applied.

b. The postoperative rate of TE depends also on patient related risk factors. Even after receiving a BHV, anticoagulation could be warranted for co-morbid conditions such as AF.

c. In elderly patients, bleeding also occurs without anticoagulation. This medication should be used with caution in any case. Since SVD of implanted BHV is slow to develop, this valve type has the preference in elderly.

9) VPPM is an important clinical problem in patients with low LVF.

Any patient has unique needs, which should be included in the decision making. This decision is a joint decision between patient, cardiologist and surgeon, after the patient has been informed about the options. It is the patient that is undergoing the risks for any postoperative complication and the cardiologist that has to take care for the patient before but also after the valve implantation.

Age and life expectancy, which are closely related to co-morbid conditions, are the most determining factors. Risk factors for TE, which makes anticoagulation therapy necessary might favour the use of MHV. Nevertheless, need to discontinue anticoagulation, for whatever reason, will become much more difficult if this type of valve is used.

ACKNOWLEDGEMENT

Declared none.

CONFLICT OF INTEREST

The author(s) confirm that this chapter content has no conflict of interest.

REFERENCES

[1] Jamieson SW, Madani MM. Editorial comment. The choice of valve prosthesis. J Am Coll Cardiol 2004; doi:10.1016/j.jacc.2004.04.021.

[2] Barrat-Boyes BG, Homograft aortic valve replacement in aortic incompetence and stenosis Thorax 1964;19:131-150.

[3] Yoganathan AP, Chandran KB, Sotiropoulos F. Flow in the prosthetic heart valves. Ann Biomedical Engineering 2005;33:1689-1694.

[4] Vesely I. Heart valve tissue engineering. Circ Res 2005;97:743-755.

[5] Siddiqui RF, Abraham JR, Butany J. Bioprosthetic heart valves: modes of failure. Histopathol 2009;55:135-144.

[6] Luciani GB, Santini F, Mazzucco A. Autografts, homografts, and xenografts: overview on stentless aortic valve surgery. J Cardiovasc Med 2007;8:91-96.

[7] Wang A, Jaggers J, Ungerleider RM, *et al.* Exercise echocardiograpic comparison of pulmonary autograft and aortic homograft replacements for aortic valve disease in adults. J Heart Valve Dis 2003;12:202-208.

[8] Böhm JO, Botha CA, Hemmer W, *et al.* Older Patients Fare Better With the Ross Operation. Ann Thorac Surg 2003;75:796-802.

[9] Rahimtoola SH. State of the art paper. Choice of Prosthetic Heart Valve for Adult Patients. J Am Coll Cardiol 2003;41:893–904.

[10] Gross C, Simon P, Mair R, *et al.* Autologous tissue cardiac valve for aortic valve replacement: technical aspects and early results. Ann Thorac Surg 1996;61:1759-1763.

[11] Staab ME, Neshimura RA, Dearani DA, Orszulak TA. Aortic valve homografts in adults: a clinical perspective. Mayo Clin Proc 1998;73:231-238.

[12] Lund O, Chandrasekaran V, Grocott-Mason R, *et al.* Primary aortic valve replacement with allografts over twenty-five years: valve related and procedure related determinants of outcome. J Thorac Cardiovasc Surg 1999;117:77-90.

[13] Dabrowska A, Sladoswki D, Krajewski P, Komender J. The quality of heart valve tissue for homograft transplantation. J Heart Valve Dis 2000;9:517-522.

[14] Hickey E, Langley SM, Allemby-Smith O, *et al.* Subcoronary Allograft Aortic Valve Replacement: Parametric Risk-Hazard Outcome Analysis to a Minimum of 20 Years. Ann Thorac Surg 2007;84:1564-1570.

[15] Waszyrowski T, Kasprzak JD, Krzeminska-Pakula M, *et al.* Early and long-term outcome of aortic valve replacement with homograft *versus* mechanical prosthesis – 8 year follow-up study. Clin Cardiol 1997;20:843-848.

[16] Grocott-Mason RM, Lund O, Elwidaa H, *et al.* Long-term results after aortic valve replacement in patients with congestive heart failure – homografts *versus* prosthetic valves. Eur Heart J 2000;21:1698-1707.

[17] Basarir S, Islamoglu F, Ozkisaik E, *et al.* Comparative analysis of left ventricular hemodynamics and hypertrophy after aortic valve replacement with homografts or mechanical valves. J Heart Valve Dis 2000;9:42-45.

[18] Maselli D, Pizio R, Bruno LP, *et al.* Left Ventricular Mass Reduction After Aortic Valve Replacement: Homografts, Stentless and Stented Valves. Ann Thorac Surg 1999;67:966-971.

[19] Gross C, Klima U, Mair R, Brücke P. Aortic Homografts *Versus* Mechanical Valves in Aortic Valve Replacement in Young Patients: A Retrospective Study. Ann Thorac Surg 1998;66:S194-197.

[20] Dossche KM, Brutel de la Rivière A, Morshuis WJ, *et al.* Cryopreserved Aortic Allografts for Aortic Root Reconstruction: A Single Institution's Experience. Ann Thorac Surg 1999;67:1617-1622.

[21] Sotiropoulos F, Borazjani I, A review of state-of-the-art numerical methods for simulating flow through mechanical heart valves. Med Biol Eng Computing 2009;47:235-256.

[22] Lund O, Pilegaard HK, Ilkjaer LB, *et al.* Performance profile of the Starr-Edwards aortic cloth covered valve, track valve, and silastic ball valve. Eur J Cardiothorac Surg 1999;16:403-413.

[23] Bach DS. Echo/Doppler Evaluation of Hemodynamics After Aortic Valve Replacement Principles of Interrogation and Evaluation of High Gradients, JACC-Cardiovasc imaging 2010;3:296-304.

[24] Kume T, Okura H, Kawamoto T, *et al.* Impact of Energy Loss Coefficient on Left Ventricular Mass Regression in Patients Undergoing Aortic Valve Replacement: Preliminary Observation. J Am Soc Echocardiography 2009;22:454-457.

[25] Jamieson WRE. Modern Cardiac Valve Devices – bioprostheses and mechanical prostheses – state of the art. J Card Surg 1993;8:89-98.

[26] Ismeno G, Renzulli A, Carozza A, *et al.* Intravascular hemolysis after mitral and aortic valve replacement with different types of mechanical prostheses. Int J Cardiol 1999;69:179-183.

[27] Josa M, Castella M, Par' C *et al.* Hemolysis in Mechanical Bileaflet Prostheses: Experience With the Bicarbon Valve. Ann Thorac Surg 2006;81:1291-1296.

[28] Mecozzi G, Milano AD, De Carlo M, *et al.* Intravascular hemolysis in patients with new-generation prosthetic heart valves: A prospective study. J Thorac Cardiovasc Surg 2002;123:550-556.

[29] Carrier M, Pellerin M, Perrault LP, *et al.* Aortic Valve Replacement With Mechanical and Biologic Prostheses in Middle-Aged Patients. Ann Thorac Surg 2001;71:S253-256.

[30] Silberman S, Oren A, Dotan M, *et al.* Aortic Valve Replacement: Choice Between Mechanical Valves and Bioprostheses. J Card Surg 2008;23:299-306.

[31] Horstkotte D, Piper C. Improvement of oral anticoagulation therapy by INR self management. J Heart Valve Dis 2004;13:335-338.

[32] Horstkotte D, Lengyel M, Mistiaen W, *et al.* Recommendations for reporting morbid events after heart valve surgery. J Heart Valve Dis 2005. 14:1-7.

[33] Milano A, Guglielmi C, De Carlo M, *et al.* Valve-Related Complications in Elderly Patients With Biological and Mechanical Aortic Valves. Ann Thorac Surg 1998;66:S82-87.

[34] Brown ML, Schaff HV, Lahr BD, *et al.* Aortic valve replacement in patients aged 50 to 70 years: Improved outcome with mechanical *versus* biologic prostheses. J Thorac Cardiovasc Surg 2008;135:878-884.

[35] Hammermeister KE, Sethi GK, Henderson WC, *et al.* Outcomes 15 years after valve replacement with a mechanical *versus* bioprosthetic valve: final report of the Veterans Affairs randomized trial. J Am Coll Cardiol 2000;36:1152-1158.

[36] Kulik A, Bédard P, Lam BK, *et al.* Mechanical *versus* bioprosthetic valve replacement in middle-aged patients. Eur J Cardio-thorac Surg 2006;30:485-491.

[37] Vicchio M, Della Corte A, De Santo LS, *et al.* Tissue *Versus* Mechanical Prostheses: Quality of Life in Octogenarians. Ann Thorac Surg 2008;85:1290-1295.

[38] Florath I, Albert A, Rosendahl U, *et al.* Mid-term outcome and quality of life after aortic valve replacement in elderly people: mechanical *versus* stentless biological valves. Heart 2005;91:1023-1029.

[39] Khan SS, Trento A, DeRobertis M, *et al.* Twenty-year comparison of tissue and mechanical valve replacement. J Thorac Cardiovasc Surg 2001;122:257-269.

[40] Logeais Y, Langanay T, Corbineau H, *et al.* Aortic Valve Replacement in the Elderly: Bioprosthesis or Mechanical Valve? Ann Thorac Surg 1998;66:S77-81.

[41] Stassano P, Di Tommaso L, Monaco M, *et al.* Aortic Valve Replacement A Prospective Randomized Evaluation of Mechanical *Versus* Biological Valves in Patients Ages 55 to 70 Years. J Am Coll Cardiol 2009;54:1862-1868.

[42] Stone PH. Current Selection of Optimal Prosthetic Aortic Valve Replacement in Middle-Aged Patients. Still Dealer's Choice. J Am Coll Cardiol 2009;54:1869-1871.

[43] Grunkemeier GL, Li H-H, Naftel DC, *et al.* Long-term performance of heart valve prosthesis. Curr Probl Cardiol 2000;25:73-156.

[44] Bloomfield P, Wheatley DJ, Prescott RJ, Miller HC. Twelve-year comparison of a Bjork-Shiley mechanical heart-valve with porcine bioprosthesis. N Engl J Med 1991;324:573-579.

[45] Neuenschwander S, Hoerstrup SP. Review: Heart valve tissue engineering. Transplant Immunology 2004;12:359-365.

CHAPTER 7

Principles of Follow-Up After Aortic Valve Replacement

Abstract: Follow-up studies have been performed for several reasons. There are minimal requirements for data collection and for follow-up techniques. These include enrolment of patients, type, frequency and mode of data acquisition. A risk profile of the preoperative patient population also allows an individual risk assessment an evaluation of the quality of care for any given institution.

The preoperative EuroSCORE has been developed as tool for such risk assessments. However, the additive as well as the logistic model tended to overestimate the risk for operative mortality. One of the reasons could be the improvements of the care since the development of this score, which have not yet been taken into account. The STS score seems more adequate, but still overestimates the operative risk.

Apart from mortality, postoperative adverse events have been listed and defined. It is, even today, not always possible to make a distinction between valve related complications and non-valvular events.

Short-term events can be represented as percentages. For long-term events, a linearized rate is usually not sufficient since the occurrence of events is not necessarily linear. Actual and actuarial analysis have to be performed.

For a risk analysis, proper statistical methods have to be applied. Identification of independent preditors for hospital events, requires the multivariate logistic regression analysis. For long-term events, this is the Cox' proportional hazard analysis.

Keywords: Cardiac events, Cox proportional hazard analysis, EuroSCORE, follow-up, Kaplan-Meier analysis, logistic regression, non-cardiac events, postoperative mortality, quality of life, STS PROM, valve related events.

1. PRINCIPLES OF FOLLOW-UP

Clinical follow-up studies after heart valve operations have been designed to describe the results of such operations. These reports have to meet some standards of quality. The purpose for follow-up can be purely scientific but can also serve other purposes, such as making a risk stratification or for use as marker for quality of care in a certain hospital or area. For the latter, hospital and 30 day postoperative mortality often have been used as marker. The ultimate goal is improvement of postoperative results, *i.e.* the reduction of mortality and adverse event as well as improvement of the postoperative QoL.

Wilhelm Peter Mistiaen

For a proper analysis of postoperative results, the preoperative condition of patients must be described adequately, *i.e.* the so-called case mix. Conditions that pose a certain risk for poor postoperative outcome can be labeled as a "risk factor" [1].

With these factors known, a risk profile can be constructed such as the European System for Cardiac Operative Risk Evaluation or EuroSCORE and the STS Predicted Risk Of Mortality or STS PROM.

Consulting reports concerning the outcome after an operation such as AVR can reveal some differences and inconsistencies. The main reasons for inconsistent results in clinical follow-up are:

- Differences in follow-up technique.
- Non-consistent reporting systems.
- Differences in classification of events.
- Differences in definitions of adverse events and difference in their grading according to the severity.

The design of the study also has its importance. For comparative studies, a RCT, is the "gold standard" but this can sometimes be difficult to implement or even be unethical. Examples are the comparison of conventional AVR and TAVI or for the effect of statins on the progression of CAVS. For both examples, an adequate treatment could be withheld in control groups. Non-randomized studies are easier to perform but these carry the risk of bias and misinterpretations of the results [2].

One cause for bias is patient selection. The risk for bias can be kept low if:

- All consecutive patients have been included in a single study.
- The study design has been a "matched pair analysis".
- Refusal of consent by the patients has remained limited.
- Inclusion and exclusion criteria have been made clear beforehand, if not all consecutive patients are enrolled.

- Inclusion of the patients has been started before the operation.

- The patient group has been large enough and hence representative for the study period.

- Interruption of enrolment and inconsistencies in patient recruitment have been stated clearly and the reasons given [2].

The follow-up technique ideally documents all postoperative adverse events precisely. Adding regularly posted questionnaires to conventional outpatient controls detects many reversible and transient events that are otherwise "forgotten". Hence self-reported events with a re-check at short intervals guarantee high quality follow-up. The less frequent the follow-up intervals and the less qualified the examiner is, the poorer the quality of the results are. The costs of such intensive follow-up must be balanced against the clinical value of the information obtained. One should be cautious with pooling data coming from studies with different follow-up techniques since the results are not necessarily comparable [2]!.

2. PREOPERATIVE RISK FACTORS: DEFINITION AND RISK STRATIFICATION

2.1. The EuroSCORE

Risk stratification in cardiac surgery is essential for the estimation of adverse events. Risk factors have to be identified. Risk adjusted results are preferable compared to the raw results [3].

Major preoperative predictors of mortality have to be identified and risk models that can accurately estimate operative mortality have to be developed. Large nationwide databases such as the STS database which contain over one million patients who have underwent cardiac surgery are valuable sources. Exclusion and inclusion criteria can define the groups (for example patients undergoing AVR for whom concomitant CABG can serve as an in or exclusion criterion) [3].

Risk scoring models can have several purposes:

- Anticipation of expected mortality.

- Comparison between different centers.
- Tool for performance improvement of individual centers/surgeons and.
- Future patient selection for surgical procedures and trials.

The accuracy of the model is of paramount importance [4]. The EuroSCORE has been developed using 19, 030 patients from 128 centres [5]. It has allowed the use of risk-adjusted mortality instead of crude mortality. These risk factors have been selected on the basis of objectivity, credibility, reliability and prevalence. Participation of heart centers has been on voluntary basis, which could create a bias, but it also guaranteed a more accurate data collection. Base line mortality has been calculated in patients who had no risk factors at all. For closure of ASD, mortality has been nil, for CABG, this has been 0.4%, for single valve replacement, this has been +/-1%. Controls have been made for accuracy and completeness.

The EuroSCORE also has been widely used as risk assessment tool in patients with severe CAVS to determine the operability. The additive score has been the first model and was simple to use [6]. The subsequently developed logistic model had an improved accuracy in high risk patients [6, 7]. A logistic EuroSCORE of 10 or less is has been considered as a low risk. A score of 20 or more is has been considered as a high risk and can be considered as an indication for TAVI.

2.2. Construction of the EuroSCORE

Following elements have been included for an EuroSCORE [5, 8]:

1) Demographic: age and gender.
2) Cardiovascular risk factors: BMI, AHT, DM.
3) Cardiovascular diseases and perioperative events, such as:
   a. PAD.
   b. Previous CABG or PCI.

c. Previous valve surgery.

d. Previous surgery of the thoracic aorta.

e. Impaired LVF, defined by LVEF<30% and NYHA class.

f. Recent AMI.

g. PAHT.

h. Active endocarditis.

i. Unstable angina, *i.e.* need for IV therapy.

j. Need for urgent or emergent surgery.

k. Need for inotropic support or IABP.

l. Need for intubation.

m. Ventricular tachycardia, especially if associated to LVH.

n. Ventricular septum rupture.

4) Non-cardiac disease: COPD, chronic renal disease, neurological dysfunction.

The preoperative risk factors as listed above must be defined as precisely as possible. Grading of the NYHA class is subjected to the interpretation of the investigator and can be influenced by co-morbidity, which can also affect exercise tolerance. The other factors must be documented objectively by medical imaging, stress tests and laboratory tests [1].

The most important factors for hospital mortality that have been identified in a multivariate analysis are:

- Ventricular septal rupture.

- Thoracic aortic surgery.

- Emergency operation.
- LVEF lower than 30% and.
- Active endocarditis.

PAD and neurological disability are also important factors [5].

2.3. Problems with the EuroSCORE

2.3.1. Incompleteness of the Listed Risk Factors

The list which contains the elements for the EuroSCORE might not be complete. Other conditions could also have an effect on the postoperative outcome [1]:

1) Concomitant heart disease or conditions indirectly related to the effect of CAVS:
    a. AF and enlarged left atrium.
    b. CD and need for PPMI.
    c. Involvement of mitral or tricuspid disease.
2) Previous heart disease/cardiac procedures:
    d. PM implant.
    e. AVR.
    f. Endocarditis.
3) Non cardiac factors [8]:
    g. Frailty.
    h. Liver disease.
    i. Previous chest irradiation.

Especially in latter condition, TAVI might become an attractive option [8].

2.3.2. Overestimation of the Risk by EuroSCORE

Overestimation of mortality after AVR by the EuroSCORE in high-risk patients (*i.e.* a score more than 20) was and still is a reason for concern. Conventional AVR might be denied in patients who would have otherwise received this procedure [8]. The EuroSCORE model as predictor could be disturbed by differences between:

- Definitions of variables.
- Institutions.
- Sensitivity in screening tools.
- Possible interdependencies.

These factors are important for patient selection for AVR and for TAVI [6, 9].

Other factors such as housing, mobility, social integration and perceived QoL also have their importance in the decision making [8].

Last but not least, crude mortality rates are not sufficient for assessment of quality of care. Long-term survival and QoL also have to be taken into consideration. However, there is some correlation between the hospital and long-term outcome. Therefore, hospital mortality can serve as main indicator for quality of care [5].

2.4. Recalibration of EuroSCORE and Remaining Problems

Recalibration of the model seems necessary since this model is based on the standards for care in 1995. These standards have improved in the recent years. Hence, the scoring system does not reflect the risk in current practice [6, 9]. Updating the data set with recalibration and recalculation of the EuroSCORE using more recent patient data seems preferable. This has been done for STS PROM [8]. But even with calibration, several errors remain [4, 7]. These could be:

1) Ignoring available variables that are associated with the risk.

2) Inclusion of variables from small patients subgroups, meaning the effect of changing risk profiles over time could be overlooked.

3) Inability of EuroSCORE to discriminate between different cardiac procedures.

4) Under-representation of variables of subgroups of patients that were not yet included in 1995.

5) Publication bias: poor results are less likely to be published.

6) Taking into account the more recent advances made in patient care.

2.5. Alternatives for the EuroSCORE

Besides the logistic EuroSCORE are the STS PROM score and Parsonnet score. These scores are also based on demographic patients characteristics, cardiac and non-cardiac status. They all have a predictive value for cardiac surgery, including AVR. By calculating these three scores for a given patient group, comparison between these scoring systems becomes possible. For all scores, Receiver Operating Characteristic curves with the area under the curve have been constructed, to summarize sensitivity and specificity for expected *versus* observed mortality [8].

The STS score seems more accurate to assess operative mortality after AVR, with a modestly higher area under the ROC curve of 71.8 *vs.* 69.9. High risk patients could be identified, who are deemed unfit for AVR. An alternative option for such patients, such as TAVI could be considered [8]. Parsonnet (additive & logistic) score, EuroSCORE (additive & logistic) and STS PROM have been used for this purpose, but this is not necessarily justified. These calculators are available on:

http://www. euroscore.org

http://66.89.112.110/STSWebRiskCalc261/de.aspx and on

http://www.sfar.org/scores2/parsonnet2.html

3. POSTOPERATIVE EVENTS: CATEGORIZATION

Postoperative events also have to be categorized and defined. This is necessary if one wants to compare the results of different patient series. Some postoperative events are related to the patient and not to the AVR or the prosthetic valve. Other postoperative events are clearly related to the valve [1, 2]. A list of these categories of events is listed below:

3.1. Complications Within the Hospital

- Mortality (all causes).
- Valve related (or supposedly valve related) events.
  - TE and PVT.
  - Bleeding (anticoagulation related).
  - PVE.
  - PPVL.
- Other cardiac events:
  - Low cardiac output syndrome, CHF.
  - CD, and need for PPMI.
  - Arrhythmias (atrial and ventricular).
  - AMI.
  - Re-exploration for surgical bleeding.
- Non-cardiac complications.
  - Acute renal function impairment.
  - Pulmonary complications: atelectasis, pneumonia, need for prolonged ventilation.
  - Pneumothorax, pleura effusion, subcutaneous emphysema.

- Wound infection, fever.
- Gastric stress ulcers and other digestive complications.

3.2. Complications During Long-Term Follow-Up

- Mortality rate (or survival as complementary to mortality).
- Valve related events.
    - TE (note: not all TE are necessarily related to the valve).
    - PVT.
    - Bleeding.
    - PVE.
    - SVD.
    - Non structural failure, including pannus and PPVL.
    - Reoperation for any of these events.
- Cardiac events:
    - AMI.
    - CHF.
    - CD and PMMI.

These events should be given as freedom of … at … years and not as linearized rates (% per patient-year), especially if these events show no linear rates such as TE and SVD.

4. POSTOPERATIVE EVENTS: DEFINITIONS

4.1. General Remarks

Every event has to be graded according to its severity. Grading of events can be done with the performance status scale according to Karnofsky, which seems appropriate for events after valve surgery. Grading according "mild", "moderate", "severe" and "fatal" must be defined properly. Fatal events which cannot be categorized should be grouped as cardiac (but not valve related) or non-cardiac related. Sudden death is listed separately [2].

4.2. Mortality [3, 10-14]

Operative and hospital mortality are the most impressive adverse events. These can be defined as:

1) All deaths occurring during the hospital period in which the operation was performed.
2) Those deaths occurring within 30 days of the procedure, unless the cause of death is unrelated to the operation [3].

One should be aware that hospital mortality, operative mortality, peri-operative mortality and early mortality are often interchangeable. The 30 days definition covers these terms and should be used. Mortality after 30 days should be labeled as mid and long-term. This applies also for non-fatal complications.

4.3. Neurological Events [15, 17-26]

Neurological events can be due to TE or to bleeding. A CT or MRI scan is helpful in the differentiation. This is important since a TE event, in contrast to bleeding, requires anticoagulation. If proper categorization is not possible, neurological events should be recorded as "**not categorized**". Embolism in other organs reveal themselves by the ischemic nature of clinical symptoms and signs.

TE events, however, can have more than one source, which is not necessarily easy to identify:

- Valvular, due to PVT and endocarditis.
- Cardiac but non-valvular: left atrial thrombosis, left ventricular thrombosis (especially if LVEF is low).
- Extracardiac: aortic arch, carotid arteries or more distally in cerebral or territorial vessels, causing lacunary infarctions.

4.4. Prosthetic Valve Thrombosis [27, 28]

PVT is a non-infective mass attached to the prosthetic ring or to the leaflets. For BHV, the risk for PVT is highest during the first three months after implantation. For MHV, the risk is continuously present, for which anticoagulating medication has to be taken. The diagnosis of PVT requires TEE.

A non-obstructive PVT can be asymptomatic. This event can go unnoticed until the next imaging is taken or when a TE occurs. The true incidence of PVT therefore is unknown. It is probably higher (up to 10%) in the early postoperative period. Risk factors for PTV are low LVF, prior TE, inadequate anticoagulation and AF.

An obstructive PVT shows are additional signs: abnormal opening and closing occluder clicks and CHF due to obstruction or to regurgitation. These events are related to limited occluder motion by thrombotic masses. Once the diagnosis is confirmed, prompt thrombolysis is needed. Surgery also could be needed, especially in presence of rapidly evolving CHF. Anticoagulation after PVT has to be followed closely [2, 16].

4.5. Pannus [28]

Pannus is growth of tissue on the stents. In some degree it could be considered as a part of a healing process. In small amounts, it forms a protective non-thrombogenic surface. If pannus reaches the adjacent parts of the leaflets, it could cause failure of the BHV. Pannus can be initiated by small amounts of thrombus, followed by an invasion of inflammatory cells, fibroblasts and myofibroblasts. When this tissue matures, collagen fibers within this pannus retract.

Leaflets can become thickened, stiffened, calcified and deformed. This results in stenosis or regurgitation. This tissue in-growth can also be responsible for obstruction of the valve. Tears can be the consequence of alterations in stress patterns posed upon the BHV. Pannus of the valve prosthesis need proper distinction from PVT by imaging (TEE, cineradiography) and Doppler techniques (determination of EOA, peak and mean transprosthetic gradient).

4.6. Bleeding [17, 18, 29-34]

Bleeding events are obvious if there are external signs. Definitions and grading system should be as uniform as possible, to make comparison between patient series possible.

For the risk-assessment of bleeding, some factors must be taken into account:

- Stability of INR and related to this, patient discipline (which can be very high with self management by appropriately trained patients).

- Co-morbid conditions (liver and renal disease, hypertension, malignancy, etc…).

- Pharmacological interaction (by NSAID).

- Age.

Cerebral hemorrhages can be distinguished from cerebral emboli by CT and MRI. The number of "not categorized" events should be kept as low as possible. The issue can be complicated by hemorrhagic transformation of a cerebral infarction. Presence or absence of mass effects can be helpful herein, but the aid of an experienced neurologist or neuroradiologist is indispensable.

4.7. Prosthetic Valve Endocarditis [35-38]

PVE is also a major complication requiring proper diagnosis which include an adequate assessment of clinical symptoms and signs, bacteriological documentation and repetitive imaging techniques comprising multiplane TEE without delay. PVE occurs more in the first two years following AVR. Previous endocarditis is a risk factor. PVE can lead to regurgitation, caused by tears within the leaflets or to stenosis, by the protruding vegetations. Treatment – including the decision to operate or not – must be performed in centres with the necessary expertise. The degree of inflammation in the explant should be graded after operation, since PVE could sometimes be mistaken for valve degeneration. Complications of PVE are paravalvular abscesses, CHF and septic emboli, which usually require surgery.

4.8. Valvular Dysfunction

When a prosthesis does not fulfills its purpose, it is said to be malfunctioning.

This can be subdivided in three ways:

- By site: structural *versus* non structural (such as PPVL).
- By hemodynamic effect: obstruction *versus* regurgitation or combined.
- By cause: PVT, PVE, pannus, interference with the occluder, material defects or metal fatigue and degeneration of tissue.

4.9. Periprosthetic Valvular Leak [39-42]

PPVL have infectious and other causes such as annulus calcification, connective tissue diseases, over-sizing and technical failures. Auscultatory murmurs, Doppler-echocardiography and cinefluoroscopy are methods for detection. Progression of dehiscence due to infection must be ruled out. Haemolytic anemia can be a result of turbulence, especially if the leak is small. Decompensated anemia is an indication for reoperation. The use of a silver impregnated stent as an attempt to prevent PVE (with a Silzone valve, in the AVERT trial) has resulted in problems in this respect.

Mechanical dysfunction can be caused by wear. Other cause for this event, such as material defects, strut fracture and leaflet escape are rare. The diagnosis in patients who survive this catastrophe long enough is cine-fluoroscopy.

4.10. Structural Valve Degeneration [43-51]

SVD is a time dependent event, typically for BHV. The tissue degenerates and dystrophic calcification occurs. This occurs sooner in younger patients who have received such a device. This early degeneration is probably related to a more active immune system at young age. Antibodies could enter the matrix of the BHV. Macrophages are deposited on the valvular surface, collagen breaks down and calcification occurs.

This calcification could be the result of reaction between the circulating calcium, phospholipids and aldehyde groups. The zona fibrosa is the most affected area. Cross linking of collagen as result of treatment of glutaraldehyde under high pressure provides a nidus of calcification. The first signs of calcification can be observed years before SVD becomes clinically evident. This process resembles somewhat the mineralization process in CAVS. Treatment of valves by surfactant and alpha oleic acid might slow down calcification of the leaflets.

SVD can result in both stenosis and regurgitation. The stenosis is the result of stiffening of the leaflets. The regurgitation is the result of tears of the leaflet at the site of calcification. Perforation of the valve is less common. Other mechanisms of regurgitation such as commissural dehiscence are rare in contemporary BHV.

Young age, presence of risk factors for atheromatosis, valve position and conditions involving calcification (such as renal failure) must be taken into account as risk factors. The hemodynamic consequences of SVD can be assessed by Doppler echocardiography. Once SVD occurs, its progress needs close follow-up in order to determine the best time for re-replacement of the valve.

Tears at the leaflets can also be the result of closing pressures and are not necessarily related to calcification. The hemodynamic stress is highest at the commissures. This is worse with low profile valves.

4.11. Intravascular Hemolysis [52-57]

Intravascular hemolysis can be detected by an elevation of serum lactate dehydrogenase or haptoglobin, as most sensitive sign for subtle cell loss. Reticulocytes, schistocytes and erythrocyte creatine also have been used as parameter for hemolysis.

Hemolysis occurs more frequently with older types of MHV. The degree of hemolysis usually remains low. Red blood cell damage due to the valve is usually subclinical. In stentless valves, no hemolysis has been detected. In cases of shear stress, such as in small periprosthetic leaks, hemolysis can become clinical. If this condition requires repeated blood transfusion, it can be labeled as severe and requires reoperation.

4.12. Congestive Heart Failure [58-62]

Hospital CHF is a serious complication after AVR and has a high mortality rate. This complication could also be labeled as low output syndrome. Few studies have been focused on the risk factors for this event. A major risk factor is need for urgent AVR, which points to an exhaustion of the left ventricle to maintain an adequate circulation [58]. Other causes could be a peri-operative myocardial infarction, especially when CAD is also present.

Long-term CHF is not easy to define in patients who have undergone AVR for stenotic CAVS. In many patients, LVH is present and LVEF is usually supranormal. An impaired relaxation of a stiff, fibrotic and hypertrophic left ventricle could serve as mechanism for postoperative CHF, especially when an AF is present.

4.13. Conduction Defects [63-68]

These events can be defined as any new postoperative CD or any postoperative worsening of a pre-existent CD. The diagnosis can be made on ECG. CD can vary from first degree AV block, without symptoms and no need for treatment to any bundle branch block and third degree AV block. Patients with the latter need a PPMI. Reversible forms need to be distinguished from irreversible blocks, since this can determine the mode of treatment. Especially after TAVI, CD have been observed.

4.14. Atrial Fibrillation [69-71]

This is one of the most frequent complications after heart surgery in general but this arrhythmia cannot be considered as innocent. Paroxysmal AF must be distinguished from the chronic form. In chronic forms, anti-arrhytmic procedures have been applied, even in patients with non mitral heart disease.

There is a wide variation in frequency of early postoperative AF, between 10 and 50%. This variation can be explained by different diagnostic methods. Proper treatment of this arrhythmia reduces length of stay within the hospital and increases the postoperative rehabilitation.

4.15. Non-Cardiac Complications [72-74]

Renal and pulmonary complications are amongst the most serious non-cardiac postoperative complications. Only a few reports have appeared in which the risk factors for these events were analyzed.

Pulmonary complications, such as a need for prolonged ventilation, atelectasis and infections have to be described adequately by clinical and radiological (plain radiography and CT of the chest) examinations. Variations in definitions of pulmonary complications can result in differences in their postoperative occurrence.

Acute postoperative renal function impairment is not easily defined. An increase of plasma creatinin with 0.3 mg% has been proposed, but this has some problems. Plasma creatinin is not the best way to assess renal function since it also depends on age, gender and muscle mass. Moreover, with a preoperative creatinin already considerably elevated, an increase of 0.3 mg% might not indicate a major postoperative decrease in renal function. This, however, certainly is the case when the preoperative creatinin is between 1 and 2 mg%. In spite of its limitations, the plasma creatinin served well as parameter in an analysis of a large cohort of patients who underwent AVR.

5. WHICH FUNCTIONS NEED TO BE SCRUTINIZED FOR FOLLOW-UP

Prosthetic valve function. After surgery, at discharge a clinical, ECG, INR and basic blood tests and TTE are necessary. Valve and ventricular function, pericardial effusion as well as pulmonary pressure can be assessed. Sometimes, a TEE is warranted if there is clinical suspicion (CHF, fever, hemolysis, inadequate anticoagulation, TE events, etc…) for an abnormal occluder motion, PVT, left atrial thrombi, PPVL or PVE [1].

Myocardial function. Postoperative LVM regression occurs in the first months. The regression of myocardial fibrosis is slower which can lead to aggravation of "diastolic CHF" [58]. Diameters of ventricles, systolic and diastolic function can be assessed by TTE. Cardio MRI can also be helpful. Exercise capacity can normalize within 3 to 12 months if there is no irreversible myocardial damage and if the postoperative course is uneventful [1].

Pulmonary artery pressure. If PAHT is the consequence of an increase in the left atrial pressure, PAHT regresses when the LV diastolic function normalizes. If PAHT is the result of an increase in resistance of the pulmonary vessels, PAHT takes more time to regress, and normal values are usually not reached. In patients with CAVS, PAHT is associated with a more severe clinical presentation and carries a poor postoperative prognosis. Therefore, these patients require a close postoperative follow up. Clinically relevant VPPM is a strong predictor for persistence of PAHT after AVR [1].

Cognitive function. Impairment of cognitive function has been observed after cardiac surgery and can be due to the use of an ECC (cerebral micro-emboli of gas or solids, systemic inflammation, side effect of the general anaesthesia, perioperative hypotension) as well as to the cardiovascular disease itself. Definitions of cognitive impairment and test batteries vary considerable, hence studies cannot always be compared. However, restoration of cognitive function is usually expected 3 months after operation. Long-term cognitive impairment can be found in a considerable portion of patients who underwent cardiac surgery. Conditions such as Alzheimer disease and other newly occurring cerebral disease as well as the effect of aging have to be taken into account.

Small gas emboli can appear in patients who have received a mechanical valve. These are the consequence of cavitation effect due to local pressure gradients and shear stress at the mechanical valve. The number of these "HITS" seems to be correlated with cognitive impairment in the first period after valve surgery. With diffusion-weighted MRI, small cerebral emboli can be detected in up to half of the patients after cardiac surgery [1].

Postoperative **medical treatment** needs to be tailored. After-load reducing therapy should not be discontinued too soon after AVR. ACE inhibitors can be useful if there are symptoms or signs of systolic dysfunction. Spironolactone can be helpful in the regression of myocardial fibrosis. Beta-blocking agents have their use in control of heart rate and arrhythmias. Statins can be administered in case of hypercholesterolemia.

Postoperative anticoagulation and antiplatelet medication is the most important issue and depends not only on the type of valve but also on co-morbid conditions that increase the risk for TE events. These include AF, low LVEF, hypercoagulability, previous TE events, etc... For biological valves, a three month regimen of peroral anticoagulation is recommended, after which antiplatelet therapy can be started. For mechanical valves, lifelong peroral anticoagulation is required. One should aim for the lowest effective INR. Not only the height but also the stability of INR is important in the reduction of postoperative TE events. Patient self-management reduces the number of TE events and of mortality considerably.

6. APPROPRIATE STATISTICAL TECHNIQUES

6.1. General Remarks

Data collection can be prospective or retrospective. Results of the latter should be interpreted cautiously since these have their limitations. A prospective clinical trial requires a follow up protocol, including full information regarding:

1) Follow up techniques.

2) Time intervals.

3) All parameters that have been documented.

Information concerning "intention-to-treat" or explorative data analysis must be provided.

The former should be used when there is some drop-out [2].

6.2. Actual *vs.* Actuarial Analysis

Proper statistical analysis takes the time relationship of events into account: many events occur in the first postoperative months (such as PPVL), other events increase with time (such as SVD, which occurs mostly after 10 years) or have a constant hazard rate (such as PVE). Hence, a linearized rate is not the appropriate way to represent results. Distinction between actual *versus* actuarial rates also has to be made [1, 2].

Unlike cumulative incidence, Kaplan-Meier method attempts to predict what the latent failure probability would be if death were eliminated. To do this, the Kaplan-Meier method assumes that the risk of dying and the risk of failure are independent. But this assumption is not true for many cardiac applications in which the risks of failure and death are negatively correlated, *i.e.*, patients with a higher risk of dying have a lower risk of failure, and patients with a lower risk of death have a higher risk of failure.

The Kaplan-Meier method calculates the freedom from death or any other complication after an operation such as AVR. As all statistical methods, it possesses some pitfalls. This analysis provides interesting information, provided some important requisites, such as adequate duration of follow up and sufficient high number of events in a population, are present. The number of events is the factor that really makes the difference. In a study with a very low rate of a complication, presenting the Kaplan-Meier curve for that complication does not provide any more valuable information than does the crude percentage. Therefore, applying the Kaplan-Meier method is worthwhile only with adequate duration of follow-up in a large population and number of events.

The 'actual' method has been created as alternative to the Kaplan-Meier method. This method documents the true rate of failure and reoperation in patients with BHV as opposed to the Kaplan-Meier method. For non-fatal events such as SVD, Kaplan-Meier estimates the SVD-free curve by censoring patients who are still alive without SVD, or have already died without SVD. Censoring means that patients are added back into the calculations, as future events distributed over future time. By assuming that patients without SVD, whether currently alive or dead, could have SVD in the future, the Kaplan-Meier method overestimates the number of events.

On the other hand, the actual analysis censors only those patients who are alive without SVD, and estimates the percentage who will actually suffer an event. In this analysis, death eliminates patients from the risk pool. So there are some very important facts to keep in mind when including the actual method in the statistical analysis:

1) The number of deaths is fundamental because a population with a low rate of late mortality will show very little difference between the actual and Kaplan-Meier method.

2) The actual method applies to analysis of complications only.

The actual method in the statistical analysis should be used when this method enables the authors to generate more accurate outcomes than by applying the Kaplan-Meier calculations only, thus improving the quality of the inferences. On the contrary, when the actual method adds no information to those obtained by the life-table analysis, then the actual method is a redundancy [75-77].

6.3. Risk Factor Analysis

Risk factors include demographic variables, cardiac and non-cardiac co-morbid conditions, current and previous cardiac procedures. Some are universally used, such as age, gender or LVEF. Some are included for the study of specific complications (*e.g.* small valve size for VPPM, previous endocarditis for PVE). Risk factors can be presented as a dichotomy (absence or presence of a factor), as categories (such as the NYHA functional class) or as a continuous distribution.

For early (operative, hospital or 30 day) events, risk factors can be screened by an univariate analysis. For dichotomous and categorical variables, a chi-square analysis (or a variant, such as a Fisher-exact method) can be used. For mid or long-term outcome, a Kaplan-Meier analysis is appropriate to identify the risk factors. Subsequently, in a stepwise logistic regression (for early events) or in a Cox' proportional hazard analysis (for long-term events), the significant variables can be entered and independent predictors can be identified [3]. Models can be created for missing values.

Following studies (the examples are not exhaustive) are possible:

- Comparative studies between procedures (AVR, AVR+CABG, AVR+MV repair, *etc.*).
- Comparative study for two or more types of valve.
- Comparative study for the effect of the position (mostly AVR *versus* MVR *versus* DVR) [3].

These results can be used to set standards for quality of care. With a given mix of risk factors, a bench mark for "acceptable outcome" can be developed. For any given institution, a predicted operative mortality can be calculated. The actual operative mortality can be compared to the predicted operative mortality. If the actual results are significantly worse, a detailed examination is warranted, but this not always an indicator for substandard care. With certain limitations, the STS database allows to determine the impact on risk factors on the outcome for cardiac surgery [3].

CONCLUSIONS

Follow-up studies have been performed for various reasons. These studies can be designed as a risk assessment for the individual patient but also as an analysis of the quality of care for any given situation.

Several risk scores have been developed for this purpose, such as the EuroSCORE and the STS PROM. These scores have been developed for CABG, in an earlier era. These scores tend to overestimate the mortality, especially in high risk patients. Hence, they should be applied with great caution in the patient selection for AVR or for alternatives such as TAVI.

Apart from mortality, an analysis can be made from non-fatal valve related events, other cardiac events and non-cardiac events. These events all need a proper definition. The data acquisition for these events also requires a minimal standard of quality.

Last, but not least, proper statistical methods have to be applied to reach meaningful conclusions.

ACKNOWLEDGEMENT

Declared none.

CONFLICT OF INTEREST

The author(s) confirm that this chapter content has no conflict of interest.

REFERENCES

[1] Horstkotte D, Lengyel M, Mistiaen WP, *et al.*, on behalf of the Working Group 'Infection, Thrombosis, Embolism and Bleeding' of the Society of Heart Valve Disease.

Recommendations for Post-Discharge Patient Follow Up after Cardiac Valve Interventions: A Position Paper. J Heart Valve Dis 2007;16:575-589.
[2] Horstkotte D, Lengyel M, Mistiaen WP, *et al.*, on behalf of the Working Group 'Infection, Thrombosis, Embolism and Bleeding' of the Society of Heart Valve Disease. Recommendations for Reporting Morbid Events after Heart Valve Surgery. J Heart Valve Dis 2005;14:1-7.
[3] Edwards FH, Peterson ED, Coombs LP, *et al.* Prediction of Operative Mortality After Valve Replacement Surgery. J Am Coll Cardiol 2001;37:885-892.
[4] Dewey TM, MA Herbert. Editorial comment. Predicting operative risk: a worthy task — an elusive goal. Eur J Cardiothorac Surg 2009;36:797.
[5] Roques F, Nashef SAM, Michel P, *et al.* Risk factors and outcome in European cardiac surgery: analysis of the EuroSCORE multinational database of 19030 patients. Eur J Cardio-thorac Surg 1999;15:816-823.
[6] Kalavrouziotis D, Li D, Buth KJ, Légaré. JF. The European System for Cardiac Operative Risk Evaluation [EuroSCORE] is not appropriate for withholding surgery in high-risk patients with aortic stenosis: a retrospective cohort study. J Cardiothorac Surg 2009, 4:32 doi:10.1186/1749-8090-4-32.
[7] Ranucci M, Castelvecchio S, Menicanti LA, *et al.* An adjusted EuroSCORE model for high-risk cardiac patients. Eur J Cardio-thorac Surg 2009;36:791-798.
[8] Wendt D, Osswald BR, Kayser K, *et al.* Society of Thoracic Surgeons Score Is Superior to the EuroSCORE Determining Mortality in High Risk Patients Undergoing Isolated Aortic Valve Replacement. Ann Thorac Surg 2009;88:468-475.
[9] Leontyev S, Walther T, Borger MA, *et al.* Aortic Valve Replacement in Octogenarians: Utility of Risk Stratification With EuroSCORE. Ann Thorac Surg 2009;87:1440-1445.
[10] Kolh P, Lahaye L, Gerard P, Limet R. Aortic valve replacement in the octogenarians: perioperative outcome and clinical follow-up. Eur J Cardio-thorac Surg 1999;16: 68-73.
[11] Florath I, Rosendahl UP, Mortasawi A, *et al.* Current Determinants of Operative Mortality in 1400 Patients Requiring Aortic Valve Replacement. Ann Thorac Surg 2003;76:75-83.
[12] Mistiaen W, Van Cauwelaert Ph, Muylaert Ph, *et al.* Risk factors and survival after aortic valve replacement in octogenarians. J Heart Valve Dis. 2004;13:538-544.
[13] Alsoufi B, Karamlou T, Slater M, *et al.* Results of concomitant aorta valve replacement and coronary artery bypass grafting in the VA population. J Heart Valve Dis 2006;15:12-18.
[14] Hannan EL, Samadashvili Z, Lahey SJ, *et al.* Aortic Valve Replacement for Patients With Severe Aortic Stenosis: Risk Factors and Their Impact on 30-Month Mortality. Ann Thorac Surg 2009;87:1741-1750.
[15] Mistiaen W, Van Cauwelaert Ph, Muylaert Ph, *et al.* Thrombo-embolism after aortic valve replacement in elderly with a Carpentier-Edwards perimount TM bioprosthesis. J Thorac Cardiovasc Surg. 2004;127:1166-1170
[16] Lengyel M, Horstkotte D, Voller H, Mistiaen WP. Recommendations for the management of prosthetic valve thrombosis.J Heart Valve Dis 2005;14:567-575.
[17] Casselman FP, Bots ML, Van Lommel W, *et al.* Repeated Thromboembolic and Bleeding Events After Mechanical Aortic Valve Replacement. Ann Thorac Surg 2001;71:1172-1180.
[18] Cromheecke ME, Levi M, Colly LP, *et al.* Oral anticoagulation self-management and management by a specialist anticoagulation clinic: a randomised cross-over comparison. Lancet 2000;356:97-102.
[19] Dauphin C, Legault B, Jaffeux P, *et al.* Comparison of INR stability between self-monitoring and standard laboratory method: Preliminary results of a prospective study in 67 mechanical heart valve patients. Arch Cardiovascular Dis 2008;101:753-761.

[20] Eckman MH, Levine HJ, Pauker SG. Effect of Laboratory Variation in the Prothrombin-Time Ratio on the Results of Oral Anticoagulant Therapy. NEJM 1993; 329:696-702.

[21] Eitz T, Schenk S, Fritzsche D, *et al.* International Normalized Ratio Self-Management Lowers the Risk of Thromboembolic Events After Prosthetic Heart Valve Replacement. Ann Thorac Surg 2008;85:949-955.

[22] Floyd TF, Shah PN, Price CC, *et al.* Clinically Silent Cerebral Ischemic Events After Cardiac Surgery: Their Incidence, Regional Vascular Occurrence, and Procedural Dependence. Ann Thorac Surg 2006;81:2160-2166.

[23] Gulbins H, Florath I, Ennker J. Cerebrovascular Events After Stentless Aortic Valve Replacement During a 9-Year Follow-Up Period. Ann Thorac Surg 2008;86:769-773.

[24] Filsoufi F, Rahmanian PB, Castillo JG, *et al.* Incidence, Imaging Analysis, and Early and Late Outcomes of Stroke After Cardiac Valve Operation. Am J Cardiol 2008;101:1472-1478.

[25] Ruel M, Masters RG, Rubens FD, *et al.* Late Incidence and Determinants of Stroke After Aortic and Mitral Valve Replacement. Ann Thorac Surg 2004;78:77-84.

[26] Valle HA, Alvarez CF, Garcıa-Palomo JD, *et al.* The Topography of Aortic Atherosclerosis Enhances Its Precision as a Predictor of Stroke. Ann Thorac Surg 2007;83:2087-2092.

[27] Lin SS, Tiong IYH, Asher CR, *et al.* Prediction of Thrombus-Related Mechanical Prosthetic Valve Dysfunction Using Transesophageal Echocardiography. Am J Cardiol 2000;86:1097-1101.

[28] Rizzoli G, Guglielmi C, Toscano G, *et al.* Reoperations for acute prosthetic thrombosis and pannus: an assessment of rates, relationship and risk. Eur J Cardio-thorac Surg 1999;16:74-80.

[29] Ansell JE. Editorial. Empowering Patients to Monitor and Manage Oral Anticoagulation Therapy. JAMA 1999;281:182-183.

[30] Butchart EG, Payne N, Li HH, *et al.* Better anticoagulation control improves survival after valve replacement. J Thorac Cardiovasc Surg 2002;123:715-23.

[31] Gadisseur APA, Kaptein AA, Breukink-Engbers WGM, *et al.* Patient self-management of oral anticoagulant care *vs.* management by specialized anticoagulation clinics: positive effects on quality of life. J Thromb Haemost 2004;2:584-591.

[32] Hamad MAS, van Eekelen E, van Agt T, van Straten AHM. Self-management program improves anticoagulation control and quality of life: a prospective randomized study. Eur J Cardio-thorac Surg 2009;35:265-269.

[33] Jackson SL, Bereznicki LR, Peterson GM, *et al.* Accuracy, reproducibility and clinical utility of the CoaguChek S portable international normalized ratio monitor in an outpatient anticoagulation clinic. Clin Lab Haem 2004;26:49-55.

[34] Koertke H, Zittermann A, Wagner O, Koerfer R. Self-Management of Oral Anticoagulation Therapy Improves Long-Term Survival in Patients With Mechanical Heart Valve Replacement. Ann Thorac Surg 2007;83:24-29.

[35] Chirouze C, Cabell CH, Fowler VG Jr., *et al.*, and the International Collaboration on Endocarditis Study Group. Prognostic Factors in 61 Cases of *Staphylococcus aureus* Prosthetic Valve Infective Endocarditis from the International Collaboration on Endocarditis Merged Database. Clinical Infectious Diseases 2004;38:1323-1327.

[36] Habib G, Tribouilloy C, Thuny F, *et al.* Prosthetic valve endocarditis: who needs surgery? A multicentre study of 104 cases. Heart 2005;91:954-959.

[37] Habib G, Thuny F, Avierinos JF. Prosthetic Valve Endocarditis: Current Approach and Therapeutic Options. Progress Cardiovasc Dis 2008;50:274-281.

[38] Mahesh B, Angelini G, Caputo M, *et al.* Prosthetic Valve Endocarditis. Ann Thorac Surg 2005;80:1151-1158.

[39] Dávila-Román VG, Waggoner AD, Kennard ED, *et al.* Prevalence and Severity of Paravalvular Regurgitation in the Artificial Valve Endocarditis Reduction Trial [AVERT] Echocardiography Study. J Am Coll Cardiol 2004;44:1467-1472.

[40] Englberger L, Schaff HV, Jamieson WRE, *et al.*, for the AVERT Investigators Importance of implant technique on risk of major paravalvular leak [PVL] after St. Jude mechanical heart valve replacement: a report from the Artificial Valve Endocarditis Reduction Trial [AVERT]. Eur J Cardio-thorac Surg 2005;28:838-844.

[41] Rallidis LS, Moyssakis IE, Ikonomidis I, Nihoyannopoulos P. Natural history of early aortic paraprosthetic regurgitation: A five-year follow-up. Am Heart J 1999;138:351-357.

[42] Schaff HV, Carrel TP, Jamieson WRE, *et al.* Paravalvular Leak and Other Events in Silzone-Coated Mechanical Heart Valves: A Report From AVERT. Ann Thorac Surg 2002;73:785-792.

[43] Burdon TE, Miller DC, Oyer PE, *et al.* Durability of porcine valves at 15 years in a representative North-American patient population. J Thorac Cardiovasc Surg 1992;103:238-252.

[44] David TE, Feindel CM, Bos J, *et al.* Aortic valve replacement with Toronto SPV bioprosthesis: Optimal patient survival but suboptimal valve durability. J Thorac Cardiovasc Surg 2008;135:19-24.

[45] Jamieson WRE, Burr LH, Miyagishima RT, *et al.* Structural deterioration in Carpentier-Edwards standard and supraannular bioprosthesis. Ann Thorac Surg 1995;60:S241-S247.

[46] Jamieson WRE, Burr LH, Miyagishima RT, *et al.* Reoperation for bioprosthetic aortic structural failure – risk assessment. Eur J Cardio-thorac Surg 2003;24:873-878.

[47] Kulik A, Masters RG, Bédard P, *et al.* Postoperative lipid-lowering therapy and bioprosthesis structural valve deterioration: justification for a randomized trial? Eur J Cardio-thorac Surg 2010;37:139-144.

[48] Nollert G, Miksch J, Kreuzer E, Reichart B. Risk factors for atherosclerosis and the degeneration of pericardial valves after aortic valve replacement. J Thorac Cardiovasc Surg 2003;126:965-968.

[49] Rizzoli G, Bottio T, Thiene G, *et al.* Long-term durability of the Hancock II porcine Bioprosthesis. J Thorac Cardiovasc Surg 2003;126:66-74.

[50] Shetty R, Pibarot P, Audet A, *et al.* Lipid-mediated inflammation and degeneration of bioprosthetic heart valves. Eur J Clin Invest 2009;39:471-480.

[51] Yankah CA, Pasic M, Musci M, *et al.* Aortic valve replacement with the Mitroflow pericardial bioprosthesis: Durability results up to 21 years. J Thorac Cardiovasc Surg 2008;136:688-696.

[52] Ismeno G, Renzulli A, Carozza A, *et al.* Intravascular hemolysis after mitral and aortic valve replacement with different types of mechanical prostheses. Int J Cardiology 1999;69:179–183.

[53] Josa M, Castellá M, Paré C, *et al.* Hemolysis in Mechanical Bileaflet Prostheses: Experience With the Bicarbon Valve. Ann Thorac Surg 2006;81:1291-1296.

[54] Lu PC, Lai HC, Liu JS. A reevaluation and discussion on the threshold limit for hemolysis in a turbulent shear flow. Journal of Biomechanics 2001;34:1361-1364.

[55] Mecozzi G, Milano AD, De Carlo M, *et al.* Intravascular hemolysis in patients with new-generation prosthetic heart valves: A prospective study. J Thorac Cardiovasc Surg 2002;123:550-556.

[56] Okumiya T, Ishikawa-Nishi M, Doi T, *et al.* Evaluation of Intravascular Hemolysis With Erythrocyte Creatine in Patients With Cardiac Valve Prostheses. Cheast 2004;125:2115-2120.

[57] Suedkamp M, Lercher AJ, Mueller-Riemenschneider F, *et al.* Hemolysis parameters of St. Jude Medical Hemodynamic Plus® and Regent® valves in aortic position. Int J Cardiology 2004;95:89-93.

[58] Mistiaen W, Van Cauwelaert Ph, Muylaert Ph, *et al.* Risk factors for congestive heart failure after aortic valve replacement with a Carpentier-Edwards pericardial prosthesis in the elderly. J Heart Valve Dis 2005;14:774-779.

[59] Gaudino M, Anselmi A, Abbat A, *et al.* Myocardial apoptosis predicts postoperative course after aortic valve replacement in patients with severe left ventricular hypertrophy. J Heart Valve Dis 2007;16:344-348.

[60] Nozohoor S, Nilsson J, Lührs C, *et al.* B-Type Natriuretic Peptide as a Predictor of Postoperative Heart Failure After Aortic Valve Replacement. Journal of Cardiothoracic and Vascular Anesthesia 2009;23:161-165.

[61] Ruel M, Al-Faleh H, Kulik A, *et al.* Prosthesis–patient mismatch after aortic valve replacement predominantly affects patients with preexisting left ventricular dysfunction: Effect on survival, freedom from heart failure, and left ventricular mass regression. J Thorac Cardiovasc Surg 2006;131:1036-1044.

[62] Unger P, Plein D, Van Camp G, *et al.* Effects of Valve Replacement for Aortic Stenosis on Mitral Regurgitation. Am J Cardiol 2008;102:1378-1382.

[63] Calvi V, Puzzangara E, Pruiti GP, *et al.* Early Conduction Disorders Following Percutaneous Aortic Valve Replacement. PACE 2009; 32:S126-S130.

[64] Dawkins S, Hobson AR, Kalra PR, *et al.* Permanent Pacemaker Implantation After Isolated Aortic Valve Replacement: Incidence, Indications, and Predictors. Ann Thorac Surg 2008;85:108-112.

[65] El-Khally Z, Thibault B, Staniloae C, *et al.* Prognostic Significance of Newly Acquired Bundle Branch Block After Aortic Valve Replacement. Am J Cardiol 2004;94:1008-1011.

[66] Erdogan HB, Kayalar N, Ardal H, *et al.* Risk Factors for Requirement of Permanent Pacemaker Implantation After Aortic Valve Replacement. J Card Surg 2006;21:211-215.

[67] Huynh H, Dalloul G, Ghanbari H, *et al.* Permanent Pacemaker Implantation Following Aortic Valve Replacement: Current Prevalence and Clinical Predictors. PACE 2009;32:1520–1525.

[68] Limongelli G, Ducceschi V, D'Andrea A, *et al.* Risk factors for pacemaker implantation following aortic valve replacement: a single centre experience. Heart 2003;89:901-904.

[69] Banach M, Goch A, Misztal M, *et al.* Predictors of paroxysmal atrial fibrillation in patients undergoing aortic valve replacement. J Thorac Cardiovasc Surg 2007;134:1569-1576.

[70] Baranowska E, Baranowki R, Michalek P, *et al.* Prediction of paroxysmal atrial fibrillation after aortic valve replacement in patients with aortic stenosis: identification of potential risk factors. J Heart Valve Dis 2003;12:136-141.

[71] Khargi K, Lemke B, Deneke T. Concomitant anti-arrhythmic procedures to treat permanent atrial fibrillation in CABG and AVR patients are as effective as in mitral valve patients. Eur J Cardio-thorac Surg 2005;27:841-846.

[72] Mistiaen W, Vissers D. Risk factors for postoperative pulmonary complications after aortic valve replacement within the hospital: an observational study. Austr J Physiotherapy 2008;54: 119-124.

[73] Mistiaen W, Van Cauwelaert P, Muylaert P, De Worm E. 1000 pericardial valves in aortic position: risk factors for postoperative acute renal function impairment in elderly. J Cardiovasc Surg 2009;50:233-237.

[74] Weerasinghe A, Yusuf M, Athanasiou T, *et al.* Role of Transvalvular Gradient in Outcome From Valve Replacement for Aortic Stenosis. Ann Thorac Surg 2004;77:1266-1271.

[75] Grunkemeier GL, Wu YX. Actual *versus* actuarial event-free percentages. Ann Thorac Surg 2001;72:677-678.

[76] Grunkemeier GL, Jin R, Eijkemans MJC, Takkenberg JJM. Actual and Actuarial Probabilities of Competing Risks: Apples and Lemons. Ann Thorac Surg 2007;83:1586-1592.

[77] Vitale N, Nappi G, Scardone M. Should 'Actual' and 'Actuarial' Curves be Considered always Essential for any Scientific Presentation ? J Heart Valve Dis 2004;13:S20.

Send Orders of Reprints at bspsaif@emirates.net.ae

CHAPTER 8

Results Obtained by Follow-Up

Abstract: The study of postoperative results in patient series can have several purposes. This goes from a simple description of a device or a technique to the identification of risk factors and the comparison between several devices and between different techniques. RCT can be considered as the "gold standard", but even non randomized prospective and retrospective series have been used.

The main outcomes under scrutiny are:

- Hospital mortality.
- Long term mortality.
- Valve related events:
  - TE.
  - Bleeding.
  - SVD.
  - PVE.
  - PPVL.
  - Reoperation.
- Other cardiac events:
  - CHF.
  - CD.
  - AF.
- Non-cardiac events:
  - Pulmonary.
  - Renal.

For these outcomes, it is useful to make a search for risk factors and independent predictors.

Keywords: CABG, cardiac events, extracorporeal circulation, hospital mortality, independent predictors, long-term mortality, non-cardiac events, risk factor analysis, survival, valve related events.

Wilhelm Peter Mistiaen

1. PURPOSE AND DESIGN OF STUDIES

Most studies have as primary purpose the **description** of the clinical outcome of a specific device. These are usually subdivided in hospital and long-term events. Mortality is a main outcome and is expressed as a % for operative, hospital or 30-day occurrence. For long-term results, they can be represented as % patient-year, but for non-linear events, this is inappropriate. Survival in % with the standard deviation is more common. It is also useful to comment on the reason for mortality: valve related, cardiac or all causes. Unexplained sudden death can also be given separately. Other important outcomes are valve related events such as TE, bleeding, PVE and SVD, cardiac events such as AF, progression or new CD, and CHF. For hospital events, a % can be used for description, for long-term events, % freedom after some years can be used (most common are 1, 2, 5, 10, 15, 20 and sometimes more years). Most of these studies are retrospective and observational in nature. Patient series are usually consecutive.

For hospital and long-term complications, a **risk factor analysis** can be useful. With an univariate analysis, a screening be performed. These risk factors can be used in a multivariate model, to find the independent predictors. These techniques increase the knowledge about such postoperative complications.

Sometimes, several techniques and devices can be **compared**. If this is considered in its retrospect, the results are liable to bias and their interpretation should be reflected on cautiously. This is especially true if a historical series has been used for comparison with a more contemporary series. A prospective randomized trial is a much stronger tool for obtaining valid conclusions. These RCT are a prerequisite to formulate a level A recommendation. RCT are needed with the introduction of improvements, of new techniques and of new devices. Examples are the AVERT trial for the Silzone valves [1] and the comparison of TAVI with more conventional techniques [2]. The expected benefit from a new technique or device does not always materialize, as can be observed with the Silzone valves.

Another type of comparison is the study for the effect of patient related factors such as age on SVD, age and gender on survival, position of the valve on SVD and on survival, INR variability on bleeding and survival [3], *etc.* These outcomes provide insight in pathophysiological principles.

Sometimes, specific complications are the focus of attention. These are usually scrutinized with advanced techniques, not applicable in daily practice. An example is neurologically silent TE, detectable by MRI. These patient series are usually small. Other purposes are more part of clinical routine and comprise LVMI regression, TVG and EOAI.

2. RESULTS FOR FOLLOW-UP

2.1. Hospital Mortality

This is a major outcome after AVR, and is presented in virtually every patient series. Hospital mortality varies from 1.2% [4] to 24% [5]. These variations are due to large differences in age and co-morbidity in the studied patient populations. With a time span of over 20 year between the first and the last published patient series, improvement in surgical techniques and peri-operative care could also be responsible for the results.

In most series, the hospital mortality is below 10%. In series where the mortality is over 10%, risk factors usually have been present. Independent predictors for hospital mortality have been identified and confirm that the presence of co-morbid conditions increase the early postoperative risk. The main predictors have been identified as:

- Emergency need for AVR [6-8].
- Preoperative functional class NYHA IV [9, 10].
- LF-LG problem [11].
- DM [10].
- Implantation of BHV [10].
- Severe CAVS [10].
- Severe CAD and need for concomitant CABG [5-7, 10].
- Small prosthesis size [11].

- Recent AMI [6, 8].
- Renal disease [6, 7, 12].
- Previous CABG [7] and valve surgery with MVH.
- Age over 80 [5, 7, 8].

An emergency need for AVR, *i.e.* to operate on the same day as the admission, has been identified as the most important predictor, with a increase of 10 times [8]. This indicates a exhaustion of all compensatory mechanisms to maintain an adequate circulation. A need for emergent/urgent AVR has also been identified as a predictor for early postoperative CHF or low output syndrome, which is a highly lethal condition [13].

2.2. Long-Term Mortality

The long-term mortality can be described as a linearized rate in % per patient-year. This varies from less than 1% [14] to 7.5% [15, 16]. The same risk factors as for hospital mortality could be responsible for long-term mortality. A better representation, however, is the survival rate at 1, 2, 5, 10, 15 and 20 year.

- Survival at 1 year varies between 69% [17] and 98% [5]. Remarkably, both patient series consist of octogenarians!
- Survival at 2 and 3 years are not often reported and are usually over 90% [5, 18].
- Survival at 5 years is considered as an important milestone. This varies between 38% [17] and 90% [19]. Some authors report survival as relative to the general population [20].
- A second important milestone is survival at 10 years. This varies between 43% [21] and 86% [22]. It must be mentioned that many reports do not go beyond 5 years.
- Some reports go beyond 15 years and show favorable results with a survival of 70% and more [20, 22]. Other series report a survival at about 20% after 15 years or beyond [23-25].

The survival rate varies considerably, as can be seen from the abovementioned series. Many of these series cannot be compared as such, since these differ in composition for age and for co-morbidity. The type of valve used in these patient series also differed. The best way to present such result is by the search for the independent predictors for long-term mortality. Comparatively few studies have been published in this respect. Predictors that have been identified are:

- Age [8, 26-29].
- Need for urgent AVR [5, 8, 17].
- Preoperative functional class NYHA IV [20, 22, 28].
- Preoperative CHF or low LVEF [17, 22, 30, 31].
- Excessive LVH [28].
- Previous AMI [5, 8].
- Variability of INR, in case a MHV has been implanted [32].
- Length of CCT [22].
- Use of digitalis [8].
- Small valve size/postoperative EOAI [27, 30].
- Preoperative AF [20, 29, 33].
- High EuroSCORE [17].
- Preoperative stroke [17].
- Preoperative renal function impairment [22].
- Previous carcinoma [8, 31].

These predictors can be grouped into demographic, cardiac and non-cardiac factors.

The prime demographic factor is age. Its effect is obvious: an old Asian proverb states "the older one gets, the closer one is at the grave". Yet, in many patient series, a postoperative survival close to the survival of a gender and age matched healthy population could be reached. The variability of survival in the explored series might be due to the age effect for the greater part. In some series, the median age is between 50 and 60 years [19, 30, 34-37], in other, it 70 or more [8, 10, 31, 33, 38-49] and in other, octogenarians are the focus of the attention [5, 17, 50-53].

Older reports described the effect of age classes specifically [16, 54-56]. However, the use of a multivariate Cox' proportional hazard analysis for long term results is more elegant and adequate. The technique identifies age as an independent predictor for survival. Its use is important since elderly patients usually have more co-morbidity, which in itself also can be responsible of a decreased postoperative survival. The effect of age, however, does not depend on the presence or absence of co-morbid conditions.

A high functional NYHA class, preoperative CHF and low LVEF all point to a burden on the LV, with subsequent failure, due to the pressure overload. If AVR is postponed for whatever reason, this condition could culminate into a need for urgent operation. In these patients, all compensatory mechanisms to maintain an adequate circulation has been exhausted. Hospital mortality can be ten times as high and long-term survival also impairs considerably. In one series, no patients in such condition has survived 5 years after AVR [8].

AF, and probably related to it, the need for digitalis could be considered as a marker for advanced heart disease. Digitalis has also been used for CHF, but this medication has been replaced by more potent drugs, such as ACE inhibitors, angiotensin receptor blockers and renin antagonists [49]. Even as treatment for AF, digitalis plays a role as predictor for a reduced survival.

Concomitant CABG has not in all series been identified as a predictor for reduced postoperative survival. The effect of CABG might be masked by the high age of the patients at operation. Nevertheless, another marker of CAD, namely AMI has an effect. This effect has not been related to the LVEF. Atheromatosis of the coronary arteries is a progressive disease, which is not stopped by CABG. Hence, after AVR combined with CABG, one could expect CAD to have its effect on survival. An increase in the length of ECC (which can be related to a concomitant CABG) also has been identified as a predictor for long-term mortality [8, 22].

An EuroSCORE can be calculated from many co-morbid conditions. The other factors that have been identified as predictors are a decreased renal function and previous stroke. The effect of these conditions or a high EuroSCORE on the postoperative survival should be no surprise [17]. The effect of a previously treated carcinoma on survival after AVR is a matter for debate. One should only refer patients for cardiac surgery who are expected to be cured of cancer. The larger the time interval between the cancer treatment and the AVR, the higher the chance of cure of the tumor. This time dependent effect has clearly been demonstrated [57].

2.3. Thromboembolic Events

TE events are one of the most important and devastating complications after AVR. As has been shown for survival, these events can be given as a %. For long-term follow up, a linearized rate, given as % per patient-year is not adequate, since it has not been proven that these events occur at a linear rate. Display of a event free rate curve could clarify a lot. For this section, no distinction has been made for severe, moderate of mild effects of TE.

In most series, TE events occur at a rate below 1% per patient-year, [14, 19, 25, 26, 36, 37, 58-61]. Other series report an incidence up to 1.8% per patient-year [26, 62, 63]. TE seem to occur for MHV and BHV equally [62].

Multivariate studies for identification of independent predictors are few in number. The predictors identified are:

- Preoperative CVA [33, 64-66].
- Hospital TE [66].
- Endocarditis [66].
- Age [26, 33, 51, 65].

- "Cardiac related factors" [26].
- AF [62], but this could always not be confirmed [33].
- CAD [62].
- Use of MHV [62].
- Female gender [65].
- Low LVEF [65].
- Calcification of the ascending aorta or the carotid artery [33, 65], but this could not always be confirmed [66].
- Diabetes [33, 65].
- Long ECC time [65].

A previous event such as a preoperative CVA and TE within the hospital are important predictors for future events [33, 64-66].

Previous endocarditis is also a predictor, but this might be a different disease, in which septic emboli are the source of the events. A damaged endocardium after endocarditis might create procoagulant conditions [66].

Age also has been identified as an independent predictor. The age distribution of any given patient population should be made known to appreciate fully the effect of this factor. Age might be related, however to co-morbid conditions such as diabetes and atheromatosis of the aorta and of the cerebral vessels. A long ECC time might indicate the need for an associate procedure, which mostly is a CABG. This could point to atheromatous vessels as a possible source for TE events. These events cannot be considered as entirely valve related. A "smoking gun", however, is often not found. And CABG itself has not been identified as a predictor for TE.

The effect of AF on the occurrence of TE events is a matter for debate: it is probably a risk factor. However, both TE events and AF are reasons for anticoagulation. This might cloud the effect of AF. In some series, AF has been identified as a predictor [62], in others not [33, 66].

The effect of carotid artery disease on TE events is also a matter for debate. The definition of this disease can vary according the % of stenosis. In some series [33, 65], it has been identified as a predictor for TE, in other series, this has not been the case [66]. A Doppler-duplex investigation is a reliable tool for the detection of lesions and is routinely performed in some institutions. It cannot, however detect atheromatosis of the intracranial vessels.

A low LVEF also has been identified as predictor for postoperative TE events. CHF and a dilated ventricle are known risk factors for TE. Damage to the ventricular wall as well as an abnormal flow of blood, and possible stasis, can promote intra-ventricular thrombosis and hence embolization. If the LVEF is below 30%, life-long anticoagulation is required [3].

All these predictors indicate that the sources of TE are multiple. Hence TE cannot be considered as entirely valve related [66, 67]. One also has to keep in mind that many TE events go unnoticed. In one small patients series, MRI after cardiac surgery could document silent events in 6 of 34 patients, a percentage that is rather high [68].

To prevent TE events after implantation of a BHV, anticoagulant medication is given for the first three postoperative months. Thereafter, it can be replaced by acetyl salicylic acid, with good results [66], provided there is no other reason for a continued treatment with anticoagulants. A RCT to support this strategy does not exist [3]. The guidelines from ACC/AHA in this respect differ from those of the ESC [69].

For MHV, a life-long anticoagulant treatment is necessary. The target level for INR is determined by the valve position (for aortic this is lower than for mitral) and by the type of MHV. Older types such as cage ball devices are more thrombogenic and require deeper anticoagulation. A strict classification for thrombogenicity is not available. Moreover, there are too many patient related factors involved [3].

Even more important is the variability of the INR. The lower this variability is, the better. A tight control, if possible through self-monitoring by educated and disciplined patients is of vital importance to prevent TE. The results in terms of QoL and survival are encouraging [70-72]. Poor control of anticoagulation with high variability of INR is a predictor for increased postoperative mortality [3].

2.4. Bleeding Events

Bleeding events are the other side of the coin of anticoagulation with vitamin K antagonists. The higher the INR, the safer it is for a TE event, but the higher is the risk for bleeding. There is a continuous balancing between the risk for TE and the risk for bleeding. The INR does not only depend on the dose of vitamin K antagonists, but also on the adsorption of vitamin K by the mucosa of the colon and on its processing by the liver. Digestive and liver diseases can have undesirable effect on the stability of INR.

For bleeding events after heart valve replacement, fewer reports appeared than for TE. The linearized rate varies between 0.3% [14] and 2.3 % [19] per patient year.

Event free rates at 5 year has been 89% for a mechanical valve [19] and 99% for a porcine valve [64]. Event free rates at 10 years have been between 85% and 99% [26, 32, 36, 64]. Some even report an event free rate at 15 years between 72% and 96% [32, 36, 64, 73]. Differences between MHV and BHV have been small [32]. The highest reported event free rate of 96% has been reported for porcine valves [64], the lowest rate has been reported for the SJM mechanical device [26].

There has been a tendency to aim for a lower level of anticoagulation after implantation of more "modern" MHV. This trade-off might not be beneficial: severe TE is more common than severe bleeding. Hence a low level anticoagulation might not be warranted [26].

Age and increased cardiothoracic index, as parameter for CHF, have been identified as predictors in one study by a multivariate analysis [26]. Fragility in elderly might be another important reason. In other series, no predictors or risk factors could be identified [73, 74].

2.5. Structural Valve Degeneration

SVD is the most important valve related event for BHV. The modes of failure have been discussed earlier. Age is the most important determinant for all positions. Hence, it is not advisable to use BHV in younger patients or in patients with a long life expectancy. The use of linearized rates is inappropriate since SVD occurs only years after implantation. The first signs of SVD, *i.e.* calcification, could already occur within a few years. SVD becomes usually clinically relevant after 10 or more years.

Many series have reported on SVD [19, 21, 22, 25, 39-45, 60, 64, 73, 75-84], mostly at 10 and at 15 years.

The current 10 year freedom for SVD ranges between 64 and 100%, largely depending on age and type of device such as CE-supra annular, CE standard, Mitroflow, Hancock II, Biocor BHV, Freestyle stentless and Sorin Bicarbon BHV [19, 21, 22, 25, 36, 40, 54, 64, 78].

The 15 year freedom for SVD ranges between 49% for a porcine valve [22] and 95% for a Hancock II in patients over 65 [73] to 97% for the CE supra-annular valve in patients over 70 years [24]. The 7 year freedom of SVD for a supra-annular implantation of a CE device has been somewhat superior to the CE-standard, but only in patients younger than 65 years [24].

In another series that has reported freedom of SVD at 10 years, age has been a major factor: in patients over 70, the freedom of SVD has been 99%; in patients between 60 and 69, this was still 96%. In younger patients, this was 84-85% [85].

In three studies over 15 years [23, 24, 79], it has been confirmed that older patients fare better with a BHV. This effect has been gradual: the worst results have been in patients between 21 and 40 years and the best in patients over 70 years. The CE supra-annular valve has performed better compared to the CE standard device in all age groups. The difference only has been significant in the younger age group.

Female gender, DM and plasma cholesterol have been identified as predictors for SVD, especially in younger patients. This suggests that risk factors for atheromatosis are also risk factors for SVD. In the past, it has seemed that treatment of these risk factors might become valuable in postponing SVD, especially younger patients [81], but in a recent investigation, the results of lipid lowering treatment had no effect on the progress of SVD [86]. Therefore, statins should not be used solely for the purpose of slowing down SVD.

2.6. Non Structural Deterioration

These events point to a failure, in which the valve itself is not affected. One of the most common event is PPVL. It should be considered as a technical failure. These events are very rare with a linearized rate of zero or almost zero [19, 25, 26, 37, 39, 58, 60].

In some series, a higher incidence of PPVL has been recorded with use of the silzone coating [87]. The frequency of this event has decreased after two years [61] and has disappeared after 4 years [88]. This trend has been confirmed in another series, but at the same time, a suture technique with pledgets has been identified as the only independent factor in the protection against PPVL [88]. Some other studies could not confirm the adverse effect of the silver coating [1].

Silzone coating consisted of a layer of metallic silver bonded to each strand of the cuff fabric has been introduced to prevent bacterial colonization and PVE. Such a coating however might not only reduce bacterial colonization but could also influence endothelialization of the sewing ring. This coating could increase the frequency of PPVL. The interim analysis of the data in the AVERT trial have discovered such an complication [89].

2.7. Hemolysis

Hemolysis is a result of PPVL [37, 90, 91]. If it is severe, a re-replacement of the valve might be indicated. Hemolysis, documented by serum LDH, serum haptoglobin, schistocytes and reticulocytes also depends on the type of MHV [92]. Hemolysis could be the result of damaged red blood cells by turbulences. It is not related to the size of the prosthesis or to EOA [91]. In BHV, hemolysis is infrequent in stented devices and absent in stentless devices [93]. Decompensated hemolysis could be a reason for re-replacement of a valve prosthesis.

2.8. Prosthetic Valve Endocarditis

The current linearized rate for PVE is low and mostly under 1% per patient year [14, 19, 25, 26, 36, 37, 45, 51, 58, 60, 76, 77]. The most event free rates after 5 to 25 year are well over 90%. This is true for MHV [32, 35, 37, 76] as well as for the different types of BHV: stented [45, 73, 80, 82], stentless [51, 77, 94] as well as for homografts [4]. No risk factors could be identified, although a previous endocarditis could arouse some suspicion. PVE carries a high risk for mortality, especially if Staphylococcus aureus is involved [95]. These micro-organisms often lead to ring abscesses and PPVL. The occurrence of CHF with PVE is the main indication for reoperation [96, 97].

2.9. Reoperation

The reoperation rate is determined by the occurrence of several complications:

- Pannus, which occurs mostly in MHV [98-101].
- PVT, which also occurs mostly in MHV [35, 98, 99].
- PVE [35, 77].
- PPVL [35, 98, 102].
- SVD and cusp tear [77].

Since some of these events do not occur linear in time, calculation of a linearized event rate is not sufficient. This simple method, shows, however some surprises. In most series, reoperation rate is below 1% per patient-year [19, 25, 26, 45, 60, 98]. Two series have shown a much higher rate: 3.3% [56] and 4.1%/patient-year [78]. Young age at implantation and SVD of the porcine valve have been responsible. Currently, the 5 year freedom of SVD is almost 100% [19, 64]. Those for 10 years vary between 76% [21] and 100% [22]. One series shows an exceptionally low event free rate of 48% [83]. Most series show an event free rate between 90 and 100 [25, 40, 82, 86, 103].

Age is an important predictor for reoperation if a BHV has been implanted. A caged ball and smaller size of the MHV implant are also predictors for reoperation

[21, 36-38]. Occurrence of PPVL after the implantation of the silzone SJM, can also be a reason for reoperation [102].

2.10. Congestive Heart Failure

Postoperative hospital CHF or low output syndrome is a highly lethal complication [13, 104], but only a few studies have reported on its predictors.

In one series, hospital CHF has occurred in 2.6% of the patients, with need for urgent AVR as the sole independent predictor. Need for an urgent AVR points to an exhaustion of all compensatory mechanisms to maintain an adequate circulation. Therefore, an AVR should not be postponed, once aortic valve stenosis has become symptomatic [13]. In another study, the level of BNP has also been identified as a predictor [104]. Apoptosis or programmed cell death of cardiomyocytes could be an important event in these patients [105].

CHF on long-term could also be a debilitating event, but this seemed less fatal. Preoperative CD, postoperative AF and CAD have been identified as independent predictors for this event. A small valve size (19 mm CE-p) and concomitant CABG only have been significant in an univariate analysis. Remarkably, almost half of the patients with this complication had a normal LVEF [13].

LVH is a common finding in patients with CAVS. Cardiomyocytes are enlarged but also fibrosis has been documented. After regression of the muscle mass, this fibrosis persists for a longer time. This stiffens the LV wall and impairs its relaxation [106]. The LVEF remains often normal. Hence, this is labeles as a "diastolic" form of CHF [13].

CD leads to perfusion defects and wall motion abnormalities, even if CAD is absent [107]. This worsens the effect of postoperative CHF. Correction by biventricular pacing often corrects CHF [108, 109].

AF results in the loss of the atrial systole and, hence impairs the filling of the LV further. This worsens the diastolic type of CHF [13].

CAD is progressive disease. During long-term postoperative follow-up, this progression can lead to ischemia and hence LV dysfunction. This also helps to explain the occurrence of CHF. Concomitant CABG, however, has not been identified as a predictor for postoperative CHF [13]. The intra-myocardial strain increases when LVH regresses after AVR. In patients who also have CAD, this effect is not observed, which could add to the LV dysfunction [110].

A small valve size is not necessarily a predictor for CHF [13]. Even with an EOAI of 0.64 cm^2/m^2, a considerable regression of LVH has been observed [42]. Hence, in patients with a small aortic root, it is not always necessary to enlarge the root or to implant a stentless valve. These surgical techniques are more demanding, and might not be necessary, provided the LVF is normal.

However, it is important to obtain a sufficiently large EOAI in patients with a low LVEF. When, in such patients, a small valve size leads to an even moderate VPPM, this might result in CHF and an increased mortality [111]. Implantation of stentless devices might be helpful to avoid VPPM in these patients [28].

Last but not least, AHT is a risk factor for heart failure. In order to obtain a good regression of LVH after AVR, it is important to treat AHT, if present, properly [28, 112].

2.11. Atrial Fibrillation

Atrial fibrillation and other non-sinusal rhythms has occured in 20% of the postoperative patients [25]. In other series, this has been 40% or more [113, 114]. The definition and the diagnostic method for detection of AF also have an effect on its incidence [114, 115]. A postoperative AF is not innocent: this event could lead to other complications and an increased length of stay within the hospital. There is a higher incidence of postoperative CHF, of renal function impairment, of infection and of neurologic events in patients with postoperative AF [113]. Postoperative AF increases also mortality [114].

The risk factors for postoperative AF are a history of previous paroxysmal AF, an enlarged left atrium, a prolonged P wave on ECG, previous episode of CHF, a high age, a low LVEF and a LVH [34, 115, 116]. The effect of age, however is a matter for debate: postoperative AF does not occur more frequently in octogenarians after AVR [51].

It seems that a postoperative AF is preventable, at least in part. Pacing could half the frequency of postoperative AF [113]. Timely and adequate treatment of AF could increase the speed of rehabilitation and reduce the stay within the hospital [115].

2.12. Conduction Defects

Conduction defects such as complete atrio-ventricular block, and hence PPMI, has occured in almost 10% of the patients who have received AVR [117]. The occurrence of all new CD is reported to be 15% [118]. Other reports have stated a lower incidence for PPMI, since not all CD need this treatment. Sometimes, a new onset CD can be reversible [117]. Development of such a new CD leads to an increased monitoring and hence a longer hospital stay [119].

The main predictor for PPMI has been preoperative CD [117, 120-122]. Other predictors that have been identified were female gender, annular calcification, a bicuspid aortic valve, a previous CD, AHT, a previous AMI, an electrolyte imbalance and a prolonged CCT [119, 123, 124]. Aortic regurgitation might also play a role since this condition usually requires implantation of larger valves [117].

Preoperative changes in the conduction system might be due to older age, to ischemia and mechanical factors. The latter might be the result of an increased LV pressure [117].

Some factors such as a calcified annulus could lead to trauma of the conduction system during surgery. The link with a congenital bicuspid aortic valve is less clear. AHT could lead to calcification but also to increased septal LVH, which makes the conduction system more difficult to protect during cross-clamping [119]. Other traumas of the conduction system could be due to impingement by the prosthetic valve or by suturing [117].

Development of a new CD such as left BBB in the postoperative period has been a marker for other adverse events, such as sudden death [118]. Therefore, appearance of such CD is not innocent.

2.13. Non Cardiac Hospital Complications

Respiratory complications after AVR are a common observation [5, 12, 27, 125] but few reports have appeared with a description of their predictors. The rate of pulmonary complications depends largely on the criteria used: need for prolonged ventilation, respiratory failure or pulmonary infection.

The basic mechanisms of these complications involve:

- Lack of lung inflation due to postoperative pain, resulting in a shallow, monotonous breathing pattern without periodic sighs.
- Prolonged recumbent positioning.
- Temporary diaphragmatic dysfunction.
- Impaired postoperative mucociliary clearance.
- Decrease in cough effectiveness.

The latter two can result in retained pulmonary secretions [126]. When airways are obstructed by these secretions, the air becomes trapped and is absorbed by the blood. The affected part of the lung collapses, which is called atelectasis. This also could lead to an infection. Occurrence of such pulmonary complications lead to an increased stay in ICU [127, 128].

The use of an ECC during cardiac operations certainly has side effects on the respiratory system [129]. The use of an ECC can induce systemic inflammation as well as an imbalance of oxidant/antioxidant and protease/antiprotease status. These changes have been implicated in pulmonary complications [130].

There is also a possible interaction between the ECC and the effect of body mass: in small patients, hemodilution is usually greater since the circuit primer represents a greater fraction of the circulating blood-prime mixture. This might increase the oncotic gradient, extravasation, the appearance of pulmonary edema and of pneumonia. Injury of the EC could worsen these problems [131]. Pulmonary edema is also a hallmark of postoperative CHF, which has clearly been identified as a risk factor for postoperative pulmonary complications.

In a large cohort of 1000 consecutive patients, who underwent AVR following predictors have been identified:

- Preoperative pacemaker implant.
- COPD and
- Early postoperative CHF [125].

The production of mucus often has increased in patients with COPD. This in turn increases the risk for atelectasis and infection. Early postoperative CHF, and hence pulmonary edema increase the need for ventilator support and prolong the stay on ICU. This also could contribute to postoperative pulmonary complications [125].

Renal and cardiovascular disease are linked in two ways. On one hand, renal function impairment, even if this modest, is an established element in the risk profile for atheromatosis and thus for CAD and for CAVS [132, 133]. On the other hand, renal function impairment can be the result of atheromatosis of the renal arteries. Renal complications have been observed after major cardiovascular surgery such as AVR. Postoperative decrease of the renal function is a serious complication with an increased mortality rate.

The predictors, which have been identified for this complication were:

- Preoperative decreased renal function.
- Preoperative AF.
- Age over 80.
- Previous myocardial infarction.

Other risk factors which have been observed, are hypertension, PAD, timing of surgery, CPB time over 70 minutes, severe angina an non elective surgery [27, 134].

The estimation of renal function has some difficulties: plasma creatinin, as a routine clinical procedure is not sufficient to replace glomerular filtration rate as parameter. Hence, values of plasma creatinin should be interpreted cautiously. The estimation of glomerular filtration rate requires a 24-h urine collection, but this method is liable to errors. As alternative, plasma creatinin, age, gender and body weight can be introduced in a formula, to calculate glomerular filtration rate.

In one series, a cut-off level of 2.0 mg% for plasma creatinin was used [134], in another series, this was 1.4 mg% [12]. These differences in cut-off values, as well as differences in patient population could explain differences in postoperative findings.

Moreover, defining a worsening of renal function by an increase of plasma creatinin [135] also has its difficulties: in patients with a plasma creatinin between 1 and 2 mg% and hence, a moderate degree in renal function impairment, an additional increase with 0.3% could mean a serious additional renal damage. The slope of the relationship between glomerular filtration rate and plasma creatinin is high. In patients with higher preoperative plasma creatinin, and thus with a more extensive renal damage, such an increase does not mean necessarily a major additional damage: the slope of the relation between glomerular filtration rate and plasma creatinin in this area is much lower.

The ECC could have a damaging effect on the glomeruli, especially if the kidney already has been injured. Mechanism inflicting renal damage are non-pulsatile perfusion, renal hypoperfusion, hypothermia, and increased levels of circulating catecholamines, cytokines, enzymes, free radicals and of free hemoglobin. The effect of ECC, however cannot be studied in patients who undergo AVR, since this operation always require such a device. An effect on renal function, however has been shown in patients who underwent CABG with and without ECC [136]. Keeping the cross-clamp time as short as possible or installing a minimal ECC could be helpful to reduce renal complications after AVR [137, 138].

Age over 80 is associated with an increase in atheromatosis and a previous myocardial infarction is certainly a marker for this vascular disease. If atheromatosis also affects the renal arteries, a postoperative decrease in renal function could be expected [120].

Endothelial dysfunction of patients with CAVS could be a link with renal function impairment. This could help explaining the observed association between preoperative AF and postoperative renal complications. There are, however, several confounding factors [139, 140].

CONCLUSIONS

Postoperative mortality and valve related complications have received much attention in most patients series. Thromboembolism and structural valve degeneration are most important valve related complications.

Recently, other cardiac postoperative complications such as heart failure, conduction defects and atrial fibrillation also have been scrutinized.

Survival rates and freedom of events give important information. The usual milestones are 1, 5 and 10 years. For SVD, 15 and even 20 years are also important data.

More important, however, is the identification of risk factors and independent predictors for every event. Most predictors are patient related factors such as high age and co-morbid conditions.

Progression of CAVS to a condition where urgent AVR is needed also has its importance, especially since this increases operative mortality ten times.

Knowledge of these risk factors is helpful in selecting the patients for AVR and is necessary to tailor the peri and postoperative care to the individual patient.

ACKNOWLEDGEMENT

Declared none.

CONFLICT OF INTEREST

The author(s) confirm that this chapter content has no conflict of interest.

REFERENCES

[1] Dávila-Román VG, Waggoner AD, Kennard ED, *et al.* Prevalence and Severity of Paravalvular Regurgitation in the Artificial Valve Endocarditis Reduction Trial [AVERT] Echocardiography Study. J Am Coll Cardiol 2004;44:1467-1472.

[2] Leon MB, Smith CR, Mack M, *et al.* for the PARNTER trial investigators. Transcatheter Aortic-Valve Implantation for Aortic Stenosis in Patients Who Cannot Undergo Surgery. New Engl J Med 2010; doi 10.1056/NEJMoa1008232.

[3] Butchart EG, Payne N, Li HH, *et al.* Better anticoagulation control improves survival after valve replacement. J Thorac Cardiovasc Surg 2002;123:715-723.

[4] Hickey E, Langley SM, Allemby-Smith O, *et al.* Subcoronary Allograft Aortic Valve Replacement: Parametric Risk-Hazard Outcome Analysis to a Minimum of 20 Years. Ann Thorac Surg 2007;84;1564-1570.

[5] Kolh P, Lahaye L, Gerard P, Limet R. Aortic valve replacement in the octogenarians: perioperative outcome and clinical follow-up. Eur J Cardio-thorac Surg 1999;16:68-73.

[6] Edwards FH, Peterson ED, Coombs LP, *et al.* Prediction of Operative Mortality After Valve Replacement Surgery. J Am Coll Cardiol 2001;37:885-892.

[7] Florath I, Rosendahl UP, Mortasawi A, *et al.* Current Determinants of Operative Mortality in 1400 Patients Requiring Aortic Valve Replacement. Ann Thorac Surg 2003;76:75-83.

[8] Mistiaen W, Van Cauwelaert Ph, Muylaert Ph, *et al.* Risk factors and survival after aortic valve replacement in octogenarians. J Heart Valve Dis. 2004;13:538-544.

[9] Jamieson WRE, Burr LH, Miyagishima RT, *et al.* Reoperation for bioprosthetic aortic structural failure – risk assessment. Eur J Cardio-thorac Surg 2003;24:873-878.

[10] Alsoufi B, Karamlou T, Slater M, *et al.* Results of concomitant aorta valve replacement and coronary artery bypass grafting in the VA population. J Heart Valve Dis 2006;15:12-18.

[11] Connolly HM, Oh JK, Schaff HV, *et al.* Severe Aortic Stenosis With Low Transvalvular Gradient and Severe Left Ventricular Dysfunction Result of Aortic Valve Replacement in 52 Patients. Circulation 2000;101:1940-1946.

[12] Mistiaen W, Van Cauwelaert P, Muylaert P, De Worm E. 1000 pericardial valves in aortic position: risk factors for postoperative acute renal function impairment in elderly. J Cardiovasc Surg 2009;50:233-237.

[13] Mistiaen W, Van Cauwelaert Ph, Muylaert Ph, *et al.* Risk factors for congestive heart failure after aortic valve replacement with a Carpentier-Edwards pericardial prosthesis in the elderly. J Heart Valve Dis 2005;14:774-779.

[14] Emery RW, Erickson CA, Arom KV, *et al.* Replacement of the Aortic Valve in Patients Under 50 Years of Age: Long-Term Follow-Up of the St. Jude Medical Prosthesis. Ann Thorac Surg 2003;75:1815-1819.

[15] Jamieson WRE, Munro AI, Miyagishima RT, *et al.* Carpentier-Edwards standard porcine bioprosthesis – clinical performance to 17 years. Ann Thoac Surg 1995;60:999-1007.

[16] Jamieson WRE, Burr LH, Tyers GFO, *et al.* Carpentier-Edwards supraannular porcine bioprosthesis – clinical performance to 12 years. Ann Thorac Surg 1995;60:S235-S240.

[17] Leontyev S, Walther T, Borger MA, *et al.* Aortic Valve Replacement in Octogenarians: Utility of Risk Stratification With EuroSCORE. Ann Thorac Surg 2009;87:1440-1445.

[18] Hannan EL, Samadashvili Z, Lahey SJ, *et al.* Aortic Valve Replacement for Patients With Severe Aortic Stenosis: Risk Factors and Their Impact on 30-Month Mortality. Ann Thorac Surg 2009;87:1741-1750.

[19] Goldsmith I, Lip GYH, Patel RL. Evaluation of the Sorin Bicarbon Bileaflet Valve in 488 Patients [519 Prostheses]. Am J Cardiol 1999;83:1069-1074

[20] Kvidal P, Bergström R, Hörte LG, Ståhle E. Observed and Relative Survival After Aortic Valve Replacement. J Am Coll Cardiol 2000;35:747-756.

[21] Le Tourneau T, Vincentelli A, Fayad G, *et al.* Ten-Year Echocardiographic and Clinical Follow-Up of Aortic Carpentier-Edwards Pericardial and Supraannular Prosthesis: A Case-Match Study. Ann Thorac Surg 2002;74:2010-2015.

[22] Fann JI, Miller DC, Moore KA, *et al.* Twenty-year clinical experience with porcine bioprosthesis. Ann Thorac Surg 1996;62:1301-1311.

[23] Jamieson WRE, Burr LH, Munro IA, Miyagishima RT. Carpentier-Edwards Standard Porcine Bioprosthesis: A 21-Year Experience. Ann Thorac Surg 1998;66:S40-S43.

[24] Jamieson WRE, Janusz MT, Burr LH, *et al.* Carpentier–Edwards Supraannular Porcine Bioprosthesis: Second-Generation Prosthesis in Aortic Valve Replacement. Ann Thorac Surg 2001;71:S224-S227.

[25] Aupart MR, Sirinelli AL, Diemont FF, *et al.* The last generation of pericardial valves in the aortic position: Ten year follow-up in 589 patients. Ann Thorac Surg 1996;61:615-620.

[26] Lund O, Nielsen SL, Arildsen H, *et al.* Standard Aortic St. Jude Valve at 18 Years: Performance Profile and Determinants of Outcome. Ann Thorac Surg 2000;69:1459-1465.

[27] Weerasinghe A, Yusuf M, Athanasiou T, *et al.* Role of Transvalvular Gradient in Outcome From Valve Replacement for Aortic Stenosis. Ann Thorac Surg 2004;77:1266-1271.

[28] Bové T, Van Belleghem Y, Francois K, *et al.* Stentless and stented aortic valve replacement in elderly patients: factors affecting midterm clinical and hemodynamical outcome. Eur J Cardio-thorac Surg 2006;30:706-715.

[29] Tjang YS, van Hees Y, Körfer R, *et al.* Predictors of mortality after aortic valve replacement. Eur J Cardio-thorac Surg 2007;32:469-474.

[30] Jamieson WRE, Koerfer R, Yankah CA, *et al.* Mitroflow aortic pericardial bioprosthesis – clinical performance. Eur J Cardio-thorac Surg 2009;36:818-824.

[31] Mistiaen W, Van Cauwelaert Ph, Muylaert Ph, *et al.* Determinants of survival after aortic valve replacement as treatment for symptomatic aortic valve disease in elderly. J Heart valve Dis 2001;10:354-360.

[32] Carrier M, Pellerin M, Perrault LP, *et al.* Aortic Valve Replacement With Mechanical and Biologic Prostheses in Middle-Aged Patients. Ann Thorac Surg 2001;71:S253-S256.

[33] Gulbins H, Florath I, Ennker J. Cerebrovascular Events After Stentless Aortic Valve Replacement During a 9-Year Follow-Up Period. Ann Thorac Surg 2008;86:769-773.

[34] Baranowska E, Baranowki R, Michalek P, *et al.* Prediction of paroxysmal atrial fibrillation after aortic valve replacement in patients with aortic stenosis: identification of potential risk factors. J Heart Valve Dis 2003;12:136-141.

[35] Borman JB, De Riberolles C. Sorin Bicarbone bileaflet valve: a 10-year experience. Eur J Cardio-thorac Surg 2003;23:86-92.

[36] Burdon TE, Miller DC, Oyer PE, *et al.* Durability of porcine valves at 15 years in a representative North-American patient population. J Thorac Cardiovasc Surg 1992;103:238-252.

[37] Torregrosa S, Gomez-Plana J, Valera FJ, *et al.* Long-Term Clinical Experience With the Omnicarbon Prosthetic Valve. Ann Thorac Surg 1999;68:881-886.

[38] Aupart MR, Mirza A, Meurisse YA, *et al.* Perimount pericardial bioprosthesis for aortic calcified stenosis: 18-year experience with 1, 133 patients. J Heart Valve Dis 2006;15:768-775.

[39] Albert A, Florath I, Rosendahl U, *et al.* Effect of surgeon on transprosthetic gradients after aortic valve replacement with Freestyle® stentless bioprosthesis and its consequences: A follow-up study in 587 patients. J Cardiothoracic Surg 2007, 2:40 doi:10.1186/1749-8090-2-40.

[40] Bottio T, Rizzoli G, Thiene G, *et al.* Hemodynamic and clinical outcomes with the Biocor valve in the aortic position: An 8-year experience. J Thorac Cardiovasc Surg 2004;127:1616-1623.

[41] Ennker JAC, Ennker IC, Albert AA, *et al.* The Freestyle Stentless Bioprosthesis in more than 1000 Patients: A Single-Center Experience over 10 Years. J Card Surg 2009;24:41-48.

[42] Freed DH, Tam JW, Moon MC, *et al.* Nineteen-Millimeter Prosthetic Aortic Valves Allow Normalization of Left Ventricular Mass in Elderly Women. Ann Thorac Surg 2002;74:2022-2025.

[43] Luciani GB, Viscardi F, Cresce GD, *et al.* Seven-Year Performance of the Edwards Prima Plus Stentless Valve with the Intact Non-Coronary Sinus Technique. J Card Surg 2008;23:221-226.

[44] Masters RG, Haddad M, Pipe AL, *et al.* Clinical Outcomes With the Hancock II Bioprosthetic Valve. Ann Thorac Surg 2004;78:832-836.

[45] Nakajima H, Aupart MR, Neville PH, *et al.* Twelve year experience with the 19 mm Carpentier-Edwards pericardial aortic valve. J Heart Valve Dis 1998;7:534-539.

[46] Tsialtas D, Bolognesi R, Beghi C, *et al.* Stented *versus* stentless bioprosthesis in aortic valve stenosis: effect on left ventricular remodeling. Heart Surgery Forum 2007;10:E205-E210.

[47] Mistiaen W, Van Cauwelaert Ph, Sys SU, *et al.* Role of age, gender and association of CABG on long-term results after aortic valve replacement with a Carpentier-Edwards bioprosthesis in elderly. J Cardiovasc Surg [Torino] 2003; 44:701-706.

[48] Mistiaen W, Van Cauwelaert P, Sys SU, *et al.* Timing of aortic valve replacement in elderly patients with symptomatic aortic valve disease using outpatient clinical parameters. Acta Clin Belg 2005;60:185-189.

[49] Mistiaen W, Van Cauwelaert P, Muylaert P, De Worm E. 1000 Carpentier-Edwards pericardial valves in aortic position: what changed in the last 20 years and what are the effects on hospital complications. J Heart Valve Dis 2007;16:417-422.

[50] Kirsch M, Guesnier L, LeBesnerais P, *et al.* Cardiac Operations in Octogenarians: Perioperative Risk Factors for Death and Impaired Autonomy. Ann Thorac Surg 1998;66:60-67.

[51] Ennker J, Dalladaku F, Rosendahl U, *et al.* The Stentless Freestyle Bioprosthesis: Impact of Age Over 80 Years on Quality of Life, Perioperative, and Mid-Term Outcome. J Card Surg 2006;21:379-385.

[52] Maillet JM, Somme D, Hennel E, *et al.* Frailty after aortic valve replacement [AVR] in octogenarians. Arch Gerontol Geriatr 2009;48:391-396.

[53] Rohde SL, Baker RA, Tully PJ, *et al.* Preoperative and Intraoperative Factors Associated With Long-Term Survival in Octogenarian Cardiac Surgery Patients. Ann Thorac Surg 2010;89:105-111.

[54] Burr LH, Jamieson WRE, Munro AI, *et al.* Porcine bioprosthesis in the elderly – clinical performance by age-groups and valve positions. Ann Thor Surg 1995;60:S264-S269.

[55] Jamieson WRE, Tyers GFO, Janusz MT, *et al.* Age as a determinant for selection of porcine bioprostheses for cardiac valve replacement – experience with Carpentier-Edwards standard bioprosthesis. Can J Cardiol 1991;7:181-188.

[56] Pomar JL, Jamieson WRE, Pelletier LC, *et al.* Mitroflow Pericardial Bioprosthesis Experience in Aortic Valve Replacement >60 Years of Age. Ann Thorac Surg 1998;66:S53-S56.

[57] Mistiaen W, Van Cauwelaert Ph, Muylaert Ph, *et al.* Effect of prior malignancy on survival after cardiac surgery. Ann Thorac Surg 2004;77:1593-1597.

[58] Baudet EM, Puel V, McBride JT, *et al.* Long-term results of valve replacement with the St Jude Medical prosthesis. J Thorac Cardiovasc Surg 1995;109:858-870.

[59] Pellerin M, Mihaileanu S, Couetil JP, *et al.* Carpentier-Edwards pericardial bioprosthesis in aortic position – long-term follow-up 1980 to 1994. Ann Thorac Surg 1995;60:S292-296.

[60] Li HH, Hahn J, Urbanski P, *et al.* Intermediate-Term Results With 1, 019 Carbomedics Aortic Valves. Ann Thorac Surg 2001;71:1181-1188.

[61] Chan V, Jamieson WRE, Germann E *et al.* Performance of bioprostheses and mechanical prostheses assessed by composites of valve-related complications to 15 years after aortic valve replacement. J Thorac Cardiovasc Surg 2006;131:1267-1273.

[62] Ruel M, Masters RG, Rubens FD, *et al.* Late Incidence and Determinants of Stroke After Aortic and Mitral Valve Replacement. Ann Thorac Surg 2004;78:77-84.

[63] Puvimanasinghe JPA, Takkenberg JJM, Eijkemans MJC, *et al.* Comparison of Carpentier-Edwards pericardial and supraannular bioprostheses in aortic valve replacement. Eur J Cardio-thorac Surg 2006;29:374-379.

[64] Minami K, Zittermann A, Schulte-Eistrup S, *et al.* Mitroflow Synergy Prostheses for Aortic Valve Replacement: 19 Years Experience With 1, 516 Patients. Ann Thorac Surg 2005;80:1699-1705.

[65] Filsoufi F, Rahmanian PB, Castillo JG, Bronster D, Adams DH. Incidence, Imaging Analysis, and Early and Late Outcomes of Stroke After Cardiac Valve Operation. Am J Cardiol 2008;101:1472-1478.

[66] Mistiaen W, Van Cauwelaert Ph, Muylaert Ph, *et al.* Thrombo-embolism after aortic valve replacement in elderly with a Carpentier-Edwards perimount TM bioprosthesis. J Thorac Cardiovasc Surg 2004;127:1166-1170.

[67] Horstkotte D, Lengyel M, Mistiaen WP, *et al.*, on behalf of the Working Group 'Infection, Thrombosis, Embolism and Bleeding' of the Society of Heart Valve Disease. Recommendations for Reporting Morbid Events after Heart Valve Surgery. J Heart Valve Dis 2005;14:1-7.

[68] Floyd TF, Shah PN, Price CC, *et al.* Clinically Silent Cerebral Ischemic Events After Cardiac Surgery: Their Incidence, Regional Vascular Occurrence, and Procedural Dependence. Ann Thorac Surg 2006;81:2160-2166.

[69] Sun CJC, Davidson MJ, Lamy A, Eikelboom JWE. Antithrombotic management of patients with prosthetic heart valves: current evidence and future trends. Lancet 2009; 374: 565-576.

[70] Koertke H, Zittermann A, Wagner O, Koerfer R. Self-Management of Oral Anticoagulation Therapy Improves Long-Term Survival in Patients With Mechanical Heart Valve Replacement. Ann Thorac Surg 2007;83:24-29.

[71] Sundt TM, Zehr KJ, Dearani JA, *et al.* Is early anticoagulation with warfarin necessary after bioprosthetic aortic valve replacement? J Thorac Cardiovasc Surg 2005;129:1024-1031.

[72] Hamad MAS, van Eekelen E, van Agt T, van Straten AHM. Self-management program improves anticoagulation control and quality of life: a prospective randomized study. Eur J Cardio-thorac Surg 2009;35:265-269.

[73] Rizzoli G, Bottio T, Thiene G, *et al.* Long-term durability of the Hancock II porcine Bioprosthesis. J Thorac Cardiovasc Surg 2003;126:66-74.

[74] Sundt TM, Zehr KJ, Dearani JA, *et al.* Is early anticoagulation with warfarin necessary after bioprosthetic aortic valve replacement? J Thorac Cardiovasc Surg 2005;129:1024-1031.

[75] d'Udekem Y, Pasquet A, El Khoury GA, *et al.* Early Calcific Stenosis of the Aortic Sorin Pericarbon Valve Implanted in the Elderly Ann Thorac Surg 1998;66:S139-S142.

[76] Baykut D, Grize L, Schindler C, *et al.* Eleven-Year Single-Center Experience with the ATS Open Pivot Bileaflet Heart Valve. Ann Thorac Surg 2006;82:847–52.

[77] David TE, Feindel CM, Bos J, *et al.* Aortic valve replacement with Toronto SPV bioprosthesis: Optimal patient survival but suboptimal valve durability. J Thorac Cardiovasc Surg 2008;135:19-24.

[78] Jamieson WRE, Burr LH, Miyagishima RT, *et al.* Structural deterioration in Carpentier-Edwards standard and supraannular bioprosthesis. Ann Thorac Surg 1995;60:S241-S247.

[79] Jamieson WRE, Burr LH, Janusz MT, *et al.* Carpentier-Edwards Standard and Supraannular Porcine Bioprostheses: Comparison of Technology. Ann Thorac Surg 1999;67:10-17.

[80] Neville PH, Aupart MR, Diemont FF, *et al.* Carpentier-Edwards Pericardial Bioprosthesis in Aortic or Mitral Position: A 12-Year Experience. Ann Thorac Surg 1998;66:S143-S147.

[81] Nollert G, Miksch J, Kreuzer E, Reichart B. Risk factors for atherosclerosis and the degeneration of pericardial valves after aortic valve replacement. J Thorac Cardiovasc Surg 2003;126:965-968.

[82] Poirier NC, Pelletier LC, Pellerin M, Carrier M. 15-Year Experience With the Carpentier-Edwards Pericardial Bioprosthesis. Ann Thorac Surg 1998;66:S57-S61.

[83] Pomar JL, Jamieson WRE, Pelletier LC, *et al.* Mitroflow Pericardial Bioprosthesis: Clinical Performance to Ten Years. Ann Thorac Surg 1995;60:S305-S310.

[84] Riess FC, Cramer E, Hansen L, *et al.* Clinical results of the Medtronic Mosaic porcine bioprosthesis up to 13 years. Eur J Cardio-thorac Surg 2010;37:145-153.

[85] Jamieson WRE, Burr LH, Tyers GFO, *et al.* Carpentier-Edwards supra-annular porcine bioprosthesis – clinical performance to 12 years. Ann Thorac Surg 1995;60:S235-S240.

[86] Kulik A, Masters RG, Bédard P, *et al.* Postoperative lipid-lowering therapy and bioprosthesis structural valve deterioration: justification for a 220andomized trial? Eur J Cardio-thorac Surg 2010;37:139-144.

[87] Grunkemeier GL, Jin R, Im KA, *et al.* Time-related risk of the St. Jude Silzone heart valve. Eur J Cardio-thorac Surg 2006;30:20-27.

[88] Englberger L, Schaff HV, Jamieson WRE, *et al.*, for the AVERT Investigators Importance of implant technique on risk of major paravalvular leak [PVL] after St. Jude mechanical heart valve replacement: a report from the Artificial Valve Endocarditis Reduction Trial [AVERT]. Eur J Cardio-thorac Surg 2005;28:838-844.

[89] Horstkotte D, Bergemann R. Thrombogenicity of the St Jude Medical prosthesis with and without Silzone-coated sewing cuffs. Ann Thorac Surg 2001;71:1065-1065.

[90] Suedkamp M, Lercher AJ, Mueller-Riemenschneider F, *et al.* Hemolysis parameters of St. Jude Medical Hemodynamic Plus® and Regent® valves in aortic position. Int J Cardiol 2004;95:89-93.

[91] Josa M, Castellá M, Paré C, *et al.* Hemolysis in Mechanical Bileaflet Prostheses: Experience With the Bicarbon Valve. Ann Thorac Surg 2006;81:1291-1296.

[92] Ismeno G, Renzulli A, Carozza A, *et al.* Intravascular hemolysis after mitral and aortic valve replacement with different types of mechanical prostheses. Int J Cardiol 1999;69:179-183.

[93] Mecozzi G, Milano AD, De Carlo M, *et al.* Intravascular hemolysis in patients with new-generation prosthetic heart valves: A prospective study. J Thorac Cardiovasc Surg 2002;123:550-556.

[94] Butany J, Zhou T, Leong SW, *et al.* Inflammation and infection in nine surgically explanted Medtronic Freestyle ® stentless aortic valves. Cardiovascular Pathology 2007;16:258-267.

[95] Chirouze C, Cabell CH, Fowler VG Jr., *et al.*, and the International Collaboration on Endocarditis Study Group. Prognostic Factors in 61 Cases of *Staphylococcus aureus* Prosthetic Valve Infective Endocarditis from the International Collaboration on Endocarditis Merged Database. Clin Infect Dis 2004; 38:1323-1327.

[96] Habib RH, Zacharias A, Schwann TA, *et al.* Effects of obesity and small body size on operative and long-term outcomes of coronary artery bypass surgery: a propensity-matched analysis. Ann Thorac Surg 2005:1976-1986.

[97] Fernandez-Guerrero ML, Gonzalez Lopez JJ, Goyenechea A, *et al.* Endocarditis caused by Staphylococcus aureus. A reappraisal of the epidemiologic, clinical and pathological manifestations with analysis of factors determining outcome. Medicine 2009;88:1-22.

[98] Rizzoli G, Guglielmi C, Toscano G, *et al.* Reoperations for acute prosthetic thrombosis and pannus: an assessment of rates, relationship and risk. Eur J Cardio-thorac Surg 1999;16:74-80.

[99] Aoyagi S, Nishimi M, Kawano H, *et al.* Obstruction of St Jude medical valves in the aortic position: significance of a combination of cineradiography and echocardiography. J Thorac Cardiovasc Surg 2000;120:142-147.

[100] Roudaut R, Roques X, Lafitte S, *et al.* Surgery for prosthetic valve obstruction. A single center study of 136 patients. Eur J Cardio-thorac Surg 2003;24:868-872.

[101] Sakamoto Y, Hashimoto K, Okuyama H, *et al.* Prevalence of pannus formation after aortic valve replacement: clinicalaspects and surgical management. J Artif Organs;2006:199-202.

[102] Schaff HV, Carrel TP, Jamieson WRE, *et al.* Paravalvular Leak and Other Events in Silzone-Coated Mechanical Heart Valves: A Report From AVERT. Ann Thorac Surg 2002;73:785-792.

[103] Brown ML, Schaff HV, Lahr BD, *et al.* Aortic valve replacement in patients aged 50 to 70 years: Improved outcome with mechanical *versus* biological prostheses. J Thorac Cardiovasc Surg 2008;135:878-884.

[104] Nozohoor S, Nilsson J, Lührs C, *et al.* B-Type Natriuretic Peptide as a Predictor of Postoperative Heart Failure After Aortic Valve Replacement. J Cardiothorac Vasc Anest 2009;23:161-165.

[105] Gaudino M, Anselmi A, Abbat A, *et al.* Myocardial apoptosis predicts postoperative course after aortic valve replacement in patients with severe left ventricular hypertrophy. J Heart Valve Dis 2007;16:344-348.

[106] Villari B, Sossalla S, Ciampi Q, *et al.* Persistent diastolic dysfunction alte after valve replacement in severe aortic regurgitation. Circulation 2009;120:2386-2392.

[107] Bavelaar Croon CD, Wahba FF, Van Hecke MV. Perfusion and functional abnormalities outside the septal region in patients with left bundle branch block assessed with gated SPECT. Q J Nucl Med 2001;45:108-114.

[108] Blanc JJ, Etienne Y, Gilard M. Evaluation of different ventricular pacing sites in patients with severe heart failure: Results of an acute hemodynamic study. Circulation 1997;96:3273-3277.

[109] Sciagra R, Giaccardi M, Porciani MC. Myocardial perfusion imaging using gated SPECT in heart failure patients undergoing cardiac resynchronization therapy. J Nucl Med 2004;45:164-168.

[110] Biederman RWW, Doyle M, Yamrozik J, *et al.* Physiologic compensation is supranormal in compensated aortic stenosis: Doed it return to normal or is it blunted by coexistent coronary artery disease? Circulation 2005;112:I429-I436.

[111] Ruel M, Al-Faleh H, Kulik A, *et al.* Prosthesis–patient mismatch after aortic valve replacement predominantly affects patients with preexisting left ventricular dysfunction: Effect on survival, freedom from heart failure, and left ventricular mass regression. J Thorac Cardiovasc Surg 2006;131:1036-1044.

[112] Lund O, Emmertsen K, Dørup I, *et al.* Regression of left ventricular hypertrophy during 10 years after valve replacement for aortic stenosis is related to the preoperative risk profile. Eur Heart J 2003;24:1437-1446.

[113] Greenberg MD, Katz NM, Iuliano S, *et al.* Atrial Pacing for the Prevention of Atrial Fibrillation After Cardiovascular Surgery. J Am Coll Cardiol 2000;35:1416-1422.

[114] Mariscalco G, Engström KG. Atrial fibrillation after cardiac surgery: Risk factors and their temporal relationship in prophylactic drug strategy decision. Int J Cardiol 2008;129:354-362.

[115] Banach M, Goch A, Misztal M, *et al.* Predictors of paroxysmal atrial fibrillation in patients undergoing aortic valve replacement. J Thorac Cardiovasc Surg 2007;134:1569-1576.

[116] Hayashida N, Shojima T, Yokokura Y, *et al.* P-Wave Signal-Averaged Electrocardiogram for Predicting Atrial Arrhythmia After Cardiac Surgery. Ann Thorac Surg 2005;79:859-864.

[117] Dawkins S, Hobson AR, Kalra PR, *et al.* Permanent Pacemaker Implantation After Isolated Aortic Valve Replacement: Incidence, Indications, and Predictors. Ann Thorac Surg 2008;85:108-112.

[118] El-Khally Z, Thibault B, Staniloae C, *et al.* Prognostic Significance of Newly Acquired Bundle Branch Block After Aortic Valve Replacement. Am J Cardiol 2004;94:1008-1011.

[119] Erdogan HB, Kayalar N, Ardal H, *et al.* Risk Factors for Requirement of Permanent Pacemaker Implantation After Aortic Valve Replacement. J Card Surg 2006;21:211-215.

[120] Koplan BA, Stevenson WG, Epstein LM, *et al.* Development and Validation of a Simple Risk Score to Predict the Need for Permanent Pacing After Cardiac Valve Surgery. J Am Coll Cardiol 2003;41:795-801.

[121] Huynh H, Dalloul G, Ghanbari H, *et al.* Permanent Pacemaker Implantation Following Aortic Valve Replacement: Current Prevalence and Clinical Predictors. PACE 2009; 32:1520-1525.

[122] Merin O, Ilan M, Oren A, *et al.* Permanent Pacemaker Implantation Following Cardiac Surgery: Indications and Long-Term Follow-Up. PACE 2009;32:7-12.

[123] Lewis JW Jr., Webb CR, Pickard SD, *et al.* The increased need for a permanent pacemaker after reoperative cardiac surgery. J Thorac Cardiovasc Surg 1998;116:74-81.

[124] Limongelli G, Ducceschi V, D'Andrea A, *et al.* Risk factors for pacemaker implantation following aortic valve replacement: a single centre experience. Heart 2003;89:901-904.

[125] Mistiaen W, Vissers D. Risk factors for postoperative pulmonary complications after aortic valve replacement within the hospital: an observational study. Austr J Physiotherapy 2008; 54:119-124.

[126] Overend TJ, Anderson CM, Lucy SD, *et al.* The effect of incentive spirometry on postoperative pulmonary complications: a systematic review. Chest 2001;120:971-978.

127] Lawrence VA, Hilsenbeck SG, Mulrow CD, *et al.* Incidence and hospital stay for cardiac and pulmonary complications after abdominal surgery. J Gen Int Med 1995;10:671-678.

[128] Johnson LG, McMahan MJ. Postoperative factors contributing to prolonged length of stay in cardiac surgery patients. Dim Crit Care Nurs 1997;16:243-250.

[129] Wynne R, Botti M. Postoperative pulmonary dysfunction in adults after cardiac surgery with cardiopulmonary bypass. clinical significance and implications for practice. Am J Crit Care 2004;13:384-393.

[130] Staton GW, Williams WH, Mahoney EM, *et al.* Pulmonary outcomes of off-pump *vs.* on-pump coronary artery bypass surgery in a randomized trial. Chest 2005;127:892-901.

[131] Habib G, Thuny F, Avierinos JF. Prosthetic Valve Endocarditis: Current Approach and Therapeutic Options. Progress Cardiovasc Dis 2008;50:274-281.

[132] Dellegrottaglie S, Saran R, Gillespie B, *et al.* Prevalence and predictors of cardiovascular calcium in chronic kidney disease [from the prospective longitudinal RRI-CKD Study]. Am J Cardiol 2006;98:571-576.

[133] Qunibi WY. Cardiovascular calcification in nondialyzed patients with chronic kidney disease. Seminars in dialysis 2007;20:134-138.

[134] Gaudino M, Luciani N, Giungi S, *et al.* Different profiles of patients who require dialysis after cardiac surgery. Ann Thorac Surg 2005;79:825-830.

[135] Cowie MR, Komajda M, Murray-Thomas T, *et al.*, on behalf of the POSH Investigators. Prevalence and impact of worsening renal function in patients hospitalized with decompensated heart failure: results of the prospective outcomes study in heart failure [POSH]. Eur Heart J 2006;27:1216-1222.

[136] Sajja LR, Mannam G, Chakravarthi MR, *et al.* Coronary artery bypass grafting with or without cardiopulmonary bypass in patients with preoperative non–dialysis dependent renal insufficiency: A randomized study. J Thorac Cardiovasc Surg 2007;133:378-388.

[137] Vaquette B, Corbineau H, Laurent M, *et al.* Valve replacement in patients with critical aortic stenosis and depressed left ventricular function: predictors of operative risk, left ventricular function recovery, and long term outcome. Heart 2005;91:1324-1329

[138] Remadi JP, Rakotoarivello Z, Marticho P, *et al.* Aortic valve replacement with the minimal extracorporeal circulation [Jostra MECC System] *versus* standard cardiopulmonary bypass: A randomized prospective trial. J Thorac Cardiovasc Surg 2004;128:436-441.

[139] Albahrani MJ, Swaminathan M, Phillips-Bute B, *et al.* Postcardiac surgery complications: Association of acute renal dysfunction and atrial fibrillation. Anest Analg 2003;96:637-643.

[140] Ngo DTM, Heresztyn T, Mishra K, *et al.* Aortic stenosis is associated with elevated plasma levels of asymmetric dimethylarginine [ADMA]. Nitric Oxide 2007;16:197-201.

CHAPTER 9

Aortic Valve Replacement in Patients Aged Over 80 Years

Abstract: The life expectancy in the Western societies has increased steadily. CAVS is usually occurring at a higher age, therefore its incidence is also rising. However, the diagnosis of CAVS in elderly is not always easy: the disease might be overlooked because its symptoms sometimes are not recognized. Moreover, ascertaining the valvular origin of the symptoms in elderly patients might be a challenge.

If the presence of a symptomatic CAVS has been established in an elderly patient, the optimal treatment still has to be decided. Age, frailty, co-morbid conditions and LVF all have played a role in this decision making. It has become clear that there were and still are different approaches of cardiologists in regard to the referral policy.

Unto recently, about one third of the patients has been denied AVR unjustly. The EuroSCORE overestimates the postoperative mortality, especially in high risk patients, and should be used with great caution.

The available postoperative results seem to justify a referral of octogenarians with symptomatic CAVS for AVR. Hospital and long-term adverse events in these elderly patients are more frequent, compared to their younger counterparts. There is, however, a considerable variation in postoperative results, which is probably due to differences in the baseline characteristics of the patients. This finding applies for patients of all ages, including octogenarians.

The study of risk factors has revealed that need for urgent surgery has a dominant effect on the postoperative results. This factor is more present in elderly, indicating that poor postoperative results in elderly could be a self fulfilling prophecy. Long-term postoperative results in octogenarians show that, compared to the general population, a normal age and gender matched survival might be reached, with an acceptable quality of life.

Keywords: CABG, co-morbidity, coronary artery disease, EuroSCORE, frailty, hospital mortality, independent predictors, left ventricular function, long-term mortality, octogenarians, quality of life, stentless valves.

1. INTRODUCTION

As the human lifespan increases and healthcare quality improves, more people are reaching an advanced age in which they present cardiac disorders such as CAVS. Significant CAVS seems to be present in about 3% of randomly selected people

Wilhelm Peter Mistiaen

aged between 75 and 86 years. This disease is the most frequent heart valve disease in the elderly, and increases with age [1]. With a life expectancy of 6.9 years for octogenarian men and 8.7 years for women in 2000, the share of octogenarians has reached 4% of the population in Western countries. It has been estimated that 40% of octogenarians have serious symptomatic heart disease [2]. Hence, AVR has become a common operation in elderly patients [3, 4]. A sound and scientific treatment policy has become necessary.

In determining this treatment policy, several steps have to be taken. These are:

- Establishing the presence and the severity of CAVS.
- Ascertaining the valvular origin of symptoms.
- Calculate the risk to benefit ratio for every treatment option: medical, BAV, TAVI or conventional AVR.

2. Diagnosis of CAVS in Elderly

Analysis of the patients' history is of paramount importance. Dyspnea, angina and syncope are the classical symptoms of CAVS. In elderly patients, additional problems have to be solved, by detailed anamnesis, as a first step:

- When did these symptoms start.
- When were these symptoms recognized as such, if these have started insidiously.
- Did limitation of ADL mask these symptoms.
- Is there currently any co-morbidity such as CAD, COPD *etc.*
- Could this co-morbidity be (partially) responsible for these symptoms.

It is of importance to establish the valvular origin of symptoms. For asymptomatic CAVS, there is no advantage in terms of survival for AVR. This operation is not indicated for CAVS in absence of symptoms, because of the operative risk [1].

Clinical examination is the second step. Auscultatory signs have to be detected: these include disappearance of the second sound, systolic murmur and irradiation of this murmur to the carotid arteries – especially in sitting position.

The cornerstone of diagnosis of CAVS is TTE: this technique confirms the existence of this condition and provides an estimation of its severity by measuring AVA, TVG and jet velocity. The effect of CAVS on the LVF can also be estimated. The echocardiographic findings must be correlated to the severity of the clinical signs and symptoms. Invasive evaluation for the sake of the valve disease itself is rarely needed. CAD, however, is rather frequent in elderly and its presence has an impact on the operative procedure and the postoperative outcome. A preoperative coronarography is needed to decide if a concomitant CABG should be performed. A cardiac CT can also give valuable information about the degree of calcification, the anatomy of the coronary arteries and the LVF [1].

3. FRAILTY OF THE ELDERLY

There are reasons to question the need for AVR in octogenarians with symptomatic CAVS:

1) Risk of surgical intervention in octogenarians is higher compared to younger patients. From the STS database operative mortality in cardiac surgical procedures has been 2.8% in patients aged between 50 and 79 years, 7.1% in octogenarians and 11.8% in nonagenarians [5].

2) Benefits of AVR might be reduced, because of the reduced life expectancy in patients who are already old.

The benefits of AVR are, however, still considerable: survival after AVR in octogenarians with CAVS has significantly improved, compared to medical treatment, even if CAD is present. One, 2 and 5 year survival after AVR are up to 87, 78 and 68%. For medical management of symptomatic CAVS, this is 52, 40 and 22% [6] and QoL is poor [2].

Elderly patients with valve disease often present with atheromatosis, associated co-morbidities as well as reduced defense and functional reserve of many organs.

Atheromatosis frequently involves the aorta. Protruding and mobile atheroma plaques have been documented by TEE in at least 20% of the patients aged over 75 years. Hence, this imaging technique should be used routinely in elderly patients. Gently preoperative manipulation of the aorta is the only practical way to avoid major surgical procedures such as resection and replacement of parts of the aorta, which is hazardous in elderly and frail patients [2]. Other factors such as porcelain aorta and previous radiation of the chest are usually not included in the risk analysis, but these conditions also may play a major role in the decision making [1].

A decreased perfusion of the brain during ECC is another consequence of diffuse atherosclerosis. Impaired auto-regulation of the cerebral circulation, uneven distribution of the blood flow and absence of a pulsatile flow during ECC could be held responsible for postoperative neurological events. These can be a delayed awakening, agitation, and incomplete return of cognitive function. Together, diffuse and focal neurological deficits may affect 15–20% of elderly patients after heart surgery. These events could lead to prolonged postoperative recovery and to permanent admittance to a home [2].

Calendar age and physiological age might differ for every patient. Nevertheless, co-morbid conditions and a decreased physiological reserve of vital organs could have an effect on the capacity of elderly patients to withstand a conventional AVR. Recent advances in surgical techniques, development of less traumatic ECC devices, more effective myocardial protection and improved peri and postoperative care have made it possible to shift the upper limit for AVR over 70 and even over 80 years [2]. This has been observed in a recent series, in which the share of octogenarians in patients referred for AVR has increased from 6.3% from 1986 to 25.5% in 2006 [7]. This increase has also been observed in other institutions.

4. DECISION MAKING AND SCORING FOR THE RISKS OF SURGERY IN ELDERLY PATIENTS

AVR can be considered as the reference treatment for CAVS. Although there are no formal contraindications for this operation, the decision making can be difficult. Potential benefit from the operation is the key. The risk – benefit ratio has to be calculated for every treatment option such as for conservative treatment, for AVR and for TAVI [1].

The decision to operate has to be taken by the cardiac team (surgeon, cardiologist, geriatrist, anesthesiologist) and the patient him or herself and if necessary, their relatives. However, one third to 40% of the elderly is denied AVR unjustly [1, 8]. Moreover, the adequate timing of the surgery is also an issue [1, 9, 10]. There are several difficulties in this decision making:

1) The gradual decrease in ADL could mask symptoms for longer time. Hence, AVR sometimes is performed (too) late, with an increase in hospital and long-term mortality as consequence. In advances cases, all compensatory mechanisms to maintain an adequate circulation might become exhausted. The severity and the rate of progress of symptoms are a major key in the timing for AVR [1, 9, 10].

2) Age has been a major factor in the decision making by the cardiologists, but this issue seems double-edged. Half of the cardiologists have shown a strong tendency to advise AVR, the remaining half has been more reluctant to refer for AVR. Surprisingly, the presence of co-morbid conditions – except for neurological dysfunction – has not or almost not played a part in this decision making [1, 8, 11, 12].

3) LVF has been another major issue in the decision making for referral for AVR. This factor is usually considered in combination with age. The very elderly (age > 85 years), with LVEF < 30%, who are not considered as good surgical candidates by most physicians are only a small minority of the population. In patients aged between 80 and 85 years with an LVEF between 30 and 50% might be better surgical candidates. Denial of surgery in such patients is not supported by a risk to benefit analysis [1, 8].

4) The effect of co-morbidity on hospital mortality can be estimated by using indices such as the EuroSCORE and STS PROM. These score systems have been developed for CABG but also have been applied

for AVR. In high risk patients, however, hospital mortality has been overestimated. This could be due to the improved surgical techniques and postoperative care. Furthermore, the individual contribution of every risk factor is difficult to estimate [1]. Outcome of surgery in terms of life expectancy and QoL favors the surgical option, especially when co-morbidity is absent. Most co-morbid conditions increase the operative risk and decrease the long-term postoperative survival. This is especially relevant when a malignancy has been treated only a few years before cardiac surgery [1, 7, 8, 13].

Summarized, the tendency for denial or postponement of AVR could lead to worse postoperative outcome, hence the effect of age on mortality could be considered as a self fulfilling prophecy [9].

5. CO-MORBIDITY AND SEVERITY OF CAVS IN ELDERLY

The presence of co-morbid conditions in octogenarians, who have been referred for AVR, vary considerably. In some series, co-morbidity has been less present compared to younger patients [14]. In other series, the opposite has been observed [9, 15]. These differences indicate large varieties in referral policy. This applies for co-morbid conditions such as diabetes, gender, CAD, but also to severity of symptoms and of LV dysfunction.

For example, some series have reported less diabetes in octogenarians, but a higher rate of female patients [4, 16-19]. A higher number of female patients could imply an increased presence of patients with small annuli [20, 21].

The presence of CAD in patients with CAVS is another matter. This condition can be considered separately from other co-morbid conditions, since CABG and AVR can be performed at the same time. CAD, and hence, the need for CABG varies greatly amongst series: from 19% [22], 25%-26% [19, 23], 34% [24], 42% [16, 21] to rates as high as 61% [7, 25-27]. This is important since addition of CABG to AVR has an influence on the postoperative outcome.

With increasing age, more reoperations occur for CABG as well as for valvular and combined operations [28-30]. This also could affect the postoperative outcome.

CAVS is more severe in older patients [14] with AVAI of less than 0.6 cm^2/m^2 and TVG over 50 mm Hg [8]. In elderly, a higher need for urgent AVR was also observed [9, 14] which can be up to 23% [19, 23].

Octogenarians have also more symptoms of NYHA grade III-IV [9, 15]. The presence of a high NYHA grade varies between 32% and 78% [19, 21, 23, 31]. One reason for this variability might be the subjective nature of this grading, which is notoriously difficult to estimate in elderly! However, mean LVEF is 52 to 66 % in octogenarians who are referred for AVR/CABG [6, 9, 31, 32], which is rather high. It seems that a high NYHA functional grading is not related to a decreased LVEF in these patients.

6. CHOICE OF PROSTHESIS IN OCTOGENARIANS

Since octogenarians rarely outlive a BHV, this type of valve has been (and still is) preferred. There is no need for long-term postoperative anticoagulation [1, 2], provided there are no other conditions requiring this treatment. Even a low dosage anticoagulation could lead to a serious bleeding in elderly patients. Hence, MHV has usually not been considered as a first option.

Stented BHV have a larger TVG than their MHV counterparts. In small annuli, the use of MHV could be defended [22]. Enlargement of the annulus or implantation of stentless devices are other options, but these techniques are more demanding, especially in calcified aortic roots [2].

In patients with normal LVF, smaller valves with higher TVG, and even a certain degree of VPPM could be tolerated [1, 20]. A small valve is not an independent predictor for postoperative CHF [33]. Therefore, in patients with small annuli and a normal LVF, enlargement of the annulus or the use of a stentless BHV could be avoided.

7. RESULTS OF SURGERY IN OCTOGENARIANS

7.1. Hospital Mortality and Other Events During Hospital Stay

The hospital mortality after AVR in octogenarians is about 10% in most recent series. It is 5% in favorable patients, *i.e.* in cases of elective surgery and in patients with few symptoms and preserved LVF [19, 20, 23, 27]. This result is only moderately higher compared to younger patients, who have an operative mortality of 2-3%. Hospital mortality in octogenarians, however, can be as high as 40% in patients with severe symptoms and low LVEF [1, 19, 23].

CAD shares some risk factors with CAVS. Hence both conditions could occur simultaneously. If significant CAD is present, CABG must be added to AVR [1, 2]. Lesions on the LAD are the key to decide for CABG. Concomitant CABG, however, is not always performed if CAD is present [16]. If a concomitant CABG is performed in patients referred for AVR, hospital mortality rises between 4 and 24% [16, 18-24, 27, 31, 34, 35]. Significant differences have been observed in a survey of 22 centers in whom over 65000 patients were treated, including over 4500 octogenarians.

In patients, referred for reoperation, which could be considered as a risk factor, the mortality also varies between 5.5% [29] and 16.4% [30]. The causes for hospital death were:

- Respiratory failure [55%].
- AMI [28%].
- And in a lesser degree, stroke, sepsis and renal failure [19, 23].

The complication rate in octogenarians has been 69.1% for all complications [31]. Stroke has been twice as common, compared to younger patients [14], especially if concomitant CABG has been performed. Widespread atheromatosis could be the reason [1]. Postoperative acute renal function impairment has been more present in octogenarians [5, 14], with an age over 80 as an independent predictor [26]. The need for postoperative pulmonary complications and prolonged ventilation has been more present in elderly in one series [5], but this could not be confirmed by other observations [25, 36]. A prolonged stay in ICU was not more observed for octogenarians according to some [36]. These postoperative results justify an economic use of cardiac surgery in elderly [17].

7.2. Risk Factors for Hospital Mortality

Emergency surgery and need for IABP are the most important risk factors for hospital mortality [1, 5, 9, 14, 19, 21, 23, 28, 37, 38]. This could be due to a postponed referral, with a prolonged burden on the left ventricle as a result. All compensatory mechanisms to maintain an adequate circulation could become exhausted by this delay. Related to such a delayed referral and hence to a prolonged burden on the LV are:

- Decreased preoperative LVF [1, 4, 31].
- Development of PAHT [31].
- Development of functional mitral regurgitation [5].
- Occurrence of CHF [2, 20].
- Increase of the NYHA functional class to grade IV [1, 19, 20, 23].

Prior CABG and BAV also have an adverse effect on mortality [14, 19, 23].

Small aortic annuli, which is more present in elderly female patients, is a matter for debate. Hospital mortality for patients with small aortic annuli is 12.5% if these patients receive a size 19 mm valve [20]. This seems in line with other results and does not indicate to a significant increase. If, as alternative a freestyle stentless in octogenarians valve is used, no hospital mortality increase of hospital mortality has been documented [36]. In contrast, a low BSA in female patients with small valves has been identified as predictor in another series [3].

Non-cardiac factors such as PAD and a preoperatively impaired renal function also increase hospital mortality [1, 5, 18]. Postoperative complications have also been associated to hospital mortality. These include [4, 21, 24, 30, 38]:

- Low output syndrome.
- Re-exploration for bleeding.
- Digestive complications.
- Sepsis.
- Stroke.

7.3. Long Term Survival in Octogenarians

The long-term survival for octogenarians has been comparable to a similar control group from the general population.

- The 1 year survival has ranged from 76% [30], 79% [31], 82% [21], 84% [4]; 85% [20], 86% [24], 87% [34] to 95% [2].
- The 3 year survival has varied from 71% [30], 75% [31] to 80% [2].
- The 5 year survival of different series has ranged from 51% [30], 56% [4, 21, 31], 57% [16]; 60% [20]; 65% [37], 69% [34], 70% [2] to 73% [23].
- The 10 year postoperative survival of octogenarians has been documented in only one report and was estimated at 30% [20].

These results show that long-term results after AVR in octogenarians are favourable. A reasonable milestone for this population is the 5-year postoperative survival, which is currently between 50 and 70%. These figures are comparable with those of the general population of the same age [8].

Implantation of a freestyle stentless device has resulted in a median survival time of octogenarians of 5.2 years, which is in line with the other results [36].

7.4. Predictors of Long-Term Mortality

Some predictors of long-term mortality could be related to a delayed referral. These are preoperative CHF, low LVEF, need for an urgent AVR and need for an IABP [1, 9, 20, 21, 34]. If a CAD is present, development of AMI could also become a problem if cardiac surgery is delayed [23].

Some other factors, however, are a matter for debate.

1) The type of prosthesis has been identified as a predictor for long-term survival. Patients who have received a MHV have shown a higher long-term mortality, due to TE and to anticoagulation related bleeding [34]. In contrast, improved survival has been documented after use of

MHV in another series (at 1 year 91%, at 3 year 88%, at 5 years 82%, at 8 years 70%). For BHV, these results have been at 1 year 86%, at 3 years 77%, at 5 years 58% and at 8 years 47% [22].

2) Concomitant CABG has shown an effect in some series: the 5 year survival for isolated AVR in octogenarians has been 75%, for AVR with concomitant CABG, this has been 65% [32]. This has been confirmed in several other series [20, 31, 34]. Previous AMI, as marker for CAD and need for CABG also has been identified as predictor [9]. In other series, the effect of CABG on long-term survival has not been observed [27].

3) Female gender also has been considered as a risk factor [31], but not in all series [27].

Postoperative adverse events have also been identified as predictors for long-term mortality. These events include:

- Postoperative stroke [21].
- Postoperative renal failure [21].
- Duration of ICU stay [19, 23].
- For reoperation: low cardiac output, GI complications [30].

7.5. Postoperative QoL in Octogenarians

The purpose of AVR is to reduce or abolish symptoms and increase the exercise tolerance and hence, QoL. Postoperative stroke, which could reduce the QoL, has not been significantly more present in octogenarians, but age as a continuous factor has been identified as a predictor for postoperative neurological problems [36]. This could influence the postoperative QoL of patients.

Currently, most octogenarians live at home after the operation and have an independent life. If these patients do not have co-morbid conditions, physical activity (whatever this means at this age) could be resumed after AVR [2]. Female gender, however, has been identified as a predictor for impaired autonomy [31].

The QoL improves after surgery and is comparable to that of the population of the same age [28, 36]: 64 to 81% of the patients is without disablement or has only minor function impairment. Improvement of symptoms to a NYHA functional class I or II is present in 91-93% of the patients [18, 19, 23, 32]. Sixty-five to 83% of the patients is fully satisfied with the QoL [31, 32].

Use of BHV contributes to the well being of these elderly patients [1], since no anticoagulation is required. In another series, however, the use of MHV has not affected QoL in octogenarians [22].

CONCLUSIONS

Age over 80 years as such is not a contra-indication for AVR in patients with severe and symptomatic CAVS.

Hospital mortality in these elderly patients is acceptable and even less than previously reported, especially in patients with preserved LVF and without co-morbid conditions. The postoperative morbidity can considerable, especially when preoperative co-morbidity is present.

Nevertheless, the EuroSCORE overestimates the risk for operative mortality, especially in high risk patients. This score should be used cautiously. With debilitating neuropsychiatric disorders, severe renal or pulmonary dysfunction, recently treated carcinoma (*i.e.* less than 5 years), AVR should be recommended only after careful consideration.

The long-term outcome after cardiac surgery in octogenarians who survive the operation is favorable, but early referral is mandatory to improve outcome. Postponement of AVR, until an urgent need for operation develops, is inadvisable, since this impairs the postoperative outcome.

If concomitant CABG is needed, long-term survival seems to be reduced but is still acceptable. Even reoperation in octogenarians has an acceptable outcome.

In patients with small annuli, stentless valves could be used, but they offer no major advantage. A 19 mm valve can have a good outcome in patients with normal LVF.

Improvement of the NYHA class functional status after AVR is remarkable in octogenarians and the QoL is comparable to the general population of the same age.

The decision for operation is a joint decision of many specialists.

ACKNOWLEDGEMENT

Declared none.

CONFLICT OF INTEREST

The author(s) confirm that this chapter content has no conflict of interest.

REFERENCES

[1] Iung B. Management of the elderly patient with aortic stenosis. Heart 2008;94:519-524.

[2] Prêtre R, Turina MI. Valve disease: Cardiac valve surgery in the octogenarian. Heart 2000;83;116-121.

[3] Bloomstein LZ, Gielchinsky I, Bernstein AD, *et al.* Aortic Valve Replacement in Geriatric Patients: Determinants of In-Hospital Mortality. Ann Thorac Surg 2001;71:597-600.

[4] Collart F, Feier H, Kerbaul F, *et al.* Valvular surgery in octogenarians: operative risks factors, evaluation of Euroscore and long term results. Eur J Cardio-thorac Surg 2005;27:276-280.

[5] Bridges CR, Edwards FH, Peterson ED, *et al.* Cardiac Surgery in Nonagenarians and Centenarians. J Am Coll Surg 2003;197:347-357.

[6] Varadarajan P, Kapoor N, Bansal RC, Pai RG. Survival in elderly patients with severe aortic stenosis is dramatically improved by aortic valve replacement: results from a cohort of 277 patients aged over 80 years. Eur J Cardio-thorac Surg 2006;30:722-727.

[7] Mistiaen W, Van Cauwelaert P, Muylaert P, De Worm E. 1000 Carpentier-Edwards pericardial valves in aortic position: what changed in the last 20 years and what are the effects on hospital complications. J Heart Valve Dis 2007;16:417-422.

[8] Iung B, Cachier A, Baron G, *et al.* Decision-making in elderly patients with severe aortic stenosis: why are so many denied surgery? Eur Heart J 2005;26:2714-2720.

[9] Mistiaen W, Van Cauwelaert P, Muylaert P, *et al.* Risk Factors and Survival after Aortic Valve Replacement in Octogenarians. J Heart Valve Dis 2004;13;538-544.

[10] Mistiaen W, Van Cauwelaert P, Sys SU, *et al.* Timing of aortic valve replacement in elderly patients with symptomatic aortic valve disease using outpatient clinical parameters. Acta Clin Belg 2005;60:185-189.

[11] Bouma BJ, van den Brink RBA, van der Meulen JHP, *et al.* To operate or not on elderly patients with aortic stenosis: the decision and its consequences. Heart 1999;82:143-148.

[12] Bouma BJ, van der Meulen JHP, van den Brink RBA, *et al.* Variability in treatment advice for elderly patients with aortic stenosis: a nationwide survey in the Netherlands. Heart 2001;85:196-201.

[13] Mistiaen W, Van Cauwelaert Ph, Muylaert Ph, *et al.* Effect of prior malignancy on survival after cardiac surgery. Ann Thorac Surg 2004;77:1593-1597.

[14] Alexander KP, Anstrom KJ, Muhlbaier LH, *et al.* Outcomes of Cardiac Surgery in Patients Age over 80 Years: Results from the National Cardiovascular Network. J Am Coll Cardiol 2000;35:731-738.

[15] Chukwuemeka A, Borger MA, Ivanov J, *et al.* Valve Surgery in Octogenarians: A Safe Option with Good Medium-Term Results. J Heart Valve Dis 2006;15:191-196.

[16] Bessou JP, Bouchart F, Angha S, *et al.* Aortic valvular replacement in octogenarians. Short-term and mid-term results in 140 patients. Cardiovasc Surg 1999;7:355-362.

[17] Avery GJ II, Ley SJ, Hill JD, *et al.* Cardiac Surgery in the Octogenarian: Evaluation of Risk, Cost, and Outcome. Ann Thorac Surg 2001;71:591-596.

[18] Gilbert T, Orr W, Banning AP. Surgery for aortic stenosis in severely symptomatic patients older than 80 years: experience in a single UK centre. Heart 1999;82:138-142.

[19] Kolh P, Lahaye L, Gerard P, Limet R. Aortic valve replacement in the octogenarians: perioperative outcome and clinical follow-up. Eur J Cardio-thorac Surg 1999;16:68-73.

[20] Medalion B, Lytle BW, McCarthy PM, *et al.* Aortic Valve Replacement for Octogenarians: Are Small Valves Bad? Ann Thorac Surg 1998;66:699-706.

[21] Melby SJ, Zierer A, Kaiser SP, *et al.* Aortic Valve Replacement in Octogenarians: Risk Factors for Early and Late Mortality. Ann Thorac Surg 2007;83:1651-1657.

[22] Vicchio M, Della Corte A, De Santo LS, *et al.* Tissue *Versus* Mechanical Prostheses: Quality of Life in Octogenarians. Ann Thorac Surg 2008;85:1290-1295.

[23] Kolh P, Kerzmann A, Honore C, *et al.* Aortic valve surgery in octogenarians: predictive factors for operative and long-term results. Eur J Cardio-thorac Surg 2007;31:600-606.

[24] Urso S, Sadaba R, Greco E, *et al.* One-Hundred Aortic Valve Replacements in Octogenarians: Outcomes and Risk Factors for Early Mortality. J Heart Valve Dis 2007;16:139-144.

[25] Mistiaen W, Vissers D. Risk factors for postoperative pulmonary complications after aortic valve replacement within the hospital: an observational study. Austr J Physiotherapy 2008; 54:119-124.

[26] Mistiaen W, Van Cauwelaert P, Muylaert P, De Worm E. 1000 pericardial valves in aortic position: risk factors for postoperative acute renal function impairment in elderly. J Cardiovasc Surg 2009;50:233-237.

[27] Roberts WC, Ko JM, Garner WL, *et al.* Valve Structure and Survival in Octogenarians Having Aortic Valve Replacement for Aortic Stenosis [+/-Aortic Regurgitation] With *Versus* Without Coronary Artery Bypass Grafting at a Single US Medical Center [1993 to 2005]. Am J Cardiol 2007;100:489-495.

[28] Blanche C, Khan SS, Chaux A, *et al.* Cardiac Reoperations in Octogenarians: Analysis of Outcomes. Ann Thorac Surg 1999;67:93-98.

[29] Ghosh P, Holthouse D, Carroll I, *et al.* Cardiac reoperations in octogenerians. Eur J Cardio-thorac Surg 1999;15:809-815.

[30] Eitz T, Fritzsche D, Kleikamp G, *et al.* Reoperation of the Aortic Valve in Octogenarians. Ann Thorac Surg 2006;82:1385-1391.

[31] Kirsch M, Guesnier L, LeBesnerais P, *et al.* Cardiac Operations in Octogenarians: Perioperative Risk Factors for Death and Impaired Autonomy. Ann Thorac Surg 1998;66:60-67.

[32] Huber CH, Goeber V, Berdat P, *et al.* Benefits of cardiac surgery in octogenarians-a postoperative quality of life assessment. Eur J Cardio-thorac Surg 2007;31:1099-1105.

[33] Mistiaen W, Van Cauwelaert Ph, Muylaert Ph, *et al.* Risk factors for congestive heart failure after aortic valve replacement with a Carpentier-Edwards pericardial prosthesis in the elderly. J. Heart Valve Dis 2005;14:774-779.

[34] Chiappini B, Bergonzini M, Gallieri S, *et al.* Clinical outcome of aortic valve replacement inthe elderly. Cardiovasc Surg 2003;11:359-365.

[36] Ennker J, Dalladaku F, Rosendahl U, *et al.* The Stentless Freestyle Bioprosthesis: Impact of Age Over 80 Years on Quality of Life, Perioperative, and Mid-Term Outcome. J Card Surg 2006;21:379-385.

[37] Dalrymple-Hay MJR, Alzetani A, Aboel-Nazar S, *et al.* Cardiac surgery in the elderly. Eur J Cardio-thorac Surg 1999;15:61-66.

[38] Unic D, Leacche M, Paul S, *et al.* Early and Late Results of Isolated and Combined Heart Valve Surgery in Patients >80 Years of Age. Am J Cardiol 2005;95:1500-1503.

CHAPTER 10

Valve Prosthesis Patient Mismatch

Abstract: The problem of VPPM needs to be addressed in patients with small aortic annuli. The options for such patients are implantation of stentless valves or of homografts. The enlargement of the aortic root could also be performed. These techniques, however, can be very demanding. The implantation of a stented valve is easier but carries the risk for VPPM.

The type of stentless valves and their implantation techniques are described very briefly. Of more importance are the postoperative results. These are difficult to compare for two reasons:

1) Stentless valves do not form a homogenous group.

2) Patients series can differ in age, co-morbid conditions and other characteristics.

Therefore, patients baseline characteristics should be described as completely as possible. The postoperative results for stentless valves seemed to be comparable with those of stented counterparts. For both, stented ans stentless devices, patient related factors have the most impact on the outcome.

The presence or absence of VPPM could be related to hemodynamic parameters, such as EOAI and TVG. This relationship, however, is not straightforward. Moreover, VPPM needs to be defined and graded properly. VPPM seems only to be clinically relevant in patients with a decreased LVF. In patients with a normal LVF, VPPM does not seem to affect the postoperative outcome in terms of survival, LVM regression and freedom of CHF.

The development of SVD could be held responsible for a recurrent hemodynamic burden on the LV. This burden could play a role in reappearance of LVH. SVD was thought to occur less in stentless valves, since turbulence and hence stress on the leaflets would be reduced. In some stentless devices this seems not to be the case.

Availability of 15 year results is needed, but this is not easy to obtain since the median age in patient series is rather high.

Keywords: Aortic root enlargement, effective orifice area, left ventricular function, left ventricular mass, stentless heart valves, structural valve degeneration, survival, transvalvular gradients, valve prosthesis patient mismatch, valve size.

Wilhelm Peter Mistiaen

1. PRINCIPLES

1.1. History

The first AVR have been performed with stentless homograft BHV and caged ball MHV. The homografts were scarce and the implantation technique has been demanding. MHV were readily available and the postoperative results have been predictable, but the risk for PVT and TE, however, required life-long use of anticoagulation. BHV devices, however, have been improved by the development of glutaraldehyde treated stented porcine and pericardial tisseus. Durability in the more contemporary BHV has improved [1, 2].

SVD and turbulences have been associated with a decrease in EOAI. Current stentless BHV, porcine as well as pericardial, should be able to deal with SVD and turbulence. Because of the lack of stress at the base, stentless valves were supposed to be less subjected to the risk of SVD. Stentless valves have become part of the clinical routine for only 10%, probably due to the demanding technique [1]. The questions remains, which patient could benefit from such a device.

1.2. Techniques

Several techniques exist for implantation of a stentless valve [1]:

1. The a sub-coronary position has the advantage of avoiding manipulation of the coronary arteries.

    a. The aortotomy is performed as usual and the annulus of the device is sutured to the native aortic annulus, *i.e.* the baseline suture.

    b. The commissures are fixed to the aortic wall by a second suture.

    c. The overall shape of the aortic valve is restored.

    d. The disadvantages are the difficult implantation in calcified and hence sick roots and the risk for regurgitation by distortion.

2. The total root with re-implantation of coronary arteries is more complex. The advantage is an excellent hemodynamic result with

avoidance of VPPM, since the annulus can be "upsized", which is an advantage in small aortic annuli. Torsions of the commissures can be avoided.

3. Other and rarely used techniques: the mini-root and partial root operations.

4. The choice for a technique could be made ad hoc, on the basis of the patients' anatomy and on the size of the annulus.

1.3. Types of Devices

Several devices are available and have been tested for their mid-term results:

- Toronto SPV (SJM) and Freestyle (Medtronic).
- Sorin Pericarbon Freedom [3].
- Shelhigh Super Stenless [4].
- Cryolife O'Brien [5] as well as.
- Newer pliable devices [6].

There are some differences between these devices.

The Toronto valve is prepared from a whole porcine aortic root with the possibility of a reduction of the compliance of the annulus. The increased stiffness of the para-commissural parts of the cusps is caused by the retained muscle bar at the base of the right coronary cusp and by the use of a Dacron lining.

The Cryolife O'Brien valve has no Dacron lining and is composed of 3 non-coronary cusps and therefore has no muscle bar [7].

Hence, stentless devices cannot be considered as a homogenous group. This has its importance for the postoperative hemodynamic parameters.

1.4. Results

As for all valves, the postoperative outcome [1] should include:

- Survival.
- The classic valve related events (TE, PVT, bleeding, PVE and SVD).
- Hemodynamic parameters [1, 3]. and
- The effect on LVM.

Patient description should include:

- Demographics.
- Co-morbidid conditions, including their severity.
- NYHA functional class grading.
- The need for urgent AVR.
- Factors related to the surgical procedures, such as ECC and CBP times as well as concomitant procedures [3].
- A preoperative description of LVF and LVH.

Especially for retrospective and non-randomized series, possible sources of bias should be taken into account [1]. Following question should be asked:

- Who performed the randomization (an experienced surgeon might be inclined to perform a full root technique)?
- When was the randomization performed (pre of intra-operatively)?
- What is the difference in aortic valve pathology (more stented valves have been used in complex pathology)?
- Are there differences in age between groups (stentless groups usually have been younger)?

- Are there differences in cross-clamp and bypass time (these have been longer with stentless valves)?
- What are the used techniques and what is the effect of the learning curve (mortality has increased in early cases)?
- What are the sizes of the used prosthetic valves?
- What are the preoperative LVF and LVM?
- What is the implantation technique?

1.4.1. Early Results

The perioperative mortality is comparable for both stented and stentless devices in randomized and non-randomized studies. With the total root technique, the learning effect has been more pronounced. This has resulted an increased hospital mortality in early cases. With increasing experience, this difference has disappeared [1].

In a prospective small study a stented Hancock and a stentless Toronto SPV have been compared in elderly patients. Both patient groups have been comparable. ECC and CBP time has been 10 to 12 minutes longer for the stentless device, but this has not been significant. The valve size has also been comparable. The operative mortality for both groups has been 5% and 8% [8].

Hospital TE, bleeding and AMI after implantation with stentless valves have been comparable to those with stented BHV [1].

In patients with CAVS and decreased LVF, the outcome of stentless valves has seemed superior. One reason might be the larger EOAI, especially after the use of the root replacement technique. TVG, energy loss and the risk for VPPM has been comparably lower. This advantage seems to be maintained in the comparison with the newest generation of stented pericardial BHV [1].

1.4.2. Long-Term Survival

In some series, the long-term survival for stentless valves has been comparable to stented valves. The stentless group, however, has been younger (70 *vs.* 75 years), which has introduced a bias [8, 9].

In other series of patients with small annuli, stentless valves (Freestyle/Toronto SPV) has performed better compared to stented (Mosaic/CE perimount) devices [1]. These results have been confirmed in other, randomized and case matched series [10]. In other studies, improved survival has been found at at 5 years, but not at 8 years [11].

Three issues have played a role for long-term survival: patient related factors, occurrence of SVD and hemodynamic results:

1) Patient related factors such as age, gender, concomitant CABG, LVEF, excessive LVH and the classic co-morbid conditions have been identified as predictors for long-term survival and had a confounding effect [1, 9-11].

2) The occurrence of SVD seemed not to be an issue since stentless valves have been used in patients with a high EuroSCORE. This could have interacted with the effect of SVD on postoperative outcome [12].

3) The hemodynamic results might be responsible for an improved postoperative survival. The effect of postoperative hemodynamics on LVF and on LVM could be an viable explanation for this observation [1]. Therefore, studies of long-term hemodynamic should include data of.

    a. TVG and of

    b. EOAI (and not only EOA!)

A proper definition of VPPM, based on these data should also be provided.

The mode of randomization should also be clarified, since this can have an effect on the postoperative results.

1.4.3. TVG, EOAI and VPPM

The TVG is lower in stentless devices, compared to stented devices and is about 15 mm Hg. This corresponds to an EOA/EOAI of 2.4 cm^2. This approaches the AVA after a full root technique [1, 8, 13-15].

In stented BHV (such as CE-p, Mosaic, Hancock) as well in MHV, TVG is about 25 mm Hg and corresponds to an EOA of 1.5 to 2.0 cm^2. The design of a stent also plays a role for EOAI. In a stented Mitroflow device, for example, TVG is low but not as low as in stentless devices [1, 15].

The hemodynamic differences between stented and stentless devices is more pronounced in prostheses with smaller sizes [16]. Some authors state that stented and stentless devices are equally effective in terms of postoperative TVG [11]. However, the size of the LVOT, LVEF and the surgical technique itself have to be taken into consideration, while interpreting these statements [9].

TVG usually is determined at resting conditions, but this is not the most relevant parameter. With rising cardiac output, TVG also rises. This could be measured in exercise conditions or during a dobutamine stress test, which is clinically more important. This rise in TVG is less in stentless valves compared to stented BHV and to MHV. This difference in rise has been observed in Freestyle stentless full root, compared to CE-p stented valves, but not in the comparison between the Toronto SPV device, and the CE-p stented valve [1].

Determination of EOAI is also important since this determines the degree of VPPM. The incidence of VPPM varies from "uncommon" [17], and 6% [18] to over 60% if the cut-off level of 0.75 cm^2/m^2 is used [19]. Severe VPPM has been present in 2.4%, moderate VPPM has been present in 26.7% of the patients [20]. VPPM has less been observed with stentless valves: 18% *vs.* 41% [1, 11, 20].

VPPM can be defined as EOAI < 0.75cm^2/m^2 [19] or 0.85 75cm^2/m^2 [21]. VPPM can also be graded as.

- EOAI > 0.85: clinically insignificant VPPM.
- EOAI between 0.65 and 0.85: moderate VPPM.
- EAOI < 0.60-0.65: severe VPPM [17, 20, 22].

The effect of VPPM on survival and regression on LVMI is controversial, but is nevertheless important. The degree of VPPM and the LVF are important parameters.

If VPPM is present, even in moderate degree, it increases operative and long-term mortality in patients with decreased LVF, but not in patients with a normal LVF [19, 21, 22]. The difference in results, from no effect of VPPM [17] to an observable effect [20], might depend on the definition of VPPM and on patient factors such as LVF. A uniformity in grading, therefore, is warranted if one wants to compare postoperative results.

The independent predictors for survival in these series have been age over 65 [19] or 70 years, need for emergency AVR, EuroSCORE > 10 and concomitant procedures [20]. These predictors have also been identified in series who studied only stented BHV [23-25]. Therefore, postoperative survival seems more related to patient related factors than to valve related factors.

1.4.4. EOAI versus Valve Size

The valve size which has been provided by the manufacturers is not the only determinant for the EOAI. The valve size cannot be used to predict the occurrence of VPPM, although VPPM could be suspected if a valve of a small size has been implanted. The use of small valves (*i.e.* size 17, 19 and 21) has seemed to have no serious disadvantages in elderly patients and VPPM has uncommonly been observed in such small valve sizes. The effect of valve size on TVG and on EOAI with a MHV has been estimated as follows [2, 18, 26, 27].

- 17 mm valve: a TVG of 28 mm Hg and of EOAI 0.97 cm^2/m^2.
- 19 mm valve: a TVG of 20 mm Hg and of EOAI 1.01 cm^2/m^2.
- 21 mm valve: a TVG of 16 mm Hg and of EOAI 1.09 cm^2/m^2.
- 23 mm valve: a TVG of 14 mm Hg and of EOAI 1.41 cm^2/m^2.

With implantation of a MHV size of 17 mm, VPPM has been present in only 8 of 23 patients [27]. This means that even small MHV have been effective in reducing TVG and in increasing EOAI in many patients [18, 27]. With a dobutamine stress echocardiography, a significant increase in peak TVG has been observed in 20 of 38 patients, but this has not been considered as being clinically relevant [18].

The operative mortality for small valves implanted in elderly has been 4.0 to 6.2%. This is comparable to other results [2, 26, 28-30]. In some series, operative mortality was even absent [27].

Long term-survival has not been affected by small valve size as well [28, 29]. The actuarial survival at 10 years has been 80% in elderly patiens with a mean age of 72 years in one report [2], and 83% at 12 years in another [26].

Freedom from TE, PVE and reoperation has been over 95% and comparable to larger valves [2, 28]. The use of the 19 mm valve size has had no adverse effect on the occurrence of CHF [25].

It seems that patient related factors such as age, the presence of 3VD and LVF are of more importance for survival than valve related factors such as size [23, 29].

With implantation of a MHV of 17 mm in small elderly patients, mid-term echocardiography has shown a reduction of LVMI of 200 to 124g, even if VPPM could be documented [27].

There are some alternatives for patients with small aortic roots in whom a postoperative important VPPM could be anticipated.

Bi-leaflet MHV with an increased diameter such as Carbomedics size 21 has shown a lower TVG compared to conventional 21 mm valves, such as SJM. The difference is about of +/-5 mm Hg. The TVG has remained constant during the postoperative course, at 3 and at 9 months. However, small size (21, 23 *vs.* 25 mm) and type of the valve has not influenced LV remodeling [31].

Posterior root enlargement has been tried as an alternative for AVR in patients with small aortic roots in order to prevent a high postoperative TVG. Pericardial and Dacron patches have been used for this purpose. Operative mortality has remained within limits (6.4%). Only concomitant CABG has been identified as its predictor. Low cardiac output syndrome and occurrence of PVE have been documented as predictors for long-term mortality [32].

In conclusion, implantation of small valves are a reliable option in elderly patients [2, 28, 29]. Enlargement of the aortic annulus could be avoided by using a perimount BHV [26].

1.4.5. LVM/LVMI Regression

Trials and series studying the effect of stented and stentless devices on LVM regression are not easy to compare. These series differ in several ways:

- Different method of detection of LVM: by MRI [33] or by TTE [15, 34].
- Difference in inclusion of hemodynamic data [15].
- Difference in patients baseline characteristics: age, preoperative LVEF and LVM, AHT and other co-morbid conditions with an effect on LVM.
- Difference in study design: case matched [10], prospective [8] and retrospective.
- Different types of stentless devices which do not have necessarily the same effect on hemodynamic parameters:
    - Toronto SPV [7, 8, 14], for which larger EOAI have been observed.
    - Medtronic Freestyle [33].
    - Cryolife O'Brien [32], for which smaller EOAI have been documented [7].
    - Prima plus stentless [1].
    - Shellhigh Super.
- Different types of stented devices, for which pericardial valves seem superior to porcine ones:
    - Hancock [8].
    - Mosaic [32].

    - Ultracor [32].
    - MHV such as ATS [32].
- Different types of surgical techniques:
    - A supra-annular position, as for CryoLife [7, 34].
    - Positioned at the annulus, as for the Toronto valve [7, 34].

In some series, the difference between stented and stentless devices has been called "not significant" [8, 11, 14, 33]. Although reduction of LVMI after implantation of stentless devices has been more rapid compared to their stented counterparts, both types BHV have been considered effective [1]. In contrast, some differences between those devices have been found in other series. Moreover, a prognostic significance has been attributed to these differences [13, 15].

On the long term, some other conditions such as AHT [11] could have an effect on the reduction of LVMI. Furthermore, a developing SVD, 10 years after implantation of the Toronto SPV stentless valve, could be responsible for a recurrent increase in LVM [1].

The baseline LVF also has had an effect on LVM regression and on freedom of postoperative CHF: with a normal LVF, no adverse effect of a small EOAI has been observed. In contrast, in patients with a reduced LVF, LVMI regression has been hampered, even when the degree of VPPM has been considered as moderate [17, 21, 22].

An excessive LVH also could lead to an incomplete regression of LVMI [11]. In accordance with this observation, diastolic dysfunction in patients with VPPM has been associated with an increase in postoperative adverse events and in mortality [35].

A high TVG could be a risk factor for impaired mobility [9], decreased QoL and could be associated with arrhythmias [19]. The use of stentless devices in elderly did not seem to affect the QoL in a negative way, hence the device could be used in this population [36].

1.4.6. SVD in Stentless Devices

It has been postulated that favorable hemodynamic properties of stentless valves would lead to lower rates of SVD. This could be due to the lower mechanical stress placed on the leaflet tissues.

This postulation is still unproven, for several reasons:

- The high mean age at implantation made it difficult to have sufficient numbers of patients at risk for SVD after 15 year.
- Stentless valves have been implanted rather recently.
- SVD has to be defined in a standardized way: it should not only be judged on results after explantation of the device but also by echocardiography.

Following observations have been made concerning SVD:

- 10 year freedom for SVD after implantation of a Freestyle device has been 95% [1, 12]. This is comparable to the results obtained with the stented counterparts.
- For Toronto SPV, good results have been documented at 8 years, but results for SVD at 10 to 12 years have seemed disappointing and could lead to a recurrent increase in LVM [1].
- The Medtronic freestyle device has had a freedom for SVD of 100% at 6 years [9]. This period, however, is short to draw definitive conclusions.
- Although the hemodynamic profile of Cryolife O'Brien valves has been good in elderly patients, the rate of SVD and reoperation has increased considerably after 8 years. These results are in contrast to previously published results [12].

Other factors could have played a role in the development of SVD [12].

- Dilatation of the STJ and hence increased stress.
- Immunological reactions against the graft.
- Reactions to the glutaraldehyde.
- A demanding implantation technique.
- Additional anti-mineralization treatment as in Freestyle device but not in others.
- Age of the patient.

The appearance of a SVD can be held responsible for a recurrence of a hemodynamic burden on the LV. For this reason, LVH can recur during the long-term follow-up, with all its undesirable consequences.

The rate of SVD has been similar in Toronto SPV, Biocor PSB and Cryolife O'Brian devices. This suggests that one common mechanism might be responsible for this event. Low pressure fixation of porcine tissue in glutaraldehyde leads to loss of the transversal ridges in the cusps and crimp of collagen. In contrast to stented valves, SVD in stentless devices has mainly been characterized by stiffening. Tears in the cusps at the commissures and micro-calcifications have not always been observed. The occurrence of SVD has not been dependent on the type of preoperative valve disease (stenosis *vs.* regurgitation, bicuspid *vs.* tricuspid) or on pre-discharge echocardiographic findings [12].

SVD has been a major determinant for the reoperation rate. The Medtronic freestyle has a freedom of reoperation of 96% at 6 year [9]. In other series, a comparable freedom of reoperation has been found: 94% at 5 year and 57% at 10 year [12].

PVE can be another reason for reoperation. No advantage for stentless valves has been shown yet. The Medtronic freestyle device has a freedom of PVE at 6 year 97% [9], but the results after implantation with MHV have also seemed excellent. A RCT for this purpose is not yet available. Hence, a recommendation cannot be made [1].

CONCLUSIONS

Some conclusions concerning stentless valves can be drawn.

- Stented valves are more often used, compared to the stentless counterparts. This is probably due to the demanding technique.
- Longer ECC and CPB times might be an issue in high risk and elderly patients.
- Yet, excellent results in these patients have been obtained.
- The long-term durability (> 15 years) still has to be determined.
- Postoperative LVM reduction seems faster compared to the stented counterparts. The clinical significance of this observation is still uncertain.
- A SVD could be responsible for a subsequent burden on the LV (> 5 years) and for a recurrent increase in LVM.
- The hemodynamic results of stentless devices are excellent: TVG is low EOAI is high, especially during physical exercise. The level of physical exercise, is usually low in elderly.
- Stentless valves seem to be more beneficial in active patients but this observation still needs confirmation.
- Stentless valves are beneficial in patients with small aortic roots.
- There is a survival benefit in patients with a reduced preoperative LVF but this has to be confirmed with larger patient series (the patient factors are confounders); in patients with normal LVF, this effect has not been observed.

ACKNOWLEDGEMENT

Declared none.

CONFLICT OF INTEREST

The author(s) confirm that this chapter content has no conflict of interest.

REFERENCES

[1] Gulbins H, Reichenspurner H. Review article. Which Patients Benefit From Stentless Aortic Valve Replacement? Ann Thorac Surg 2009;88:2061-2068.

[2] Aupart M, Simonnot I, Sirinelli A, *et al.* Pericardial valves in small aortic annuli: ten years' results. Eur J Cardio-thorac Surg 1996;10:879-883.

[3] D'Onofrio A, Aurigemma S, Magagna P, *et al.* Aortic valve replacement with the Sorin Pericarbon Freedom stentless prosthesis: 7 years' experience in 130 patients. J Thorac Cardiovasc Surg 2007;134:491-495.

[4] Cattaneo P, Bruno VD, Mariscalco G, *et al.* Early Hemodynamic Results of the Shelhigh SuperStentless Aortic Bioprostheses. J Card Surg 2007;22:379-384.

[5] Gelsomimo S, Da Col G, Morocutti R, *et al.* Stentless aortic valve replacement in elderly Patients. Cardiovasc Surg 2002;10:233-237.

[6] Grubitsch H, Linneweber J, Kossagk C, *et al.* Aortic valve replacement with new-generation stentless pericardial valves: short-term clinical and hemodynamic results. J Heart Valve Dis 2005;14:623-629.

[7] Chambers JB, Rimington HM, Rajani R, *et al.* A randomized comparison of the Cryolife O'Brien and Toronto stentless replacement aortic valves. J Thorac Cardiovasc Surg 2007;133:1045-1050.

[8] Santini F, Bertolini P, Montalbano G, *et al.* Hancock *Versus* Stentless Bioprostheses for Aortic Valve Replacement in Patients Older Than 75 Years. Ann Thorac Surg 1998;66:S99-S103.

[9] Albert A, Florath I, Rosendahl U, *et al.* Effect of surgeon on transprosthetic gradients after aortic valve replacement with Freestyle® stentless bioprosthesis and its consequences: A follow-up study in 587 patients. J Cardiothorac Surg 2007, 2:40 doi:10.1186/1749-8090-2-40.

[10] David TE, Puschmann R, Ivanov J, *et al.* Aortic valve replacement with stented and stentless porcine valves: a case match study. J Thorac Cardiovasc Surg 1998;116:236-241.

[11] Bové T, Van Belleghem Y, Francois K, *et al.* Stentless and stented aortic valve replacement in elderly patients: factors affecting midterm clinical and hemodynamical outcome. Eur J Cardio-thorac Surg 2006;30:706-715.

[12] Pavoni D, Badano LP, Ius F, *et al.* Limited Long-Term Durability of the Cryolife O'Brien Stentless Porcine Xenograft Valve. Circulation 2007;116:I307–I313.

[13] Borger MA, Carson SM, Ivanov J, *et al.* Stentless Aortic Valves are Hemodynamically Superior to Stented Valves During Mid-Term Follow-Up: A Large Retrospective Study. Ann Thorac Surg 2005;80:2180-2185.

[14] Tsialtas D, Bolognesi R, Beghi C, *et al.* Stented *versus* stentless bioprosthesis in aortic valve stenosis: effect on left ventricular remodeling. Heart Surgery Forum 2007;10:E205-210.

[15] Thomson HL, O'Brien MF, Almeida AA, *et al.* Haemodynamics and left ventricular mass regression: a comparison of the stentless, stented and mechanical aortic valve replacement. Eur J Cardio-thorac Surg 1998;13:572-575.

[16] Goetzenich A, Langebartels G, Christiansen S, *et al.* Comparison of the Carpentier-Edwards Perimount™ and St. Jude Medical Epic™ Bioprostheses for Aortic Valve Replacement—A Retrospective Echocardiographic Short-Term Study. J Card Surg 2009;24:260-264.

[17] Vicchio M, Della Corte A, De Santo LS, *et al.* Prosthesis-patient mismatch in the elderly: survival, ventricular mass regression and quality of life. Ann Thorac Surg 2008;86:1791-1798.

[18] Sezai A, Kasamaki Y, Abe K, *et al.* Assessment of the St. Jude Medical Regent Prosthetic Valve by Continuous-Wave Doppler and Dobutamine Stress Echocardiography. Ann Thorac Surg 2010;89:87-92.

[19] Mannacio VA, De Amicis V, Di Tommaso L, *et al.* Influence of prosthesis–patient mismatch on exercise-induced arrhythmias: A further aspect after aortic valve replacement. J Thorac Cardiovasc Surg 2009;138:632-638.

[20] Walther T, Rastan A, Falk V, *et al.* Patient prosthesis mismatch affects short-and long-term outcomes after aortic valve replacement. Eur J Cardio-thorac Surg 2006;30:15-19.

[21] Ruel M, Al-Faleh H, Kulik A, *et al.* Prosthesis–patient mismatch after aortic valve replacement predominantly affects patients with preexisting left ventricular dysfunction: Effect on survival, freedom from heart failure, and left ventricular mass regression. J Thorac Cardiovasc Surg 2006;131:1036-1044.

[22] Mohty D, Dumesnil JG, Echahidi N, *et al.* Impact of Prosthesis-Patient Mismatch on Long-Term Survival After Aortic Valve Replacement. Influence of Age, Obesity, and Left Ventricular Dysfunction. J Am Coll Cardiol 2009;53:39-47.

[23] Mistiaen W, Van Cauwelaert Ph, Muylaert Ph, *et al.* Risk factors and survival after aortic valve replacement in octogenarians. J Heart Valve Dis. 2004;13:538-544.

[24] Mistiaen W, Van Cauwelaert Ph, Muylaert Ph, *et al.* Thrombo-embolism after aortic valve replacement in elderly with a Carpentier-Edwards perimount TM bioprosthesis. J Thorac Cardiovasc Surg. 2004;127:1166-1170.

[25] Mistiaen W, Van Cauwelaert Ph, Muylaert Ph, *et al.* Risk factors for congestive heart failure after aortic valve replacement with a Carpentier-Edwards pericardial prosthesis in the elderly. J. Heart Valve Dis 2005;14:774-779.

[26] Vitale N, Clark SC, Ramsden A, *et al.* Clinical and Hemodynamic Evaluation of Small Perimount Aortic Valves in Patients Aged 75 Years or Older. Ann Thorac Surg 2003;75:35-40.

[27] Okamura H, Yamaguchi A, Tanaka M, *et al.* The 17-mm St. Jude Medical Regent Valve Is a Valid Option for Patients With a Small Aortic Annulus. Ann Thorac Surg 2009;87:90-94.

[28] Carrier M, Pellerin M, Perrault LP, *et al.* Experience With the 19-mm Carpentier-Edwards Pericardial Bioprosthesis in the Elderly. Ann Thorac Surg 2001;71:S249-S252.

[29] Medalion B, Lytle BL, McCarthy PM, *et al.* Aortic Valve Replacement for Octogenarians: Are Small Valves Bad? Ann Thorac Surg 1998;66:699-706.

[30] Freed DH, Tam JW, Moon MC, *et al.* Nineteen-Millimeter Prosthetic Aortic Valves Allow Normalization of Left Ventricular Mass in Elderly Women. Ann Thorac Surg 2002;74:2022-2025.

[31] Albes JM, Hartrumpf M, Rudolph V, *et al.* Are Mechanical Valves With Enhanced Inner Diameter Advantageous in the Small Sized Aortic Annulus? Ann Thorac Surg 2003;76:1564-1570.

[32] Ardal H, Toker ME, Rabus MB, *et al.* Does Aortic Root Enlargement Impair the Outcome of Patients With Small Aortic Root? J Card Surg 2006;21:449-453.

[33] Sensky PR, Loubani M, Kal RP, *et al.* Does the type of prosthesis influence early left ventricular mass regression after aortic valve replacement? Assessment with magnetic resonance imaging. Am heart J 2003;146:e13.

[34] de Arenaza DP, Lees B, Flather M, *et al.*, on behalf of the ASSERT [Aortic Stentless *versus* Stented valve assessed by Echocardiography Randomized Trial] Investigators. Randomized Comparison of Stentless *Versus* Stented Valves for Aortic Stenosis. Effects on Left Ventricular Mass. Circulation 2005;112:2696-2702.

[35] Brown J, Shah P, Stanton T, Marwick TH. Interaction and Prognostic Effects of Left Ventricular Diastolic Dysfunction and Patient-Prosthesis Mismatch as Determinants of Outcome After Isolated Aortic Valve Replacement. Am J Cardiol 2009;104:707-712.

[36] Ennker J, Dalladaku F, Rosendahl U, *et al.* The Stentless Freestyle Bioprosthesis: Impact of Age Over 80 Years on Quality of Life, Perioperative, and Mid-Term Outcome. Card Surg 2006;21:379-385.

Send Orders of Reprints at bspsaif@emirates.net.ae

CHAPTER 11

TAVI: Trans-Catheter Aortic Valve Implantation

Abstract: For patients deemed unfit to undergo AVR, BAV has been tried as a less traumatic alternative. Recurrence of stenosis within months has been observed, however. BAV has been abandoned, and alternatives have been explored.

Implantation of a valve through a catheter has proven experimentally feasible and has been performed for the first time in a patient in 2003. The more cumbersome trans-septal technique has been replaced by the trans-arterial technique. This procedure has not always been applicable in patients with atheromatosis of the femoral and iliac arteries or of the aorta. As alternative, a trans-apical approach has been developed. TAVI might also become attractive as "valve-in-valve" procedure, for patients with a degenerated BHV.

The current procedure needs an elaborate imaging system, with a pre-procedural study of the anatomy of the aortic root. Interference with anatomical structures such as the coronary arteries and the conduction system needs to be avoided. Attachment and anchoring systems needs to be adequate, to avoid secondary displacement.

The selection of patients is problematic: the EuroSCORE tends to overestimate operative mortality of conventional AVR, especially in high risk patients. Such patients might be denied this operation unjustly. A RCT, comparing TAVI with medical treatment and with conventional AVR might seem desirable.

The early clinical and hemodynamic results in terms of TVG and AVA seem acceptable but PPVL could be a problem. A recently published RCT, which compared medical treatment or BAV with TAVI, showed superior clinical and hemodynamic results for the latter. PPVL has been considered as acceptable and has not worsened after one year. Vascular complications, bleeding an stroke have been troubling. Technical improvements with smaller delivery systems might offer relief. A second RCT has shown the non inferiority of TAVI, compared to conventional AVR, at least for the first postoperative year. TAVI offers the advantage of being less traumatic, compared to open surgery.

These results make clear that TAVI is here to stay.

Keywords: Balloon aortic valvotomy, bleeding, conventional aortic valve replacement, EuroSCORE, exclusion criteria, imaging, life expectancy, paravalvular leak, percutaneous devices, quality of life, randomized controlled trial, stroke, transapical, transarterial, vascular complications.

Wilhelm Peter Mistiaen

1. HISTORY

Once CAVS has become symptomatic, the prognosis becomes poor. With medical treatment, one and 5-year survival are 60% and 32%. AVR is the only option that prolongs life and improves QoL. The operative mortality is about 4% in the best series. Even today, many patients are not referred for AVR for reasons of high age, clinically important co-morbidity and poor LVF [1]. A recent retrospective analysis of 179 patients with symptomatic CAVS has shown that the two year survival in the surgical group has been significantly higher compared to the medical group (90% *vs.* 69%). The medically treated group, however, has been older and has had a higher EuroSCORE compared to patiens who underwent TAVI or conventional AVR. Reasons for medical treatment have been high operative risk, or symptoms considered mild, or stenosis considered as mild, or patient preference [1].

It should be noted, however, that the EuroSCORE overestimates hospital mortality after AVR considerably. Moreover, a recent series has shown that patients, treated with AVR have become older and sicker, but without increase in postoperative mortality or cardiovascular complication rate [2]. In elderly patient, the symptomatic status might be severly underestimated. Last but not least, with poor LVF, the severity of CAVS might be underestimated, because of a LF-LG conundrum.

Another aspect has been the conviction that ACE inhibitors are contra-indicated in patients with CAVS. There has seemed a risk for profound peripheral vasodilation and hemodynamic collapse. However, a surprisingly large part of the patients with asymptomatic (and often at that time unknown) CAVS took this medication for other reasons. A survival benefit has seemingly been recognized, but this still warrants further study [3].

Use of ACE inhibitors has not changed aortic jet velocity, calculated TVG, blood pressure, heart rate and cardiac output in patients with mild-to-moderate CAVS. ACE inhibitors have been well tolerated in such patients [4]. In patients with asymptomatic CAVS and hypertension, a single blinded study has shown 1) no difference in NYHA class, 2) a lower blood pressure, 3) a higher mean TVG and

4) a higher ventricular SWL, if ACE inhibitors have been used. Other basic clinical and Doppler parameters have not been altered. During exercise, stroke volume has also been higher with ACE inhibitors. The ACE inhibitors have reduced the afterload in CAVS, but this has been blunted by a parallel increase in TVG. Since ACE inhibitors have a positive effect on hemodynamic function during exercise in such patients, this medication should not be discontinued [5].

The first alternative for AVR has been a balloon aortic valvotomy or BAV, which has been introduced in 1985. The application for CAVS has soon been abandoned since its results proved to be only limited and very temporary. The AVA has increased and the severity of symptoms has been reduced, but the stenosis has recurred within months. One and two year survival has been low: 64% resp. 31% [8]. The increase in AVA has been due to the fracture of the calcified nodules in the aortic valve leaflets. Healing of those fractures has been held responsible for the short duration of this improvement. Moreover, hospital morbidity and mortality have been high, mostly due to arrhythmias, conduction defects, stroke and problems related to the vascular access. For these reasons, BAV has been restricted as palliation or as a bridge to AVR in hemodynamical unstable patients or in patients urgently needing non-cardiac surgery [9-16].

TAVI is a procedure, which goes far beyond BAV. Since conventional AVR still can be considered as a gold standard, TAVI probably will remain restricted to patients with severe CAVS, but deemed unfit to undergo open surgery [7]. TAVI might be able to relieve symptoms and increase life expectancy.

The stent has been designed to resist the recoil of the aortic annulus or of the diseased valve itself. Such recoil has been observed after BAV. The stent also supports the valvular leaflets, on which these are sutured. Several devices have been developed, but these all had to overcome several obstacles [7].

One should bear in mind that TAVI is not a valve replacement, but a valve implantation. The original valve is not removed, as in conventional AVR. The calcified and fibrotic tissue remains in place. The distinction between implantation and replacement might be more than semantics, since the presence of the native valve could be held responsible for PPVL, stroke or other complications [10]. Especially in patients with heavy calcification, more PPVL has been observed [11].

2. EXPERIMENTS

In 2001, the first experimental implantation of a valve in a pulmonary position in an animal through a catheter technique has been performed [12, 13]. The device was a jugular vein, sutured in a stent. Echocardiographic, hemodynamic and angiographic control have shown no complications after 4 weeks. The pulmonary position has one advantage over the aortic: the absence for risk of coronary artery occlusion. However, the aortic valve is clinically more relevant, because it is the valve at risk for disease. In subsequent experiments, valves have been implanted in aortic position. It has become obvious that non-surgical implantation of a comparable device is feasible, but with aid of an orientation mechanism, to prevent obstruction of coronary arteries. Migration and major PPVL have been other problems observed [12].

A porcine valve, sutured in a self expandable nitinol stent has been tested *in vitro* in advance, to detect problems as regurgitation or stenosis. This device has also been experimentally placed in the supra-coronary position. Hemodynamic results have been favorable with low TVG, absent to mild regurgitation or PPVL [13]. Another experiment has been performed, without cardiac arrest and under guidance of TEE. Although the device has been considered as safe, failure has been observed in 2 of 6 cases. There has been no malfunction of the implant, damage to the aortic wall or coronary artery obstruction [14].

In 2005 another approach has experimentally been tested. With use of an ultrasound guidance, an off-pump transapical route has been used in pigs. This approach allows a more direct response to unexpected movements of the device. If necessary, correction can be performed. The distance to the valve is short. Mal-position with occlusion of the coronary arteries and dislodgement due to size mismatch and incorrect unfolding have been observed in 6 of 17 animals. In the remaining 11 subjects, a satisfactory valve function for several hours has been shown. These observations have made the technique potentially applicable in patients, provided the procedural obstacles can be overcome [15]. In a comparable experiment, in 8 of 24 pigs, valve migration has been observed due to several reasons and PPVL has been noticed in 14 of the 18 valves *in situ*. The antegrade approach has been considered less cumbersome and the deliver system was smaller. PPVL has remained a serious problem, however [16]. The technique has proven its feasibility [17, 18].

Experimental efforts have also been undertaken to develop a re-positionable valve/stent. The implantation in pigs has been successful but thrombus formation inside the "umbrella" valve has proven to be a problem [19].

A "valve-in-valve" technique through a trans-apical approach could also be considered as a possible advancement in the treatment of degenerated BHV, thereby avoiding a risky reoperation. A valve deployment has been successful in pigs who previously had undergone AVR or MVR using a conventional CE porcine valve. The radio-opaque stent of the first valve has been helpful in the optimal positioning of the expandable stent. There has been no migration, PPVL or obstruction of the coronary arteries which makes the "valve-in-valve" concept potentially useful in patients. *In vitro* experiments has also shown the feasibility of the technique in stenotic BHV [9, 20].

3. FIRST HUMAN CASES AND PATIENT SERIES

3.1 Antegrade Trans-Septal and Trans-Arterial Approach

The first human case with TAVI has been described in 2003 [21, 22]. Three bovine pericardial leaflets have been mounted within a balloon expandable stent. A 57 year old patient with CAVS, cardiogenic shock and multiple co-morbidities has been deemed unfit to undergo conventional AVR. The device has successfully been implanted through a trans-septal approach at the site of the native valve. An immediate hemodynamic improvement has been observed. For months, the valve has functioned satisfactory, as could be documented on TEE. Heart failure has not recured. The patient has died after 17 weeks due to non-cardiac complications.

Small patient series for TAVI treatment have been described in the following years. Immediate post-procedural reduction in mean TVG and improvement of global and regional LVF have been be documented by Doppler. The device was made of 3 leaflets of equine pericardium, mounted in a stent of stainless steel. TTE and TEE have documented proper valve function, but some PPVL has been present. In most cases, displacement has been absent, but early migration with subsequent death has occurred in some patients [23-25].

TAVI has become a valuable alternative for balloon valvotomy [26, 27]. However, conventional AVR has been and still is an established and highly successful procedure, with a low mortality rate. Conventional AVR could serve as gold standard [26]. For proper comparison, clinical end points must be the same as for conventional AVR. However, patients referred for TAVI are usually older and sicker and are denied conventional AVR [28], which makes comparisons difficult.

The first larger series of 36 patients with mid-term follow-up (up to 26 months in a phase I trial) has shown a successful implantation in 27 patients. In most cases, the antegrade trans-septal route has been preferred, since it had a higher success rate. The retrograde procedure, however, has been easier and quicker. Diseased and tortuous femoral arteries, however, could not always accommodate the large sheath. Prior to deployment, the diseased valve has been dilated, with rapid pacing during expansion of the device. This rapid pacing has resulted in an immediate and predictable decrease in stroke volume. This has been tolerated well and is necessary to prevent the left ventricle ejecting the balloon catheter carrying the device. AVA and TVG have improved significantly after implantation. Postprocedural PPVL has been mild to absent in most patients and LVF has improved in one week. This improvement has been most obvious in patients with an LVEF < 50%. In about one quarter of the patients, major adverse events have occurred within 30 days. Patients still alive have experienced a relief of symptoms with unchanged function of the implant as mid-term [29].

Comparable observations have been made in another series of 25 patients who underwent TAVI with a self expanding device. The approach has been retrograde, under general anesthesia and with aid of ECC. Procedural success has been achieved in 21 of 25 patients. The TVG has reduced markedly but major adverse events have occurred in 8 patients, with 5 fatalities [30].

These two series have indicated that TAVI is feasible for patients, who have been considered unfit for conventional AVR. The technical problems to solve for TAVI, soon after its introduction have been [7, 13, 22]:

1) Attachment of the valve into the stent.

2) The vascular access: the valve stents are larger than most other percutaneous stents and devices.

    a. Stents are in the order of 22-24 Fr and require – if a retrograde approach is used – access through femoral, iliacal or axillary arteries. This usually implies surgical exploration.

    b. Although percutaneous venous access is possible for the antegrade trans-septal approach, vascular injury is still possible due to the large size of the device.

    c. Alternatives are minimal invasive surgery for a trans-apical approach or a thoracoscopic access through the descending thoracic aorta.

3) The device could interfere with cardiac structures. Two dimensional echocardiography provides limited control, guidance and adjustments of the device. There are several anatomical structures to be safeguarded.

    d. There is a danger of obstructing the coronary arteries, although by pushing aside the native leaflets, a space is created between the wall of the stent and the sinus of Valsalva. Calcium fragments can embolize into the coronary vessels and carotid arteries.

    e. The motility of the anterior mitral leaflet can be hampered if the device is placed low in the LVOT.

    f. The conduction system can be affected by impingement, when the device is placed too low. This could cause a complete AV block.

Therefore, devices that can be retrieved and repositioned during the procedure have been developed.

4) The device must be fixed within the aortic annulus. Placement can be obtained by rapid ventricular pacing, which interrupts shortly cardiac output. Extracorporeal support through femoral vessels has been used in the first periods in order to unload the left ventricle.

5) This fixing has to be able to prevent future dislodging and embolization of the device.

6) The space created between the opening of the coronary arteries and stent by the native calcified valve carries a risk for PPVL. The devices have a round profile, which fits not necessarily to the irregular residual calcium. The latter is completely excised during open AVR

7) Durability of the material, provided the patients live long enough.

3.2. Trans-Apical Approach

The trans-apical approach has been performed in patients with extensive atheromatosis in the femoral and aortic region, and who have been considered unfit for AVR. Through a mini-thoracotomy and LV apical puncture, TAVI has been tried in a small series of patients [31].

The implantation has been successful, with an acceptable 30-day mortality. Marked reduction of mean TVG and increase in AVA has been documented after 6 months. No major PPVL has been observed. This technique has obviated the need for ECC [32]. Migration of the devices has been observed in some patients, however [33].

The clinical and hemodynamic outcomes of both procedures have been comparable [34], but some differences have also been documented. In some series, a higher 30 day mortality has been observed in the trans-apical group (27% *vs.* 8%). Co-morbidity as well as unexpected complications such as hematoma of the septum, and delayed rupture of the apex could account for this result [35, 36]. Major bleeding and tearing of the apex might be prevented by using a temporary pacing Swan-Ganz catheter and sutures with large pledgets for an apical purse-string and tension free removal of the sheath [37].

Stroke seems to be less after the trans-apical approach [38, 39]. One explanation could be that fewer procedure-related lesions in the aortic arch have been found with the trans-apical approach [40]. The trans-femoral approach could be the first choice, when no contra-indications were present [38-41]. Both techniques have certain site specific complications, which require specialized management.

Another alternative is the trans-axillary approach. This can be used in patients with severe atheromatosis and with COPD. The former condition makes the transfemoral technique impossible, the latter makes a thoracotomy hazardous. The results seemed acceptable [42, 43]. The experience is limited and the complication rate yet unknown. Hence, this approach is not (yet) recommendable as general practice [18].

3.3. The Valve-in-Valve Procedure

The valve-in-valve procedure, which has been shown to be feasible in experiments has also been applied in patients, in whom a previously implanted BHV has degenerated. In those patients, a reoperation could be considered hazardous, especially if co-morbidity can be documented. The first case reports have pointed to favorable results in patients with regurgitating stentless BHV [44-46].

In a small series of 11 high risk patients, the valve-in-valve technique has been performed off-pump through a trans-apical approach with the Edwards Sapien device. PPVL has not been observed, the mean TVG has been 11 mm Hg and patients have been well after a mean follow up of 330 days [47].

With a Core-Valve system, a similar successful outcome has also been reported. Mortality has been be related to a learning effect. Currently, the valve-in-valve procedure seems to offer reproducible results [48]. Technical improvements are still ongoing. New delivery systems are being tested and the success deploy rate and 30-day mortality rates seem favorable [49].

4. EXISTING DEVICES

Two systems have been developed before 2005: 1) the balloon expandable Cribier-Edwards (equine) which became later the Edwards Sapien (bovine) aortic valve prosthesis and 2) the self expandable CoreValve Revalving system. The latter has a nitinol cage which supports valve leaflets of porcine origin, which replaces the initially used bovine material [6, 18, 50]. These systems demonstrated the abovementioned problems [7].

4.1. The Edwards-Sapien

This device consists of three pericardial leaflets. Bovine leaflets has replaced the material from equine origin. These leaflets are mounted in a tubular slotted balloon-expandable stent made from stainless steel. The manufacturers have made a limited number of sizes available: 23 and 26 mm sizes for trans-femoral approach for 22F and 24F sheaths and 26F for trans-apical approach [6, 9]. In 2010, the 29 size also has become available in Europe.

The original **antegrade trans-venous approach** has for the first time been performed in 2002 [50]. This approach has been replaced by the trans-apical and trans-arterial route because of its technical complexity. The main advantage is the distensibility of the veins. Moreover, the procedure can be performed in patients with severe PAD. The procedure has been difficult, but has had a success rate of 75% in terms of TVG reduction and increase in AVA [6, 51].

The **trans-arterial approach** has followed suit in 2004 [50]. In an attempt to reduce PPVL, valves have been oversized. After the introduction of the 23 mm size, two more valve sizes, 26 and 29 mm have became available. Elongation of the skirt also has been tried. Sizing can be estimated using the transverse diameter of the aortic annulus at the level of the aortic leaflet insertion. Dislodging of the device has been reduced by recognizing the necessary landmarks. Non-traumatic passage of the aortic arch has been made possible using manually activated deflectable tips of the catheter. The delivery of the device has been facilitated by central positioning the guide-wire through the aortic commissures. The device for this system is not retrievable [50]. With increasing experience, procedural success rate and outcome have improved. Mortality has been considerably affected by vascular complications. These observations have demonstrated the need for proper patient selection. Improvement of long-term function has been attempted by implementing a treatment to prevent calcification. A first RCT, called PARTNER, has been published in 2010 [52].

The **trans-apical approach** has been the most recently developed approach [33]. This technique has been used in patients with severe PAD, in whom the trans-femoral approach cannot be performed [50]. Through a small left lateral thoracotomy, the apex can be visualized and the left ventricle can be punctured. Through a sheath, a guide wire can be introduced. The subsequent steps, under rapid pacing for deployment are comparable. The device can be positioned under guidance of TEE and fluoroscopy. The valve function can be tested by TEE and angiography. The clinical outcome and hemodynamic improvement in the first cases have seemed acceptable. There has been less stroke, since the aorta has been less manipulated [50]. An important explanation for the difference in outcome compared to the trans-arterial approach has been the patient selection, notably the presence of PAD [6].

4.2. The Core Valve Revalving System

This system is a porcine pericardial BHV, which has been designed for the aortic position and is only available for trans-arterial approach. The device is mounted on a self-expandable nitinol frame, which extends from the aortic root into the LVOT. The valve is sized according to the aortic root and placed in a supra-annular position. The device does not interfere with the coronary circulation. The system has the advantage of being self centering and being partly repositionable [6, 18, 50].

The device can be deployed by withdrawal of the delivery sheath. With the body temperature, the nitinol stent expands automatically into the aortic valve. Prior folding of the device into a capsule on a catheter occurs in cold water at freezing temperature. The lower portion is implanted in the annulus, the middle portion carries the valve and the upper portion fixes the valve within the ascending aorta.

- The lower portion exerts a radial force, thereby reducing PPVL, preventing recoil from the native valve and providing fixation.

- The middle portion carries the porcine pericardial BHV. The design prevents obstruction of the coronary arteries.

- The upper portion aligns the frame into the ascending aorta and provides a stable fixation [18].

PPVL can further be reduced by a second short balloon inflation [50]. The manufacturers have made a limited number of sizes available: 26 and 29 mm for 18F sheats through the trans-femoral approach [6, 9].

A reduction of the delivering sheath from 24F to 21F and even to 18F has made the conversion from a procedure with anesthesia to a fully percutaneous one possible. Need for support by ECC has been abolished and hence also thrombocytopenia and bleeding events. Deployment success has been as high as 88% and absence of major cardiac events has been 68%. Hemodynamic results has shown marked decrease in TVG, while severe PPVL has not been observed.

Hospital mortality has been 6.4%, which is comparable to that for conventional AVR. Conversion to conventional AVR has sometimes been necessary. A valve-in-valve procedure for severe regurgitation also has served as a salvage procedue. In 2007, the procedural success of 97% and a procedural mortality of 1.5% has been achieved. Hemodynamic improvements have lasted during the observation time and serious problems such as stroke, tamponade and major PPVL have been rare. PPMI has been necessary in 9.3% of the patients [6, 51-53].

Newer generations trans-catheter devices are being tested and might become available. Innovations are being designed to improve the freedom of repositioning and decrease PPVL. Arteriotomies might become smaller [6].

5. CURRENT SUPPORTING SYSTEMS FOR TAVI

For the femoral approach, sedation and local anesthesia can be sufficient. Support by ECC should be in "stand by" in case of complications. The aortic valve is crossed and dilated by a balloon. This is also a "rehearsal" for TAVI. The balloon is stabilized by a short interruption of cardiac output. This can be achieved by rapid pacing. Between two periods of rapid pacing, blood pressure must recover completely.

Periprocedural imaging is necessary and should include [9]:

- Fluoroscopy, especially in cases with severe calcification. It shows the correct level for implantation.

- Aortography, with different views at the start and if necessary when the device is in place but still undeployed; it shows the position of the valve and the plane of alignment.

- TEE, especially in patients with moderate calcification; for guidance and positioning of the device and detection of complications.

- 3D real time TEE: experience for this imaging technique needs to be acquired before it can be used.

- Real time MRI in an experimental setting provides excellent visualization during the procedure and the guidance: it identifies the critical anatomical landmarks. Moreover, it can provide information about tissue perfusion and ventricular contractility [54]. Standard use of 3D TEE has also been proposed during trans-apical approach [55].

When the correct position has been reached, the device can be released. Imaging modalities must be able to diagnose complications [9].

6. PATIENT SELECTION

TAVI is indicated in patients with aortic stenosis, due to CAVS. Patients with pure aortic regurgitation are no good candidates. Prior cardiac surgery is not a contra-indication for TAVI, since good clinical and hemodynamic results can be obtained in these patients through the trans-apical approach [56]. Degenerated BHV are also possible indications for TAVI (the so called valve-in-valve procedure) if surgical re-intervention carry a high risk. A proper patient selection requires several steps [9].

1) Establishing the severity of CAVS, especially in presence of the LFLG conundrum.

2) Exclusion of rheumatic valve disease and of aortic valve regurgitation due to annular dilatation [1].

3) Evaluation of symptoms, and establishing their valvular origin.

4) Risk analysis in relation to a life expectancy. Clinical judgment should also include:

   a. Previous chest irradiation or burns, which makes AVR less attractive as an option.

   b. Previous CABG with patent grafts.

   c. Porcelain aorta, [1, 4, 47].

   d. Recent events such as AMI or CVA or uncontrolled AF.

   e. Symptomatic stenosis of the carotid/vertebral artery.

   f. Bleeding diathesis.

5) Assessment of feasibility of TAVI which include:

   g. Evaluation of coronary anatomy, the relation of ostia to the valvular cusps and estimation of CAD and its treatment options.

   h. Evaluation of the size and the shape of the LVOT by TTE, TTE or MDCT: the STJ should be smaller than 45 mm and the aortic annulus should be between 18 and 25 mm.

   i. Locating calcific deposits (preferably no asymmetric calcifications) and visualizing the aortic orifice area [6, 57, 58].

6) Exclusion of bicuspid valves: the valvular orifice is elliptical in these patients; this could lead to PPVL or mal-deployment [59].

7) Exclusion of contra-indications for trans-arterial approach: severe PAD, small arteries, any aortic disease and previous surgery on the aorta [50, 60].

8) For the trans-apical approach exclusion criteria are:

   a. Calcification of the pericardium.

   b. Previous surgery performed on the LV with a patch.

   c. Severe COPD and

   d. Non approachable LV apex.

Patient selection includes risk assessment and involves a multidisciplinary approach by cardiologists, surgeons, imaging specialists, anesthesiologists, etc… [9, 61].

The EuroSCORE overestimates mortality by up to almost 18%. Therefore, this instrument is not a first choice in the selection of an individual patient for TAVI [62]. Comparable findings have been made in other large groups of patients referred for AVR [6, 50, 63-65]. The STS-PROM has proven to be a more useful method to predict overall mortality, at least for high risk patients [6, 60]. Nevertheless, the availability of TAVI has increased the number of patients, to whom one or another intervention could be offered [66].

Life expectancy and QoL depend also in a large degree on the presence of co-morbid conditions. A shift in surgical practice has been observed: in the last decades, increasingly more patients with one or several co-morbidities have been referred for AVR, without an concomitant increase in postoperative cardiac complications or hospital mortality. The number of non-fatal and non-cardiac complications have increased considerably, however. This observation could question the use of the EuroSCORE as instrument for patient selection further [67].

Use "off label" can be defined as the presence of at least one exclusion criterion. In one study "off label" use of TAVI has proved to be common, with up to 3 exclusion criteria. Procedural success rate and hemodynamic outcome has not seemed to be significantly worse. Nevertheless, further evaluation of the consequences of "off label" use is mandatory [68].

It remains to be seen if patients, who are possible candidates for conventional AVR are good candidates for TAVI. Patients younger than 70 years or with a life expectancy of less than 1 year are likely no good candidates for TAVI [9].

7. RESULTS

7.1 Hospital Complications in Early Series

- Thirty-day mortality has ranged between 2.6 and 18%. This has been higher in some trans-apical series [9, 51, 69, 70] in spite of a procedural success of 99% [18].

- Rupture of the aortic annulus, has occured during over-sizing in some elderly and frail patients [18].

- Type A aortic dissection has been observed in the same type of patients [18].

- Ventricular perforation and cardiac tamponnade has occurred in 2-10% [65], perforation of the aorta in 0-4%, especially with the node-coned Sapien device [18, 70]

- Major ventricular tachy-arrhythmia has been observed in 0-4% [70].

- AMI, with or without coronary occlusion, has occured between 0 and 15% of the patients [9, 70].

- PPVL has been documented in 50%, but usually in a mild to moderate degree. No increase has been observed in the first year after implantation [71]. The occurrence of massive PPVL has been reduced by an improved size-matching technique.

- Hemolysis, CHF and PVE have been associated to postprocedural PPVL [72].

- Displacement of the device has occurred in less than 1% of the patients.

- Vascular complication rate has been 8 to 17% [9, 70] and has contributed considerably to the morbidity and mortality.

- Stroke has ranged between 3 and 10% [9, 70] and has been more common in the trans-femoral approach; silent cerebral emboli on MRI have even been more common: over 70%-80% in several studies [73, 74].

- Complete AV block with need for PPMI has been documented in 4 to 20%, [18, 39, 75], for LBBB this has been in over 45% of the patients. In some series, transient CD has been observed, without increased need for PPMI. This could be attributed to a lower valve positioning and greater over-sizing [76]. Predictors for PPMI have been pre-existing CD, narrow LVOT and severe mitral annulus calcification [77, 78].

- A need for conversion to open surgery has been observed in 0-8% of the patients [70].

- Need for re-intervention (*i.e.* any surgical and percutaneous procedure that repairs, adjust, replaces or adjusts in any sense the implanted valve prosthesis), has been observed in 30-35 % of the patients who underwent TAVI [71].

- Acute renal injury has occured in 11.7% of the patients and has been associated with increased mortality. Three predictors of this complication have been identified: AHT, COPD and the need for blood transfusion [79]. Use of large doses of contrast could also have been responsible [50].

Improvement of the results have been obtained by [9]:

- Experience as individuals and as team, preceded by proper training, simulations, animal laboratories, hands-on training. The 30 day mortality has been 33% in the first 15 patients, and dropped to 12.5% thereafter [80].

- Cooperation between specialists in multidisciplinary teams with cross-fertilization of expertise, including echocardiographists, interventional cardiologists, surgeons with expertise in handling complex valvular pathology and in vascular access repair, anesthesiologists with expertise in cardiology. This also applied for the postoperative care.

- Equipment: spacious and sterile environment, high quality imaging devices [81], facility to perform immediate rescue surgery.

- Proper patient selection.

Both approaches, femoral and apical, have shown comparable complication rates. In the apical approach, more concomitant PAD has been present. Conversion to conventional AVR has been low. There have been, up to 2008, no comparative studies available.

Before TAVI can be compared to AVR, some more technical developments have to be realized [9, 18]. These developments include:

- Lower profile of the device, if possible 16 and even 14 F.

- Possibility to reposition the device.

- Steerable delivery catheters.

- Retrievable and reloadable devices and delivery systems.

- More durable valves.

- 3D imaging & stereotaxis modalities.

7.2. Mid-Term Results in Early Series

Mortality at 3 or at 6 months have ranged from 10 to 25% after the trans-femoral approach and from 26 to 43% after the trans-apical approach [51]. In a larger multicentre study of 345 trans-femoral and trans-apical procedures in 339 patients, a procedural success of 93.3% has been observed. Thirty-day mortality has been 10.4% and mortality after a median follow-up of 8 months has been 22.1%. The survival at 1 month, 6 months and 1 year have been 92, 74 and 71% in another series. These results can be compared to the trans-femoral approach [34].

The predictors of long-term mortality have been:

- A peri-procedural sepsis.
- A need for hemodynamic support during the procedure.
- Presence of PAHT.
- Presence of chronic renal disease.
- Presence of COPD.
- Experience of the operator [41].

Frailty or a porcelain aorta has not affected the outcome [82, 83].

Results can be considered adequate if AVA has reached a value between 1.5 and 1.8 cm². Long-term studies have still been limited in 2008. A two year survival of 70 to 80% has been reached, with improvement in clinical status. Mortality has mostly been due to co-morbidity. Prosthetic valve function on echo has remained consistently well, without occurrence of SVD.

As for January, 2008 [9], over 1000 patients with high risk and symptomatic severe CAVS have received a TAVI. Most patients have been over 80 years and have had a logistic EuroSCORE of over 20.

In spite of a considerable postprocedural improvement in hemodynamic parameters and without worsening of PPVL after one year, TAVI has a potential for serious complications. The results of this procedure must be evaluated in RCT, which has become only recently available.

7.2.1. Comparative Studies & RCT

The specific selection of patients influences outcome of TAVI in a major degree. The results of the procedure are difficult to compare with those of conventional AVR. The currently available scoring systems might be inappropriate, since these overestimate the risk. For this moment, the proof of concept for TAVI has been delivered, the applied techniques are feasible and the clinical and hemodynamic outcome after 2 years shows improvement [9].

A rigorous RCT, such as the PARTNER trial, is the only way to compare the safety and efficacy with other treatment models. Conventional AVR could be considered as "gold standard" in this respect, with predicable low mortality and morbidity [56]. However, this makes comparison of TAVI with AVR (which is still the best available treatment) difficult to defend in an ethical way: on the one hand, patients with a favorable risk profile should not be denied AVR. On the other hand, patients should not be subjected to AVR when this operation is considered as being to hazardous.

Another way is to compare TAVI with medical treatment or with the natural development of CAVS. These data can only be derived from historical series and are not fully known. Nevertheless, it is clear that AVR improves the survival of patients with symptomatic CAVS drastically [84].

In any case, the pre-procedural patient data must be described as completely as possible. The effects of CAD, if present, must also be taken into account since this condition can have an adverse effect on immediate and long-term outcome. An equal distribution of CAD in both arms of a trial would be advisable [85].

Even for TAVI, the pre-procedural mortality plays an important role: one of the most important reason for "no intervention" was death while being on the waiting list [86]. Timely intervention, either TAVI or conventional AVR is of critical importance!

The outcome in such trails should also be defined in a clear and standardized way, as for conventional AVR, and should include the same parameters as for conventional AVR. These are:

1) The classical adverse events (valve related, other cardiac and non-cardiac) as well as reinterventions (such as a "valve-in-valve procedure).

2) QoL, and a possibility to have an independent life outside any institution.

3) Hemodynamic parameters: AVA, trans-prosthetic TVG, PPVL.

4) The effect on the LVEF and LVM.

The long-term durability is still an open question, but series with a 2 year follow-up seems to show satisfactory results [23].

A provisional comparison between TAVI and conventional AVR with stented and stentless BHV has revealed that the TVG after 6 months has been lower in the TAVI group (10 *vs.* 13 and 14 mm Hg), but mild regurgitation has occurred more often (42% *vs.* 10 and 12%). For moderate regurgitation, this has been 8% *vs.* 0%.

Severe VPPM also has been lower in the TAVI than in the surgical group (6% *vs.* 28 and 20%). It seems that TAVI offers superior hemodynamics in terms of TVG and prevention of VPPM, but not in regurgitation. Over-sizing of the device with 2 to 3 mm is a common practice and could explain these results. The radial force are helpful in to achieve a stable position after implantation.

The clinical relevance of these hemodynamic differences is still unclear. After one year, TVG after TAVI has been comparable to a TVG after implantation of stentless valve. Probably, with sufficient hemodynamic improvement, regression of LVH can be anticipated. The hemodynamical results after TAVI might even exceed these after conventional AVR [72].

Trans-apical TAVI and minimally invasive AVR through upper sternotomy have been compared in a small patient series. In a non randomized way, high risk patients with mean EuroSCORE 35 or more, have received one of both treatment modalities. Early morbidity and mortality have been comparable, but operative time, ventilation time, stay in ICU and hospital have been in favor of TAVI [70, 87].

When comparing TAVI with more standard techniques, the approach needs to be taken into account. In the Sapien Aortic Bioprosthesis European Outcome (SOURCE) study, the trans-femoral appraoch, which has received approval in the EU in 2007, has been compared with the trans-apical approach, which has received approval in 2008.

Patients treated with the trans-apical approach have shown significantly more preprocedural co-morbidity (EuroSCORE 29.1% *vs.* 25.7%). The 30 day mortality has been low in either group: 10% in the trans-apical group, and 6% in the trans-femoral group. Both approaches can be considered as successful, with low complication rates [88]. But with the differences in EuroSCORE, these results have to be interpreted with caution.

From these results, it has become clear that, whenever it would become ethically acceptable to compare TAVI with conventional AVR in an RCT, patient populations have to be subdivided:

- For the TAVI arm:
    - Trans-femoral approach *vs.* trans-apical approach to account for the difference in co-morbidity.
- For the AVR arm:
    - Stentless *vs.* stented valves to account for the hemodynamic effects, especially in patients with poor LVF, in whom VPPM has adverse effects.
    - Minimally invasive *versus* full sternotomy approach.

7.2.2. The First RCT: BAV versus TAVI

A major RCT in which TAVI and BAV are compared has been published in 2010 (PARTNER B). In both groups, 179 patients have been included. Characteristics of both groups have been comparable in most aspects. In the medical treatment/BAV group, logistic EuroSCORE has been higher, but extensive calcification of the aorta has been less present. Clinical outcomes have been mortality for all causes and for cardiac causes at different times: peri-procedural, 30 day and at 1 year after the procedure. Major stroke, vascular problems, repeat hospitalization and bleeding events have been the other outcomes. The population also has been divided into subgroups, according to 10 criteria. As a whole and for each of the 10 subgroups, TAVI has scored better than BAV. One-year composite outcome (death from any cause and repeat hospitalization) has been far better for TAVI than for BAV or medical treatment: 71.6% *vs.* 42.5%.

Six conclusions can be drawn from the study [52].

1) BAV has not altered the natural history of CAVS.

2) The results after TAVI have been superior to those after BAV, with a marked reduction of death from any cause, from cardiovascular origin and of repeat hospitalization.

3) 30 day mortality after TAVI has not differed significantly compared to BAV, even if early generation systems and effects of the learning curve were included.

4) NYHA classification and 6 minutes walk test have shown superior results after TAVI.

5) Strokes, major vascular complications and bleeding (at 30 day as well after 1 year) have occurred more after TAVI; bleeding and vascular complications can be attributed to the large femoral access sheaths. These complications might be reduced with the development of a lower profile valve and a supporting frame. Strokes after TAVI are still "troublesome" and are the result of atherothrombotic emboli. Smaller devices and improved protection of the cerebral circulation might be helpful herein.

6) Echocardiography has shown excellent hemodynamic performance ofter TAVI, without evidence of deterioration after 1 year. PPVL has frequently been observed, but this usually has been mild and has not worsened within the first year. Treatment for worsening symptoms rarely has been required.

Some issues still need to be addressed:

1) What is the effect of the learning curve and of the operator experience [80].

2) What is the effect of the introduction of newer and smaller systems on the adverse effects such as stroke, vascular complications and bleeding.

3) How can the need for conversion to conventional AVR be reduced.

4) What is the long-term outcome of TAVI after two years (the current results are limited to a follow-up of 2 to 3 years with an overall survival at 36 months of almost 70% [80]).

5) What is the proper definition of a number of terms such as non-structural valve dysfunction, re-intervention, "repositionable", "retrievable" [66].

6) The viability of the trans-apical approach needs also exploration, especially in patients with severe PAD.

7) If the use of TAVI will be expanded to patients who are deemed fit to undergo conventional AVR, this has to be preceded by an RCT, comparing those two procedures.

8) What is the long-term durability of the valve implanted through TAVI [61]. Hemodynamic parameters such as AVA and TVG seem stable, but this observation is limited to 36 months [80].

9) What is the long-term effect of PPVL on work load of LV or energy loss [89].

10) What is the long-term effect of TAVI on QoL [18].

In spite of the study limitations, one can safely state that the introduction of TAVI has been major advance in the treatment of CAVS in patients who are deemed unfit for conventional AVR. The procedure widens the armamentarium of treatment for a very specific group of patients with symptomatic CAVS [17, 52]. One can expect that the use of TAVI in patients with CAVS will increase in the future [90]. TAVI, however, should not replace a well established treatment such as conventional AVR in a broad group of patients [18].

There are some more issues to resolve:

- Is it ethical to "soften" the indication of TAVI towards high risk patients who still might be candidate for conventional AVR [61].

- Results "less than perfect", which have unacceptable for conventional AVR some years ago, have nowadays become acceptable for patients considered a risk too high to operate [60]. In this respect one can say that cardiac surgeons have been instructed to judge PPVL as a complication of surgery, while for TAVI, PPVL is considered as acceptable collateral damage, intrinsic to the procedure itself. What the long-term effects will be has still to be awaited [72].

7.2.3. The Second RCT: BAV versus Conventional AVR

In 2011, a second RCT has been published (the so-called PARTNER A trial), in which TAVI has been compared to conventional AVR in 699 patients with severe symptomatic CAVS [91]. The EuroSCORE had to be at least 15 (or an STS score of at least 10). The inclusion criteria has been the same as for the first trial [52]. The patients had a high age. For TAVI, transapical as well as transfemoral approach were treatment options.

Results (mortality, stroke, bleeding, vascular complications and atrial fibrillation) after 30 day and one year have been studied. The end point was non-inferiority for one-year mortality after TAVI and conventional AVR.

- Thirty-day mortality has shown a trend in favour for TAVI compared to surgical AVR (3.4% *vs.* 6.5%, p=0.07).

- Thirty-day major stroke in the TAVI group has been 3.8% and in the surgical group 2.1% (p=0.20).

- Major vascular complications have been significantly more frequent after TAVI (11.0% *vs.* 3.2%, p<0.001).

- Major bleeding (9.5% *vs.* 19.5%) and new onset atrial fibrillation (8.6% *vs.* 16.0%, p=0.006) have been significantly more frequent after surgical AVR.

The one-year mortality in the TAVI group has been 24.2%. For surgical AVR, this has been 26.8% (p=0.44), which demonstrates the non-inferiority of TAVI. Stroke after one year has shown a trend in favour for surgical AVR (5.1% *vs.* 2.4%, p=0.07). The symptomatic status has been comparable for both groups.

The PARTNER B trial has shown a significant decrease in mortality at 1 and 2 years after TAVI, compared to medical treatment/BAV. The PARTNER A trial has shown only a divergence in mortality curve between 0 and 6 months, in favour of TAVI. A convergence has been reached before 6 months. At 1 and 2 years, the mortality curves in the PATRNER B trial have shown no real difference. To summarize, TAVI is superior to medical treatment or BAV and is not inferior to surgical AVR.

The results after 30 days have indicated that the procedural trauma is less after TAVI, compared to surgery. Moreover, TAVI offers a viable alternative for conventional AVR at mid-term, but the increased risk for a major stroke after TAVI must be balanced carefully against the benefits.

This trial demonstrates that not all inoperable patients are automatically candidates for TAVI. Exclusion criteria have been a limited life expectancy (less than one year), poor left ventricular function and severly impaired renal function. The trial also demonstrates the need for an appropriate patient selection and for a multidisciplinary cardiac team. Accurate multi-modal imaging remains also mandatory. The question remains, however, if it is unethical to withhold AVR with its known long-term results of favour of TAVI, for which only short to mid-term results exist. AVR seems an option, even in elderly patients with multiple co-morbid conditions [2].

CONCLUSIONS

Implantation of an aortic valve through a catheter has proven to be feasible in animal experiments. This has been confirmed by the first patient cases. The initial trans-venous trans-septal approach has been replaced by the retrograde trans-femoral approach. The feasibility of the technique depends on the anatomy of the aortic root: the size of the annulus, the LVOT and the STJ. Presence of a pure regurgitation and of a bicuspid aortic valve are exclusion criteria.

Contra-indications are small arteries and atheromatosis of aortic and iliofemoral vessels. Vascular surgery and other aortic diseases are also contra-indications. Complications, such as stroke have been observed. As alternative, the trans-apical approach has been developed for these patients. Complications such as tears of the ventricular apex have been observed.

Currently, major obstacles are complications caused by interference with the coronary arteries and the conduction system. Adequate real-time imaging techniques are required for correct positioning and deployment of the device. Migration of the device should be prevented by anchoring.

A major problem is the patient selection for TAVI. This technique should be applied in patients who are deemed unfit for a conventional AVR. The EuroSCORE overestimates the operative risk, especially in high risk patients. This score should be used with great caution. TAVI can be used as a valve-in-valve procedure for high risk patients with a degenerated BHV.

The first series have shown favourable hemodynamic results: an increase in AVA and a decrease of TGV. Currently, PPVL seems limited and is not increasing with time. Procedural mortality, complication rate and mid-term outcome seem acceptable in these patient groups with high risk.

The first RCT (PARTNER B) has compared TAVI with BAV and medical treatment. The clinical and hemodynamic superiority of TAVI over BAV is considerable. Stroke, bleeding and vascular complications after TAVI are frequent and can be related to the large delivery systems.

The PARTNER A trial has compared TAVI with AVR. A non-inferiority of TAVI after one year has been demonstrated. This does not mean that indications for this procedure should be expanded. Moreover, PPVL, which is considered as a technical failure in conventional AVR seems to be accepted as collateral damage in TAVI. The long-term effects of PPVL still need investigation. Conventional AVR is still a valid solution for elderly patients, even if they have multiple co-morbid conditions.

ACKNOWLEDGEMENT

Declared none.

CONFLICT OF INTEREST

The author(s) confirm that this chapter content has no conflict of interest.

REFERENCES

[1] Van Geldorp MWA, van Gameren M, Kappetein AP, *et al.* Therapeutic decisions for patients withsymptomatic severe aortic stenosis: room for improvement? Eur J Cardiothorac Surg 2009;35:953-959.

[2] Mistiaen W, Van Cauwelaert P, Muylaert P, De Worm E. 1000 Carpentier-Edwards pericardial valves in aortic position: what changed in the last 20 years and what are the effects on hospital complications. J Heart Valve Dis 2007;16:417-422.

[3] Newby DE, Cowell SJ, Boon NA. Emerging medical treatments for aortic stenosis: statins, angiotensin converting enzyme inhibitors or both? Heart 2006;92:729-734.

[4] O'Brien KD, Zhao XQ, Shavelle DM, *et al.* Hemodynamic effects of the angiotensin-converting enzyme inhibitor ramipril in patients with mild to moderate aortic stenosis and presereved left ventricular function. J Invest Med 2004;52:185-191.

[5] Jimenez-Candil J, Bermejo J, Yotti R, *et al.* Effects of angiotensin converting enzyme inhibitors in hypertensive patients with aortic valve stenosis: a drug withdrawal study. Heart 2005;91:1311-1318.

[6] Zajarias A, Cribier AG. Outcomes and Safety of Percutaneous Aortic Valve Replacement. J Am Coll Cardiol 2009;53:1829-36.

[7] Davidson MJ, White JK, Baim DS. Review. Percutaneous therapies for valvular heart disease. Cardiovas Pathol 2006;15:123-129.

[8] To ACY, Zeng I, Coverdale HA. Balloon aortic valvuloplasty in adults: a 10 year review of Auckland's experience. Heart Lung Circ 2008;17:486-474.

[9] Vahanian A, Alfieri OR, Al-Attar N, *et al.* Transcatheter valve implantation for patients with aortic stenosis: a position statement from the European Association of Cardio-Thoracic Surgery [EACTS] and the European Society of Cardiology [ESC], in

collaboration with the European Association of Percutaneous Cardiovascular Interventions [EAPCI]. Eur J Cardio-thorac Surg 2008;34:1-8.
[10] Portoghese M. Letter to the editor. Transcatheter Aortic Valve Therapy Is Not Aortic Valve Replacement. Ann Thorac Surg 2009;88:2069-2074.
[11] Roberts WC, Ko JM, Filardo G. Comparison of Heavier *Versus* Lighter Operatively Excised Stenotic Aortic Valves in Adults With Aortic Stenosis and Implications for Percutaneous Aortic Valve Implantation Without Replacement. Am J Cardiol 2009;104:393-405.
[12] Boudjemline Y, Bonhoeffer P. Steps Toward Percutaneous Aortic Valve Replacement. Circulation. 2002;105:775-778.
[13] Lutter G, Kuklinski D, Berg G, *et al.* Percutaneous aortic valve replacement: An experimental study. I. Studies on implantation. J Thorac Cardiovasc Surg 2002;123:768-776.
[14] Ferrari E, Rizzo E, Sulzer C, von Segesser LK. Case Report. Unexpected left ventricular free-wall rupture following an aortic catheter-valve implantation. Eur J Cardio-thorac Surg 2010;37:242-244.
[15] Huber CH, von Segesser LK. Direct Access Valve Replacement [DAVR] — are we entering a new era in cardiac surgery? Eur J Cardio-thorac Surg 2006;29:380-385.
[16] Dewey TM, Walther T, Doss T, *et al.* Transapical Aortic Valve Implantation: An Animal Feasibility Study. Ann Thorac Surg 2006;82:110-116.
[17] Kappetein AP, Piazza N, Laborde JC, *et al.* Transapical implantation of a self-expanding aortic valve bioprosthesis-animal feasibility study. Eur J Cardio-thorac Surg 2009;36:813-817.
[18] Linke A, Walther T, Schuler G. Clinical Decision Making: The Utility of Trans-Catheter Aortic Valve Replacement After Commercialization: Does the European Experience Provide a Glimpse Into the Future Use of This Technology in the United States? Catheterization and Cardiovascular Interventions 2010:75:511-518.
[19] Hashimoto M, Kaminou T, Ohuchi Y, *et al.* Development of a Re-Positionable Aortic Stent-Valve: A Preliminary Study in Swine. J Intervent Cardiol 2008;5:432-440.
[20] Azadani AN, Jaussaud N, Matthews PB, *et al.* Valve-in-Valve Implantation Using a Novel Supravalvular Transcatheter Aortic Valve: Proof of Concept. Ann Thorac Surg 2009;88:1864-1870.
[21] Cribier A, Eltchaninoff H, Bash A, *et al.* Percutaneous Transcatheter Implantation of an Aortic Valve Prosthesis for Calcific Aortic Stenosis First Human Case Description. Circulation. 2002;106:3006-3008.
[22] Cribier A, Eltchaninoff H, Tron C, *et al.* Percutaneous artificial cardiac valves: from animal experimentation to the first human implantation in a case of calcified aortic stenosis. Arch Malad Coeur Vaiss 2003;96:645-652.
[23] Bauer F, Lemercier M, Zajarias A, *et al.* Immediate and Long-Term Echocardiographic Findings after Transcatheter Aortic Valve Implantation for the Treatment of Aortic Stenosis: The Cribier-Edwards/Edwards-Sapien Valve Experience. J Am Soc Echocardiogr 2010;23:370-376.
[24] Bauer F, Eltchaninoff H, Tron C, *et al.* Acute Improvement in Global and Regional Left Ventricular Systolic Function After Percutaneous Heart Valve Implantation in Patients With Symptomatic Aortic Stenosis. Circulation. 2004;110:1473-1476.

[25] Cribier A, Eltchaninoff H, Tron C, *et al.* Early Experience With Percutaneous Transcatheter Implantation of Heart Valve Prosthesis for the Treatment of End-Stage Inoperable Patients With Calcific Aortic Stenosis. J Am Coll Cardiol 2004;43:698-703.

[26] Palacios IF. Editorial comment. Percutaneous Valve Replacement and Repair. J Am Coll Cardiol 2004;44:1662-1663.

[27] Vahanian A, Palacios IF. Review. Percutaneous Approaches to Valvular Disease. Circulation 2004;109;1572-1579.

[28] Fish RD. Review. Percutaneous Heart Valve Replacement Enthusiasm Tempered. Circulation 2004; 110;1876-1878.

[29] Cribier A, Eltchaninoff H, Tron C, *et al.* Treatment of Calcific Aortic Stenosis With the Percutaneous Heart Valve Mid-Term Follow-Up From the Initial Feasibility Studies: The French Experience. J Am Coll Cardiol 2006;47:1214-1223.

[30] Grube E, Laborde JC, Gerckens U, *et al.* Percutaneous Implantation of the CoreValve Self-Expanding Valve Prosthesis in High-Risk Patients With Aortic Valve Disease The Siegburg First-in-Man Study. Circulation. 2006;114:1616-1624.

[31] Kurra V, Schoenhagen P, Roselli EE, *et al.* Prevalence of significant peripheral artery disease in patients evaluated for percutaneous aortic valve insertion: Preprocedural assessment with multidetector computed tomography. J Thorac Cardiovasc Surg 2009;137:1258-1264.

[32] Ye J, Cheung A, Lichtenstein SV, *et al.* Six-month outcome of transapical transcatheter aortic valve implantation in the initial 7 patients. Eur J Cardio-thorac Surg 2007;31:16-21.

[33] Svensson LG, Dewey T, Kapadia S, *et al.* United States Feasibility Study of Transcatheter Insertion of a Stented Aortic Valve by the Left Ventricular Apex. Ann Thorac Surg 2008;86:46-55.

[34] Walther T, Chu MWA, Mohr FW. Transcatheter aortic valve implantation: time to expand? Curr Opin Cardiol 2008;23:111–116.

[35] Al-Attar N, Ghodbane W, Himbert D, *et al.* Unexpected Complications of Transapical Aortic Valve Implantation. Ann Thorac Surg 2009;88:90-94.

[36] Al-Attar N, Himbert D, Descoutures F, *et al.* Transcatheter Aortic Valve Implantation: Selection Strategy Is Crucial for Outcome. Ann Thorac Surg 2009;87:1757-1763.

[37] Dumont E, Rodés-Cabau J, De LaRochellière R, *et al.* Rapid Pacing Technique For Preventing Ventricular Tears during Transapical Aortic Valve Replacement. J Card Surg 2009;24:295-298.

[38] Bleiziffer S, Ruge H, Mazzitelli D, *et al.* Survival after transapical and transfemoral aortic valve implantation: Talking about two different patient populations. J Thorac Cardiovasc Surg 2009;138:1073-1080.

[39] Bleiziffer S, Ruge H, Mazzitelli D, *et al.* Results of percutaneous and transapical transcatheter aortic valve implantation performed by a surgical team. Eur J Cardio-thorac Surg 2009;35:615-621.

[40] Bombien RH, Appel M, Attmann T, *et al.* Percutaneous aortic valve replacement: gross anatomy and histological findings after transapical and endoluminal resection of human aortic valves *in situ*. Eur J Cardio-thorac Surg 2009;36:112-117.

[41] Himbert D, Descoutures F, Al-Attar N, *et al.* Results of Transfemoral or Transapical Aortic Valve Implantation Following a Uniform Assessment in High-Risk Patients With Aortic Stenosis. J Am Coll Cardiol 2009;54:303-311.

[42] Asgar AW, Mullen MJ, Delahunty N, *et al.* Transcatheter aortic valve intervention through the axillary artery for the treatment of severe aortic stenosis. J Thorac Cardiovasc Surg 2009;137:773-775.

[43] De Robertis F, Asgar A, Davies S, *et al.* The left axillary artery — a new approach for transcatheter aortic valve implantation. Eur J Cardio-thorac Surg 2009;36:807-812.

[44] Hofmann S, Franz N, Billion M, *et al.* Successful catheter-besed valve-in-valve implantation for a regurgitant stentless bioprosthesis. J Heart Valve Dis 2009;18:713-716.

[45] Kelpis TG, Mezilis NE, Ninios VN, Pitsis AA. Minimally invasive transapical aortic valve-in-a-valve implantation for severe aortic regurgitation in a degenerated stentless bioprosthesis. J Thorac Cardiovasc Surg 2009;138:1018-1020.

[46] Napodano M, Cutolo A, Fraccaro C, *et al.* Totally percutaneous valve replacement for severe aortic regurgitation in a degenerating bioprosthesis. J Thorac Cardiovasc Surg 2009;138:1027-1028.

[47] Kempfert J, Van Linden A, Linke A, *et al.* Transapical Off-Pump Valve-in-Valve Implantation in Patients With Degenerated Aortic Xenografts. Ann Thorac Surg 2010;89:1934–1941.

[48] Webb JG, Wood DA, Ye J, *et al.* Transcatheter Valve-in-Valve Implantation for Failed Bioprosthetic Heart Valves. Circulation 2010;121:1848-1857.

[49] Webb JG, Altwegg L, Masson JB, *et al.* A New Transcatheter Aortic Valve and Percutaneous Valve Delivery System. J Am Coll Cardiol 2009;53:1855-1858.

[50] Fassl J, Augoustides JGT. Emerging Technology Review. Transcatheter Aortic Valve Implantation—Part 1: Development and Status of the Procedure. J of Cardiothorac Vasc Anesthesia 2010;24:498-505.

[51] Van Brabandt H, Neyt M. Safety of percutaneous aortic valve insertion. A systematic review. BMC Cardiovascular Disorders 2009, 9:45 doi:10.1186/1471-2261-9-45.

[52] Leon MB, Smith CR, Mack M, *et al.*, for the PARTNER Trial Investigators. Transcatheter Aortic-Valve Implantation for Aortic Stenosis in Patients Who Cannot Undergo Surgery. New Engl J Med 2010. DOI 10.1056/nejmoa1008232.

[53] Grube E, Schuler G, Buellesfeld L, *et al.* Percutaneous Aortic Valve Replacement for Severe Aortic Stenosis in High-Risk Patients Using the Second-and Current Third-Generation Self-Expanding CoreValve Prosthesis Device Success and 30-Day Clinical Outcome. J Am Coll Cardiol 2007;50:69-76.

[54] Horvath KA, Mazilu D, Guttman M, *et al.* Midterm results of transapical aortic valve replacement *via* real-time magnetic resonance imaging guidance. J Thorac Cardiovasc Surg 2010;139:424-30.

[55] Marcos-Alberca P, Zamorano JL, Sánchez T, *et al.* Intraoperative Monitoring With Transesophageal Real-Time Three-Dimensional Echocardiography During Transapical Prosthetic Aortic Valve Implantation. Rev Esp Cardiol. 2010;63:352-356.

[56] Walther T, Falk V, Borger MA, *et al.* Transapical aortic valve implantation in patients requiring redo surgery. Eur J Cardio-thorac Surg 2009;36:231-235.

[57] Akhtar M, Tuzcu EM, Kapadia SR, *et al.* Aortic root morphology in patients undergoing percutaneous aortic valve replacement: Evidence of aortic root remodeling. J Thorac Cardiovasc Surg 2009;137:950-956.

[58] Rivard AL, Bartel T, Bianc RW, *et al.* Evaluation of aortic root and valve calcifications by MDCT. J Heart Valve D 2009;18:662-670.

[59] Zegdi R, Lecuyer L, Achouh P, *et al.* Increased Radial Force Improves Stent Deployment in Tricuspid but Not in Bicuspid Stenotic Native Aortic Valves. Ann Thorac Surg 2010;89:768-772.

[60] Manasse E. Cookies and recipes. Eur J Cardio-thorac Surg 2009;36:787-790.

[61] Kallenbach K, Karck M. Percutaneous aortic valve implantation – contra. Herz 2009;34:130-139.

[62] Brown ML, Schaff HV, Sarano ME, *et al.* Is the European System for Cardiac Operative Risk Evaluation model valid for estimating the operative risk of patients considered for percutaneous aortic valve replacement? J Thorac Cardiovasc Surg 2008;136:566-71.

[63] Kalavrouziotis D, Li D, Buth KJ, Légaré JF. The European System for Cardiac Operative Risk Evaluation [EuroSCORE] is not appropriate for withholding surgery in high-risk patients with aortic stenosis: a retrospective cohort study. Jf Cardiothoracic Surg 2009, 4:32. doi:10.1186/1749-8090-4-32.

[64] Osswald BR, Gegouskov V, Badowski-Zyla D, *et al.* Overestimation of aortic valve replacement risk by EuroSCORE: implications for percutaneous valve replacement. Eur Heart J 2009;30:74-80.

[65] Di Giammarco G, Rabozzi R, Chiappini B, Tamagnini G. Absolute and relative risk prediction in patients candidate to isolated aortic valve replacement: should we change our mind? Eur J Cardio-thorac Surg 2010;37:255-260.

[66] Descoutures F, Himbert D, Lepage L, *et al.* Contemporary surgical or percutaneous management of severe aortic stenosis in the elderly. Eur Heart J 2008;29:1410-1417.

[67] Mistiaen W, Van Cauwelaert P, Muylaert P, De Worm E. 1000 Carpentier-Edwards pericardial valves in aortic position: what changed in the last 20 years and what are the effects on hospital complications. J Heart Valve Dis 2007;16:417-422.

[68] Piazza N, Otten A, Schultz C, Onuma Y, *et al.* Adherence to patient selection criteria in patients undergoing trascatheter aortic valve implantation with the 18F CoreValveRvalving System. Heart 2010;96:19-26.

[69] Thielmann M, Wendt D, Eggebrecht E, *et al.* Transcatheter Aortic Valve Implantation in Patients With Very High Risk for Conventional Aortic Valve Replacement. Ann Thorac Surg 2009;88:1468-1475.

[70] Yan TD, Cao C, Martens-Nielsen J, *et al.* Transcatheter aortic valve implantation for high-risk patients with severe aortic stenosis: A systematic review. J Thorac Cardiovasc Surg 2010;139:1519-1528.

[71] Piazza N, Onuma Y, de Jaegere P, Serruys PW. Guidelines for Reporting Mortality and Morbidity After Cardiac Valve Interventions—Need for a Reappraisal? Ann Thorac Surg 2009;87:357-358.

[72] Walther T, Falk *vs.* Editorial. Hemodynamic Evaluation of Heart Valve Prostheses Paradigm Shift for Transcatheter Valves? J Am Coll Cardiol 2009;53:1893-1894.

[73] Ghanem A, Müller A, Nähle CP, *et al.* Risk and Fate of Cerebral Embolism After Transfemoral Aortic Valve Implantation A Prospective Pilot Study With Diffusion-Weighted Magnetic Resonance Imaging. J Am Coll Cardiol 2010;55:1427-1432.

[74] Kahlert P, Knipp SC, Schlamann M, *et al.* Silent and Apparent Cerebral Ischemia After Percutaneous Transfemoral Aortic Valve Implantation A Diffusion-Weighted Magnetic Resonance Imaging Study. Circulation 2010;121:870-878.

[75] Calvi V, Puzzangara E, Pruiti GP, *et al.* Early Conduction Disorders Following Percutaneous Aortic Valve Replacement. PACE 2009; 32:S126–S130.

[76] Gutiérrez M, Rodés-Cabau J, Bagur R, *et al.* Electrocardiographic changes and clinical outcomes after transapical aortic valve implantation. Am Heart J 2009;158:302-308.

[77] Jilaihawi H, Chin D, Vasa-Nicotera M, *et al.* Predictors for permanent pacemaker requirement after transcatheter aortic valve implantation with the CoreValve bioprosthesis. Am Heart J 2009;157:860-866.

[78] Baan J Jr., Yong ZY, Koch KT, *et al.* Factors associated with cardiac conduction disorders and permanent pacemaker implantation after percutaneous aortic valve implantation with the CoreValve prosthesis. Am Heart J 2010;159:497-503.

[79] Bagur R, Webb JG, Nietlispach F, *et al.* Acute kidney injury following transcatheter aortic valve implantation: predictive factors, prognostic value, and comparison with surgical aortic valve replacement. Eur Heart J 2010;31:865-874.

[80] Ye J, Cheung A, Lichtenstein SV, *et al.* Transapical transcatheter aortic valve implantation: Follow-up to 3 years. J Thorac Cardiovasc Surg 2010;139:1107-1113.

[81] Chin D. Echocardiography for transcatheter aortic valve implantation. Eur J Echocardiogr 2009;10: i21-29.

[82] Rodés-Cabau J, Webb JG, Cheung A, *et al.* Transcatheter Aortic Valve Implantation for the Treatment of Severe Symptomatic Aortic Stenosis in Patients at Very High or Prohibitive Surgical Risk Acute and Late Outcomes of the Multicenter Canadian Experience. J Am Coll Cardiol 2010;55:1080-1090.

[83] Rodes-Cabau J. Review. Progress in Transcatheter Aortic Valve Implantation. Rev Esp Cardiol. 2010;63:439-450.

[84] Carabello BA. Review. Is it Ever Too Late to Operate on the Patient With Valvular Heart Disease? J Am Coll Cardiol 2004;44:376-383.

[85] Dewey TM, Brown DL, Herbert MA, *et al.* Effect of Concomitant Coronary Artery Disease on Procedural and Late Outcomes of Transcatheter Aortic Valve Implantation. Ann Thorac Surg 2010;89:758-767.

[86] Kapadia SR, Goel SS, Svensson L, *et al.* Characterization and outcome of patients with severe symptomatic aortic stenosis referred for percutaneous aortic valve replacement. J Thorac Cardiovasc Surg 2009;137:1430-1435.

[87] Zierer A, Wimmer-Greinecker G, Martens S, *et al.* Is transapical aortic valve implantation really less invasive thanminimally invasive aortic valve replacement? J Thorac Cardiovasc Surg 2009;138:1067-1072.

[88] Thomas M, Schymik G, Walther T, *et al.* Thirty-day results of the SAPIEN aortic bioprosthesis European Outcome [SOURCE] registry. A European registry of transcatheter aortic valve implant using the Edwards SAPIEN valve. Circulation 2010;122:62-U130.

[89] Azadani AN, Jaussaud N, Matthews P, *et al.* Energy Loss Due to Paravalvular Leak With Transcatheter Aortic Valve Implantation. Ann Thorac Surg 2009;88:1857-1863.

[90] Walther T, Falk V, Kempfert J, *et al.* Transapical minimally invasive aortic valve implantation; the initial 50 patients. Eur J Cardio-thorac Surg 2008;33:983-988.

[91] Smith CR, Leon MB, Mack MJ, *et al.* PARTNER Trial Investigators. Transcatheter *versus* surgical aortic-valve-replacement in high-risk patients. N Engl J Med 2011;364:2187-2198.

Send Orders of Reprints at bspsaif@emirates.net.ae
"Degenerative" Aortic Valve Stenosis, its Pathogenesis and Treatment, 2013, 289-310

CHAPTER 12

TEHV – Tissue Engineering of Heart Valves

Abstract: The development of tissue engineered heart valves has seemed promising: with its development, a living tissue, capable of growth, repair and remodelling would cure the valve disease. Nevertheless, TEHV will have to compete with well established procedures and devices such as pericardial BHV.

The release of a device that can compete with currently available valves will take probably many more years. The development of TEHV is complex and requires several steps.

First, the scaffold has to be chosen: a synthetic and biodegradable device or a decellularized scaffold from biological origin. For the latter, many decellularization protocols exist, all with their pro's and con's.

Second, the decision for cell reseeding has to be made. The source for the cells has its importance. Differentiated cells of the same type but from a different region (vascular EC *vs.* valvular EC) can behave differently. Autologous mesenchymal stem cells derived from bone marrow and progenitor cells from other sources seem promising.

After reseeding, culturing in a bioreactor can improve the biomechanical properties of the device. Much depends however on the mechanical loading protocols and on the biochemical composition of the culture medium. Small differences in such protocols lead to a great variety of tissues.

It seems that the "silver bullet", leading to the desired differentiation of the seeded cells, which are capable of remodelling an repairing the ECM, still has to be found. Moreover, long-term animal studies, *in vivo* evaluation of the device and bench-to-bed series are still lacking. Attempts to implant TEHV in young patients with congenital heart disease were and still are not promising.

Keywords: Biochemical protocols, bioreactor, cell sources, collagen, decellularization, endothelial cells, extracellular matrix, glycosminoglycan, mechanical loading protocol, mesenchymal stem cells, myofibroblasts, reseeding, scaffold, smooth muscle cells.

1. INTRODUCTION

Valve replacement surgery in valvular heart disease has its proven value [1, 2]. Nevertheless, some problems remain. BHV consist of non-viable material that can

Wilhelm Peter Mistiaen

deteriorate, since it lacks the capacity to grow, to repair or to remodel. In MHV, the need for anticoagulation remains undiminished. Furthermore, not all innovations have been a success. The Carbomedics Photofix-alpha valve has suffered from cusp abrasion and perforation, the Medtronic Parallel mechanical valve has shown a higher rate of TE and the St Jude Silzone coating has resulted into tissue necrosis, with more PPVL as a result. For such reasons, manufacturers have become more conservative. The risks associated with the introduction of new devices have made it difficult for TEHV to compete with established values [2].

A device which can remodel itself could solve the problem of durability. This is becoming increasingly important since life expectancy in Western populations is increasing [1, 3]. The success of TEHV will depend on the ability of the living components (*i.e.* the seeded cells) to repair, remodel and to grow [3, 4]. While current devices palliate a heart valve disease, TEHV – as living substitute – has the potential to become curative. Hence the widespread efforts to provide for such a device that can revolutionize the current medical and surgical practice [2]. Tissue engineering is also important in a pediatric population with congenital heart disease, in which devices that can grow along are strongly desirable.

As a discipline of its own, tissue engineering is surprisingly old. The term "tissue engineering" was defined already in 1987 at a National Science Foundation workshop in Washington, DC. The different approaches for tissue engineering have appeared independently as early as the 1960s, when advanced tissue culture technologies have been used to propagate skins cells. Tissue engineering has had a number of definitions. One of these states:

> *The application of principles and methods of engineering and life sciences to obtain a fundamental understanding of structure-function relationships in novel and pathological mammalian tissues and the development of biological substitutes to restore, maintain or improve tissue function.*

Tissue engineering, relevant to heart valves, is defined as "the manipulation of biological molecules and cells for the purpose of creating new structures capable of metabolic activity" [2].

A new type of heart valve thus fabricated must, therefore, contain material of biological origin in a configuration that did not emerge naturally. Heart valves containing amounts of biological material, such as pannus overgrowth are not considered tissue-engineered valves.

Valves consisting of inert materials covered with a cellular coating, developed for the purpose of improving the performance of the valve, could be considered TEHV. The first example of TEHV dates from 1991, where EC have been successfully grown on glutaraldehyde fixed bovine pericardium. This has been only possible after inactivation of the aldehyde. This approach, however, has not been implemented any further [2].

2. CONCEPT OF TISSUE ENGINEERING [1, 4]

The principle for TEHV has been introduced in 1995 by Shinoka, for valves in pulmonary position [1].

There are currently several tissue engineering concepts for heart valves:

1) Biodegradable scaffolds, to be seeded with autologous cells.

2) Decellularized allografts/xenografts to be seeded with autolous cells.

3) Decellularized allografts/xenografts without subsequent cell seeding.

Through these concepts, a device should function as closely possible as a healthy native valve. This includes an adequate mechanical function, durability, adequate haemodynamic performance without provoking immune responses or inflammation.

Three issues determine the success for TEHV:

1) The scaffold must determine the shape and serves as temporary matrix or guiding & anchoring structure for cells to attach and for subsequent tissue formation.

2) The source of cells: EC, SMC, *etc.*

3) The culture conditions of the valve construct before implantation [1], *i.e.* the bioreactor that provides the necessary metabolic and mechanical conditions for proliferation, sorting and differentiation, which takes about 3 to 4 weeks [3, 4].

After implantation, the tissues in this device can mature further by biodegradation of the scaffold and formation of ECM by the cells. Further remodelling can occur. Some of these events can occur also *in vitro*, before implantation [3, 4].

3. SCAFFOLDS

Scaffolds can be synthetic or have a biological source.

3.1. Synthetic Scaffolds

Synthetic and biocompatible or biodegradable scaffolds can be made from polyglactin, polyglycolic acid, polylactic acid or from a co-polymer of both. Their stiffness is a disadvantage. Polyhydroxy-alkanoate has also been used because it is more compliant.

These scaffolds have been used first as tissue engineered skin [2]. Their usefulness in cardiovascular tissue engineering has also been demonstrated. Poly-4-hydroxybuyrate can serve as coat for polyglactin. This results in thermoplasticity and allows moulding into more complex three dimensional shapes such as aortic valves. Moreover, the biodegradation properties and biomechanics can be chemically designed to meet the requirements of the particular application. Growth factors and other proteins may be incorporated into the scaffold structure, which allows the promotion of tissue growth [1].

Polyhydroxy-alcanoate based devices with three leaflets have shown simultaneous opening, without development of thrombi. Stenosis and regurgitation have been mild. The biodegradation has been prolonged, however, and its replacement by autologous tissue has not been observed. The use of polyglycolic acid matrix has resulted in better development of the ECM, but it has proved impossible to maintain the necessary structure under flow conditions. Coating of polyglycolic acid matrix by poly-4-hydroxybuyrate, which is a thermoplastic elastomer, has shown better mechanical results and a biodegradation with 6 to 8 weeks after implantation. These TEHV have resembled the morphology and the function of healthy native heart valves in sheep [1].

Although cell seeding on "inert" substrates has been successful in vascular grafts, this has not been the case in TEHV, because of material fatigue, development of microscopic cracks with insudation of plasma proteins and of subsequent calcification. For these reasons, glutaraldehyde fixated BHV nowadays dominate the valve field. Although these devices cannot be reseeded without inactivation of the aldehyde, TE events and other adverse reaction do seem not to occur frequently [1].

By 2005 none of these abovementioned scaffolds have been tried in patients. Valves are life-sustaining class III devices. Therefore, they must be taken through the full set of preclinical and clinical trials before market approval. Biological matrices do not degrade through hydrolysis, but rather through proteolysis. Hydrolysable matrices therefore are clearly not biomimetic and their use as biodegradable substrates should give rise for concern. Modes of failure of these devices have not been published and no good histological pictures of failed valves have appeared in the literature. Hence, little can be learned from the 10 years of experience with this approach. Some difficult questions remain: are biodegradable materials inherently inappropriate or have they been used improperly in the past? Are future research designs a waste of time? Do competitive motives play a role in a booming market? Are unfavourable results going to be published? This is the only way to learn from past mistakes [2]!

Some alternatives have also been tried. By electro-spinning techniques, polyester urethane urea elastomeres can be constructed, in which fibre diameter, fibre alignment, porosity, anistropic mechanical properties and degradation rate can be controlled [5]. Electro-spinning is also used to fabricate hybrid polymer scaffolds which can be coated with basic fibroblast growth factor, as attempt to improve recellularization with mesenchymal stem cells [6].

3.2. Scaffold of Biological Origin

The homograft scaffold has received the most attention. It has all the biomechanical properties of a normal aortic valve. The homograft is very durable, probably due to the interconnected sheets of collagen, the layers and tubes of elastin, the biomechanical properties, anisotropy and visco-elasticity [2].

Aortic valve homografts need to be decellularized before implantation in the recipient. This process reduces the immune response and hence rejection, inflammation and degeneration. A rat model has shown that damage to the ECM after a two-step decellularizing process with gentle detergents and enzymes was much less than inflammation after implantation of grafts which were not decellularized [7-9].

In spite of these advantages, enzymes as trypsin fragment and distort elastin, change collagen distribution and remove GAG, laminin an fibronectin, which are adhesion molecules. Detergents such as Triton X-100 have a comparable effect. This could lead to problems in valve functioning after implant of the grafts [7]. Some detergents and decellularization protocols might show better results concerning the quality of the tissues [10]. Cryopreservation has shown extensive disruption between collagen and inter-fibrillar proteoglycan associations within the ECM of decellularized tissues. Structural and mechanical properties have been altered, which raises questions concerning the durability after implant [11].

4. CELL SEEDING

4.1. Principles of Cell Seeding

To seed or not to seed is one of the major issues in the use of xenograft matrix. Human matrices are considered to be the ideal matrix for repopulation with cells. They provoke less immune response than porcine material and have the right mechanical properties. Nevertheless, some report that homografts fail to repopulate with cells of the recipient, and worse, implants become completely a-cellular, months after implantation. Therefore, attempts to reseed before implantation in animal models have been performed. Reliance on cells contributing to long-term durability makes it more difficult to have a device approved by the Drug and Food Administration [2]. Nevertheless, without a autologous blood-tissue barrier of EC, damage to the graft may be higher compared to seeded grafts. Seeded EC are capable of synthesis of ECM components which are lost during the decellularization process [7].

In a **first** approach, these homografts/xenografts scaffolds can be reseeded by autologous vascular EC and myofibroblasts. Reseeding with EC has the advantage of reducing the risk of calcification and of TE events. The model has been tested in sheep [1]. Attempts to accelerate *in vivo* re-colonization of the graft through mobilizing bone marrow cells by granulocyte colony-stimulating factor have been leading to increased valve degeneration and should be avoided [12]. In porcine valves, the use of hepatocyte growth factor associated to fibronectin have seemed more successful for cell growth after seeding [13].

An interesting result has been obtained with an intra-peritoneal preseeding of a TEHV device, before its implantation in pulmonary position in sheep. This device has been constructed as a photo-oxidized decellularized cross-linked bovine pericardial TEHV. Compared to non-seeded devices, these seeded valves had more matrix and have been thicker, with a concomitant decrease in the length of the leaflet. Furthermore, the observed immune response has been low. Infiltration of mesenchymal stem cells with appropriated differentiation into myofibroblasts and spontaneous re-endothelialization has been observed. Cellular covering of the surface trough intra-peritoneal seeding has been significantly increased, compared to spontaneous reseeding, one month after implantation in pulmonary position. The matrix has seemed biomechanically reliable and the cells viable. The mediators for these results have remained largely unknown [14].

Five months after implantation, the valve functioning has been acceptable with a mildly increased TVG and regurgitation. Intra-peritonelly re-seeded valves have been thicker and shorter, the re-cellularization has been excessive and the ECM has been partially degraded with loss of the organization of collagen fibres. The strength and stiffness have decreased accordingly. More cells had contractile properties. The valve remodelling has been considered as inadequate [15].

Coating with fibronectin has been helpful for homing in of stem cells. No calcification has been observed in such valves and the amount of cells has been comparable to those of native valves. These cells have been capable of producing a new matrix and of covering the surface of the leaflets. An improvement has been obtained by double coating: the presence of fewer contractile myofibroblasts has resulted in less shortening of the leaflets [16].

These results, however, still are very preliminary and imply an additional procedure, *i.e.* an opening of the peritoneal cavity. Moreover, the pulmonary position is not necessarily representative for the aortic position, since its pressures are lower. The animal model has to be chosen with care. Calcification in a sheep model also has its predictors: a younger age, a mitral position, a stentless device (more than in stented one), a porcine valve (more than in a pericardial one) and omission of treatment with surfactant [17, 18].

In a **second** approach, biological scaffolds from human or animal origin have been implanted in patients, without reseeding. Decellularization has been achieved by detergents such as Sodium dodecyl sulphate, accompanied by enzymes. Various elaborate protocols have been developed, followed by mechanical testing of the remaining matrix.

The histological features have varied greatly, however, indicating that conventional investigation techniques do not reveal all properties of the material [1, 2]. In contrast to valves of porcine origin, it has not been necessary to cross-link valves of human origin with glutaraldehyde before implantation. Matching according to the major histocompatibility complex has not been performed either. It might be that due to high flow, immune-competent cells can not attach the wall of the graft [2].

A gentle decellularization protocol has allowed *in vitro* repopulation with VIC and EC [19]. Those cells have been capable of synthesizing ECM in a bioreactor [20]. Moreover, *in vivo* repopulation with cells has been expected to occur spontaneously, since there has been no prior fixation in glutaraldehyde. Cell sources for this repopulation could have been from circulating EPC and from circulating mesenchymal stem cells, which originate from the bone marrow [4]. A repopulated and enveloped graft by an EC monolayer [21] would become "invisible" for immune-competent cells.

As the porcine ECM becomes completely remodelled, it would become entirely "self" to the recipient. This approach has been feasible in principle. No follow-up studies have been available, except in children. In these series, disastrous inflammatory responses with structural failures have been observed [1, 2, 4].

Furthermore, the results in animal experiments have shown inflammation, detachment and formation of obstructive masses [22].

A risk of transmission of human diseases such as Creutzfeldt-Jacob disease (for homografts) and porcine endogenous retroviruses (for xenografts) has to be considered. The latter has been documented [1]. In a-cellular porcine valves, processed with detergents and enzymes, no porcine endogenous retrovirus has been detected, what makes these grafts safe in this respect [23].

In a **third** approach, the biological matrices have been treated with glutaraldehyde for chemical fixation and cross-linking of ECM proteins. This process sterilizes the matrices, reduces their antigenic potential with its immunological complications and also reduces transmission of infectious diseases. Treatment with glutaraldehyde makes seeding with EC impossible. Several detoxification procedures using urazole and citric acid have been tried. Adherence of EC in these detoxified matrices has been improved by pre-seeding with fibroblasts. Alternatives for glutaraldehyde have also been tested but all procedures have resulted into non-living and non degrading ECM, which is incapable of growth [1].

4.2. Cell Sources

Cells can be derived from the cardiovascular system and from the bone marrow.

Cardiovascular cells can be harvested from the mammary artery, the radial artery or from the saphenous vein, which are routinely used in heart surgery. It implies the sacrifice of intact vascular structures. The availability of these structures might be limited! Cells from atherosclerotic vessels are not suitable. Pure EC and myofibroblast cell lines can be selected from the mixed vascular cell populations, by labelling the cells with a LDL marker. Subsequently, the desired cells can be sorted by fluorescence techniques. As alternative, biopsies can be treated with collagenase in order to detach EC from the surface. The remainder of the vessel can be cultured until primary myofibroblasts grow out. Formation of ECM has increased when venous cells have been cultured in three dimensional structures. However, these cells may express a considerable different phenotype compared to natural VIC [1].

EC were thought to be able to provide both interstitial and endothelial functions. Therefore, these cells could potentially serve as a single-cell source for construction of autologous heart valves [24]. One has to be aware of the different behaviour of the same cell type, but from a different source. For example, in a laminar flow, aortic valve EC align perpendicularly while aortic wall EC align parallel to the flow. This observation indicates that not all cells of the same type might be suitable for constructing TEHV [25].

Mesenchymal stem cells, bone marrow stem cells, umbilical cord cells and progenitor cells, derived from peripheral blood can be attractive as alternative. The use of mesenchymal stem cells offers several advantages: these cells should be able to:

1) Be obtained easily, with less invasive procedures.
2) Show an extensive *in vitro* proliferation capacity.
3) Have a potential to differentiate into EC and VIC or myofibroblasts.
4) Provide for a well developed ECM.

Mesenchymal stem cells can be collected by a simple puncture of the iliac crest under local anaesthesia. Centrifugation in a solution, within a density gradient and the capacity to adhere to plastic surfaces allows selection of the desired cells. This selection still needs improvement by specific antibodies.

After proper culturing, the cells can be seeded in the scaffolds. Mesenchymal stem cells already have shown a capacity to differentiate into vascular cells such as myofibroblast-like cells. The tissue engineering concept suggests that the application of a favourable microenvironment will guide cellular differentiation towards phenotypes that are appropriate for autologous tissue replacement. The mechanics of differentiation, however, are poorly understood [1].

TEHV from stem cells and biodegradable scaffolds have been implanted in sheep in pulmonary position. This has shown acceptable TVG, EOAI and minimal regurgitation over 4 months. Microscopic investigation after explantation has demonstrated an ECM and a distribution of cell phenotypes comparable to native pulmonary valves [26].

Cells such as myofibroblasts derived from umbilical cord vessels and whole umbilical cord have shown excellent growth properties, comparable to those of the saphenous vein. ECM formation by these cells has been promising. Harvesting of these juvenile cells has made invasive procedures to procure cells from arteries or veins unnecessary [27, 28]. Cryopreserved cells from the umbilical cord have shown a myofibroblast-like morphology in culture, with excellent growth potential and ability to form ECM [29].

EPC is a second cell type, which also can be selected from umbilical cord blood. These cells have shown good proliferation capacities. Stable EC phenotype has been obtained after seeding in a biodegradable scaffold. These sources seem appropriate for pediatric populations with congenital heart defects [28, 29].

In elderly patients, growth, migration and differentiation capacities of several cell types have been reduced. Harvesting, growth and differentiation of bone marrow derived mesenchymal stem cells of elderly patients have seemed more successful [30]. This has to be kept in mind, if in the future, cells will be harvested in elderly patients with CAVS, who are referred for implantation with a TEHV.

The use of the two main stem cells, mesenchymal stem cells and circulating EPC, have posed some problems. After harvesting, growth and seeding on substrates, fibrotic overgrowth and failure of valvular matrixes has been observed. It is doubtful that stem cells will behave in a "intelligent" way in valve substrates.

Probably, efforts to guide stem cells along the desired differentiation path before seeding and implantation will be needed. It seems worthwhile to proceed in this direction: cell seeding has shown a therapeutic advantage for the implanted matrices. Stem cells, once differentiated to the proper end point, are expected to provide a broader source of autologous cell lines. For manufactures, legal regulatory, marketing and financial issues are much simpler with a-cellular devices with the promise of autologous stem cells [2].

5. COLLAGEN GELS: ECM AND CELLS IN ONE

The use of collagen gels also implies the use of cells, which classifies these gels as a separate entity. Entrapment of appropriate cells in collagen gels is one of the least explored area's but this technique requires the greatest amount of engineering. Cells entrapped in a collagen gel cause contraction and compaction of this gel. The soluble collagen interacts with the cells and is rearranged as insoluble fibrils. The desired direction and alignment of these collagen fibres can be obtained by constraints. In this way, a highly compacted and aligned collagen construct can be fabricated. This procedure results in one dimensional strings, which can be used as building blocks for the development of the aortic valve. When elastin and GAG are added, a complete device might have following properties:

- The collagen tissue bears the diastolic tensile load.
- The elastin returns the collagen to the resting state between the loading cycles.
- GAG maintains the hydration and the visco-elastic properties of the valve.

Hyaluronan, a macromolecular GAG, holds water molecules and can resist compressing forces. Hyaluronan is compatible between species. These properties makes hyaluronan easily applicable as scaffold for TEHV.

A reproducible complex of cross-linked sheets can be made. The cell types and the details of protocols are important for the outcome. The standardization of these protocols has still not been finalized and animal implants have not yet been performed in 2005.

Co-culturing myofibroblast and EC have produced considerable amounts of collagen and proteoglycans. These entrapped cells, however, synthesize MMP and also undergo apoptosis. Chitosan, obtained from crustacean shells and mixed with collagen yields better results than either alone [2].

The quality of collagen gels could be improved by adding chondroitin-sulphate. This has resulted in a more porous model, which influenced the activity of seeded

VIC and EC in a favourable way. Synthesis of a basement membrane, formation of cell junctions and enhanced production of ECM, collagen, elastin and laminin have been documented [31].

Hyaluronic acid hydrogels can easily be altered in such a way that VIC produce ECM. A synergism between chondroitin sulphate and hyaluronic acid has been demonstrated by the increased production of elastin by VIC [32].

Dermal fibroblasts trapped in a fibrin gel in an appropriate mould and under proper conditions have resulted in collagen fibres aligned with the fibrin. This tissue has been able to withstand pressures comparable with aortic porcine valves [33, 34].

Microgrooves in substrates can be used to align collagen fibres. Also, open pores in three dimensional constructs can affect the orientation of collagen fibres. Rectangular pores seem to be able to guide cell and collagen orientation more effectively than diamond shaped pores. This can influence tensile strength and stiffness of the produced collagen [35].

Since the ECM is arranged in a tissue specific three-dimensional ultra-structure, it can serve

1) As a structural support.
2) As attachment sites for cell through surface receptors, and
3) As a reservoir for signalling factors, which modulate biological processes such as angiogenesis, cell migration and proliferation.

This allows the ECM to serve as an appropriate biological scaffold for tissue repair and reconstruction [1].

6. THE USE OF A BIOREACTOR

All pulsatile bioreactors function in generally the same manner [36]. A bioreactor for conditioning TEV has six components.

1) A driving force or pump for fluid movement, which is controlled by a computer program; the flow as well as the shape of the wave form can be controlled, in order to create a laminar flow through the valve.

2) A reservoir containing cell culture media.

3) A test section containing the heart valve or component of heart valve.

4) A fluid capacitance to store and release energy at every pump cycle, to forward and reverse the flow.

5) A resistance element, to control the overall system pressure.

6) The possibility for gas exchange and hence oxygenation, by active bubbling or simple diffusion.

A bioreactor provides the necessary chemical environment (pH, pO_2, pCO_2, Lactate, Glucose, Insulin, etc…) and mechanical stimuli (laminar flow, cyclic stress, etc…) for cells to proliferate and to form the elements for the ECM. In some protocols, more complex factors such as TGF-beta 1 have been added [33].

The use of a diastolic loading protocol in a bioreactor has resulted in an improved tensile strength of the matrix. This strength has reached that of the native valves. By use of incremental cyclic strength, collagen fibre alignment has been improved and the SMC have been developed better. Thes cells have produced more collagen, but the matrices have remained comparatively stiff [35, 37, 38].

The use of a range of strain ratios (circumferential *vs.* radial directions) has been important for obtaining the necessary mechanical properties of the engineered tissues [34, 35, 37].

Only with a bioreactor, such results can be obtained [39]. A bioreactor also allows variations in loading protocols and a real time quality check of TEHV [40, 41]. These quality checks are not easy: long test periods for biomechanical properties carry the risk for contamination, while accelerated tests with high frequency cycles are not physiologic and unrepresentative [3]. Moreover, optimal loading protocols have not been developed yet. Fine tuning of protocols could be very important, since small differences can yield widely varying results [36].

Ideally, when tissue engineering techniques will be introduced in future clinical routine, the schedule for a patient diagnosed for valvular disease may be:

1) Cell harvest by a bone marrow puncture under local anaesthesia.

2) Differentiation and expansion of these cells and tissue engineering of a heart valve prosthesis *in vitro.*

3) Before implantation, seeding the matrix with EC [1, 4].

4) Implantation of a living autologous prosthesis into the patient after a time period of 6–8 weeks, after the necessary quality check, for which there are no criteria yet [1].

This concept avoids the problems associated with the use of cells from other sources and with calcification due to glutaraldehyde treatment [4].

7. EVALUATION OF TEHV DEVICE

The animal models have shown that the concept of TEHV is potentially applicable. However, the use of biodegradable scaffolds for TEHV cannot be translated into clinical practice yet. For this purpose, quality markers for the function of TEHV are needed, which should be obtained in large long-term animal series. These quality markers include:

- Durability.
- Biocompatibility.
- Biomechanical properties.
- The capacity to grow, which is important for a pediatric population.
- To repair and to remodel the device after implantation.

Adverse events such as TE, immunologic and inflammatory reactions with breakdown of the construct should be avoided at all costs. The number and the quality of VIC, EC, fibres and ECM, as well as their organisation, degradation, calcification and the remodelling can be studied by IHC. This technique, however, implies killing the animal and only an one-time measurement is possible.

Repeatable *in vivo* evaluation techniques have been developed, such as multiphoton fluorescence excitation techniques. These can be combined with MRI, CT, and molecular imaging. These techniques allow a high resolution imaging of deep tissues. Hemodynamic parameters such as TVG, jet velocity, EOAI, valvular motion and regurgitation as well as LVEF and LVM can be evaluated by Doppler-echocardiography [3].

8. TEHV IN THE MOST RECENT YEARS

The development of TEHV is ongoing in 2010 and 2011, but long-term animal studies are still awaited. Major problems still have to be solved. These problems include the "*in vitro*" as well as the "*in vivo*" stages of tissue engineering.

- Immune reactions against matrices, especially in native and decellularized matrices can lead to inflammatory reaction [42].

- Decellularization protocols still need improvement since the available methods could alter the mechanical properties of the ECM [43].

- Mechanical properties of matrices still pose a problem: even with various loading protocols in a bioreactor, the material has been much stiffer compared to native valves [44, 45].

- The reduction by cyclic strains on the expression of pro-inflammatory genes is a very complex process, that is still being unraveled [46].

- Animal experiments (bone marrow derived mesenchymal cells on a bioresorbable scaffold, implanted in sheep, in pulmonary position), have resulted in a decrease in leaflet mobility on MRI and an increasing regurgitation at 12 weeks [47].

- RVOT reconstruction in young patients with TEHV have shown failure due to inflammation, fibrosis and obstruction within one year. These TEHV, seeded with viable autologous vascular EC have been considered as valuable alternatives for cryopreserved pulmonary homografts [48].

- Unraveling homing-in mechanisms for stem cells to repopulate valves still are not completely understood [16].

These results clearly indicate that many of the basic processes for the development of TEHV are poorly understood. The "silver bullet", which is needed for this development, if it exists at all, still remains to be found!

9. CONVERGING OF TEHV WITH TAVI

TAVI has been tried as method for delivery and deployment of TEHV devices [49, 50].

A porcine valve has been prepared for implantation in pulmonary position in sheep. The stent has been covered with intestinal submucosa. The scaffold has been seeded by autologous myofibroblasts. After a first culturing in a dynamic bioreactor for 16 days, EC have been seeded, followed by a second culturing for 4 days. The device has been delivered in the animal by a TAVI technique [49].

In another attempt, a biodegradable synthetic scaffold has been integrated in a self expanding stent. This device has been seeded with vascular or bone marrow derived autologous cells. After culturing, the device has been implanted through a trans-apical approach [50].

Procedural success has been achieved. Echocardiography and angiography at 4 to 8 weeks has shown normal valve function. These results seem promising for the reconstruction of the RVOT as well as for re-interventions [49]. Layers of new tissue with endothelialized surfaces have been documented. Higher values for collagen and GAG have also been demonstrated. The leaflets were less pliable, however [50].

The combination of the development of TEHV with TAVI procedures is principally feasible, but long-term studies in larger animal series and in aortic position are needed.

It must be repeated, that if the "silver bullet", for the development of TEHV is not found, new delivery and deployment techniques will be unhelpful in dealing with CAVS.

CONCLUSIONS

The production of TEHV requires several steps, which are not fully standardized yet. These steps include:

- The choice of the matrix.
    - Biodegradable synthetical material.
    - Homograft.
    - Xenograft.
- The type of fixation (glutaraldehyde or more gently with detergents) and of decellularizing.
- The decision for or against cell reseeding.
- The choice for the chemical and biomechanical protocols in the bioreactor for the promotion of cell growth, cell attachment and formation of ECM.
- The long-term evaluation in an animal *in vitro* and *in vivo.*

The introduction of TEHV for clinical use can take a long time. There are several sources for a such a delay:

1. None of the existing protocols has been proven to be superior. Once a superior protocol has been found, it will quickly prevail. This might

take a long time, however, since many challenges still have to be met. This has still been the focus in very recently published studies!

2. The TEHV devices have to be studied for their durability by IHC methods, after explantation. This type of study is still a minority!

3. The *in vivo* long-term animal studies will also require time, once a superior protocol has been designed. Such studies have not been published yet.

4. TEHV has to compete with thoroughly evaluated BHV and MHV devices. These have a very predictable outcome. Moreover, not every past innovation has been successful, which makes the manufacturers rather conservative. The only real clinical experience was in children and these efforts were less than successful.

5. Even when a device enters the market as treatment for CAVS, it has to be compared with existent devices for at least 15 to 20 years, which is more or less the durability of a modern BHV such as the CE-p in elderly [2, 3].

The most recent TEHV studies still focus on biochemical and mechanical protocols in bioreactors, computational models, decellularization techniques, electrospinning techniques and cell seeding protocols. Translational research, from bench to bed and animal studies are less in number. This indicates that the development of TEHV still has a long way to go and that the "silver bullet" might not be found. New techniques for delivery and deployment of the device, such as TAVI, will not be helpful if the basic requirements are not met!

ACKNOWLEDGEMENTS

Declared none.

CONFLICT OF INTEREST

The author(s) confirm that this chapter content has no conflict of interest.

REFERENCES

[1] Neuenschwander S, Hoerstrup SP. Review article. Heart valve tissue engineering. Transpl Immunol 2004;12:359-365.

[2] Vesely I. Review article. Heart Valve Tissue Engineering. Circ Res 2005;97:743-755.

[3] Hjortnaes J, Bouten CVC, Van Herwerden LA, *et al.* Review article. Translating Autologous Heart Valve Tissue Engineering from Bench to Bed. Tissue Engineering Part B 2009;15:307-317.

[4] Schoen FJ. Review Article. Cardiac valves and valvular pathology. Update on function, disease, repair, and replacement. Cardiovascular Pathology 2005;14:189-194.

[5] Courtney T, Sacks MS, Stankus J, *et al.* Design and analysis of tissue engineering scaffolds that mimic soft tissue mechanical anisotropy. Biomaterials 2006;27:3631-3638.

[6] Hong H, Dong N, Shi J, *et al.* Fabrication of a Novel Hybrid Heart Valve Leaflet for Tissue Engineering: An *In vitro* Study. Artif org 2009;33:554-558.

[7] Grauss RW, Hazekamp MG, van Vliet S, *et al.* Decellularization of rat aortic valve allografts reduces leaflet destruction and extracellular matrix remodeling. J Thorac Cardiovasc Surg 2003;126:2003-10.

[8] Ketchedjian A, Linthurst Jones A, *et al.* Recellularization of Decellularized Allograft Scaffolds in Ovine Great Vessel Reconstructions. Ann Thorac Surg 2005;79:888-896.

[9] Meyer SR, Nagendran J, Desai LS, *et al.* Decellularization reduces the immune response to aortic valve allografts in the rat. J Thorac Cardiovasc Surg 2005;130:469-476.

[10] Rieder E, Kasimir MT, Silberhumer G, *et al.* Decellularization protocols of porcine heart valves differ importantly in efficiency of cell removal and susceptibility of the matrix to recellularization with human vascular cells. J Thorac Cardiovasc Surg 2004;127:399-405.

[11] Narine K, Claeys E, Cornelissen M, *et al.* Readily available porcine aortic valve matrices for use in tissue valve engineering. Is cryopreservation an option? Cryobiology 2006;53:169-181.

[12] Juthier F, Vincentelli A, Gaudric J, *et al.* Decellularized heart valve as a scaffold for *in vivo* recellularization: Deleterious effects of granulocyte colony-stimulating factor. J Thorac Cardiovasc Surg 2006;131:843-852.

[13] Ota T, Sawa Y, Iwai S, *et al.* Fibronectin-Hepatocyte Growth Factor Enhances Reendothelialization in Tissue-Engineered Heart Valve. Ann Thorac Surg 2005;80:1794-1802.

[14] De Visscher G, Vranken I, Lebacq A, *et al.* *In vivo* cellularization of a cross-linked matrix by intraperitoneal implantation: a new tool in heart valve tissue engineering. Eur Heart J 2007;28:1389-1396.

[15] De Visscher G, Blockx H, Meuris B, *et al.* Functional and biomechanical evaluation of a completely recellularized stentless pulmonary bioprosthesis in sheep. J Thorac Cardiovasc Surg 2008;135:395-404.

[16] De Visscher G, Lebacq A, Mesure L, *et al.* The remodeling of cardiovascular bioprostheses under influence of stem cell homing signal pathways. Biomaterials 2010;31:20-28.

[17] Flameng W, Meuris B, De Visscher G, *et al.* Trilogy Pericardial Valve: Hemodynamic Performance and Calcification in Adolescent Sheep. Ann Thorac Surg 2008;85:587-592.

[18] Flameng W, Meuris B, Yperman J, *et al.* Factors influencing calcification of cardiac bioprostheses in adolescent sheep. J Thorac Cardiovasc Surg 2006;132:89-98.

[19] Bertipaglia B, Ortolani F, Petrelli L, *et al.* Cell Characterization of Porcine Aortic Valve and Decellularized Leaflets Repopulated With Aortic Valve Interstitial Cells: The VESALIO Project [Vitalitate Exornatum Succedaneum Aorticum Labore Ingenioso Obtenibitur]. Ann Thorac Surg 2003;75:1274-1282.

[20] Ku CH, Johnson PH, Batten P, *et al.* Collagen synthesis by mesenchymal stem cells and aortic valve interstitial cells in response to mechanical stretch. Cardiovascular Research 2006;71:548-556.

[21] Lichtenberg A, Tudorache I, Cebotari S, *et al. In vitro* re-endothelialization of detergent decellularized heart valves under simulated physiological dynamic conditions. Biomat 2006;27:4221-4229.

[22] Conconi MT, Rocco F, Spinazzi R, *et al.* Biological fate of tissue-engineered porcine valvular conduits xenotransplanted in the sheep thoracic aorta. Int J Molec Med 2004;14:1043-1048.

[23] Gu C, Wei X, Wang Y, *et al.* No infection with porcine endogenous retrovirus in recipients of acellular porcine aortic valves: a two-year study. Xenotransplantation 2008;15:121-128.

[24] Sales VL, Mettler BA, Engelmayr GC Jr., *et al.* Endothelial Progenitor Cells as a Sole Source for *Ex vivo* Seeding of Tissue-Engineered Heart Valves. Tissue Engin 2010 Part A;16:251-261.

[25] Butcher JT, Penrod AM, Garcıa A, Nerem RM. Unique Morphology and Focal Adhesion Development of Valvular Endothelial Cells in Static and Fluid Flow Environments. Arterioscler Thromb Vasc Biol. 2004;24:1429-1434.

[26] Sutherland FWH, Perry TE, Yu Y, *et al.* From Stem Cells to Viable Autologous Semilunar Heart Valve. Circulation 2005;111:2783-2791.

[27] Kadner A, Zund G, Maurus C, *et al.* Human umbilical cord cells for cardiovascular tissue engineering: a comparative study. Eur J Cardio-thorac Surg 2004;25:635-641.

[28] Schmidt D, Mol A, Neuenschwander S, *et al.* Living patches engineered from human umbilical cord derived fibroblasts and endothelial progenitor cells. Eur J Cardio-thorac Surg 2005;27:795-800.

[29] Sodian R, Lueders C, Kraemer L, *et al.* Tissue Engineering of Autologous Human Heart Valves Using Cryopreserved Vascular Umbilical Cord Cells. Ann Thorac Surg 2006;81:2207-2216.

[30] Xin Y, Wang YM, Zhang H, *et al.* Aging Adversely Impacts Biological Properties of Human Bone Marrow-derived Mesenchymal Stem Cells: Implications for Tissue Engineering Heart Valve Construction. Artif Organs, Vol. 34, No. 3, 2010:215-222.

[31] Flanagan TC, Wilkins B, Black A, *et al.* A collagen-glycosaminoglycan co-culture model for heart valve tissue engineering applications. Biomat 2006;27:2233-2246.

[32] Masters KS, Shah DN, Leinwand LA, Anseth KS. Crosslinked hyaluronan scaffolds as a biologically active carrier for valvular interstitial cells. Biomat 2005;26:2517-2525.

[33] Robinson PS, Johnson SL, Evans MC, *et al.* Functional Tissue-Engineered Valves from Cell-Remodeled Fibrin with Commissural Alignment of Cell-Produced Collagen. Tissue Engin Part A 2008;14:83-95.

[34] Robinson PS, Tranquillo RT. Planar Biaxial Behavior of Fibrin-Based Tissue-Engineered Heart Valve Leaflets. Tissue Eng Part A 2009;15:2763-2772.

[35] Engelmayr GC Jr., Rabkin E, Sutherland FWH, *et al.* The independent role of cyclic flexure in the early *in vitro* development of an engineered heart valve tissue. Biomat 2005;26:175-187.

[36] Berry JL, Steen JA, Williams KJ, *et al.* Bioreactors for Development of Tissue Engineered Heart Valves. Ann Biomed Engin 2010;38:3272-3279.

[37] Engelmayr GC Jr., Sales VL, Mayer JE Jr., Sacks MS. Cyclic flexure and laminar flow synergistically accelerate mesenchymal stem cell-mediated engineered tissue formation: Implications for engineered heart valve tissues. Biomat 2006;27:6083-6095.

[38] Syedain ZH, Weinberg JS, Tranquillo RT. Cyclic distension of fibrin-based tissue constructs: Evidence of adaptation during growth of engineered connective tissue. PNAS 2008; vol. 105; 18: 6537-6542.

[39] Balguid A, Mol A, van Vlimmeren MAA, *et al.* Hypoxia Induces Near-Native Mechanical Properties in Engineered Heart Valve Tissue. Circulation 2009;119:290-297.

[40] Kortsmit J, Rutten MCM, Wijlaars MW, Baaijens FPT. Deformation-Controlled Load Application in Heart Valve Tissue Engineering. Tissue Engin Part C 2009;15:707-716.

[41] Kortsmit J, Driessen NJB, Rutten MCM, Baaijens FPT. Nondestructive and Noninvasive Assessment of Mechanical Properties in Heart Valve Tissue Engineering. Tissue Engin Part A 2009;15:797-806.

[42] Bayrak A, Tyralla M, Jadhoff J, *et al.* Human immune responses to porcine xenogeneic matrices and their extracellular matrix constituents *in vitro*. Biomat 2010;31:3793-3803.

[43] Gui L, Chan SA, Breuer CK, Niklason LE. Novel Utilization of Serum in Tissue Decellularization. Tissue Engin Part C 2010;16:173-184.

[44] Cox MAJ, Driessen NJB, Boerboom RA, *et al.* Mechanical characterization of anisotropic planar biological soft tissues using finite indentation: Experimental feasibility. J Biomechan 2008;41:422-429.

[45] Cox MAJ, Kortsmit J, Driessen N, *et al.* Tissue-Engineered Heart Valves Develop Native-like Collagen Fiber Architecture. Tissue Eng part A 2010;16:1527-1537.

[46] Smith KE, Metzler, SA, Warnock JN. Cyclic strain inhibits acute pro-inflammatory gene expression in aortic valve interstitial cells. Biomech Model Mechanobiol 2010;9:117-125.

[47] Gottlieb D, Kunal T, Emani S, *et al. In vivo* monitoring of function of autologous engineered pulmonary valve. J Thorac Cardiovasc Surg 2010;139:723-731.

[48] Rüffer A, Purbojo A, Cicha, *et al.* Early failure of xenogenous de-cellularised pulmonary valve conduits – a word of caution! Eur J Cardio-thorac Surg 2010;38:78-85.

[49] Lutter G, Metzner A, Jahnke T, *et al.* Percutaneous Tissue-Engineered Pulmonary Valved Stent Implantation. Ann Thorac Surg 2010;89:259-264.

[50] Schmidt D, Dijkman PE, Driessen-Mol A, *et al.* Minimally-Invasive Implantation of Living Tissue Engineered Heart Valves. A Comprehensive Approach From Autologous Vascular Cells to Stem Cells. J Am Coll Cardiol 2010;56:510-520.

Index

A

B

C

D

E

F

G

H

I

J

L

M

N

O

P

Q

R

S

T

U

V

X

Made in the USA
Las Vegas, NV
03 November 2026

57422845R00200